DANCING IN MY DREAMS

DANCING IN MY DREAMS

CONFRONTING THE SPECTRE OF POLIO

KERRY HIGHLEY

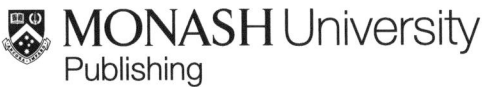

© Copyright 2016 Kerry Ann Highley
All rights reserved. Apart from any uses permitted by Australia's *Copyright Act 1968*, no part of this book may be reproduced by any process without prior written permission from the copyright owner. Inquiries should be directed to the publisher.

Monash University Publishing

Matheson Library and Information Services Building
40 Exhibition Walk
Monash University
Clayton, Victoria 3800, Australia
www.publishing.monash.edu

Monash University Publishing brings to the world publications which advance the best traditions of humane and enlightened thought.

Monash University Publishing titles pass through a rigorous process of independent peer review.

www.publishing.monash.edu/books/dmd-9781922235848.html

Design: Les Thomas

Cover image: Fairfield Hospital patient, circa 1937. Reproduced with permission from the Fairfield Hospital archives.

National Library of Australia Cataloguing-in-Publication entry:
Creator: Highley, Kerry Ann, author.
Title: Dancing in my dreams : confronting the spectre of polio / Kerry Highley.
ISBN: 9781922235848 (paperback)
Series: Australia history.
Notes: Includes bibliographical references and index.
Subjects: Poliomyelitis.
                Poliomyelitis--Treatment.
                Poliomyelitis--Prevention.
                Poliomyelitis--Vaccination.
                Poliomyelitis vaccine--Social aspects.
                Poliovirus--Research--History.
Dewey Number: 616.835062

Printed in Australia by Griffin Press an Accredited ISO AS/NZS 14001:2004 Environmental Management System printer.

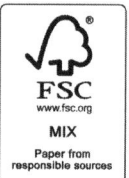

The paper this book is printed on is certified against the Forest Stewardship Council ® Standards. Griffin Press holds FSC chain of custody certification SGS-COC-005088. FSC promotes environmentally responsible, socially beneficial and economically viable management of the world's forests.

CONTENTS

List of Illustrations vii
Acknowledgments viii
About the Author ix
Prologue x

1 Introduction 1
2 I'm Afraid It's Polio 10
3 Staying Alive: Life in Hospital 21
4 Silent Traveller: Polio in Australia 39
5 Pushing the Boundaries: Polio Treatment and Elizabeth Kenny . . 65
6 Sister Kenny Goes to America 94
7 Dancing in My Dreams: Confronting the Spectre of Polio 110
8 A Tale of Brains, Guts, and a Virus 144
9 Polio: Retrospect and Prospect 169

Annex 178
Notes 181
Bibliography 225
Index 257

LIST OF ILLUSTRATIONS

Children in gendered iron lungs in the Royal Children's Hospital.
Children in Thomas splints on the balcony at Fairfield Hospital.
Molly and Jean Macnamara.
Children having heliotherapy at Frankston Convalescent Hospital.
Jean Macnamara.
Polio patients, Warm Springs.
Concert given by polio patients, Warm Springs.
Physical therapists, Warm Springs.
Splint workshop, Warm Springs.
Child in splints, Warm Springs.
Hydrotherapy, Warm Springs.
Child in splints to correct knock-knees.
Elizabeth Kenny in nurse's uniform.
Sister Elizabeth Kenny.
Sister Ella Morphett and Staff Nurse Kenny at Harefield Hospital.
Picnic to celebrate the first anniversary of the Townsville clinic.
Nursing staff at 'Experimental Muscle Rehabilitation Clinic'.
Sister Kenny demonstrating her therapy techniques, Minneapolis.
Sister Kenny meets President Roosevelt at the White House.
Poster for the President's Birthday Ball.
Students in training at the Elizabeth Kenny clinic in Brisbane.
Sister Kenny demonstrating her therapy in the Brisbane clinic.
Elizabeth Kenny Clinic on the corner of George and Charlotte Streets.
Sister Kenny Institute patients celebrate the Institute's first birthday.
Sister Kenny with her secretary, Miss Betty Brennan, at 'Struan'.
Elizabeth Kenny waving from the deck of the *Queen Mary*.
Patients achieving short-term goals at Fairfield Hospital.
Sister Kenny and Kenny nurses at Hampton Convalescent Hospital.
The Little White House, Warm Springs.
President Roosevelt celebrates his birthday at Warm Springs.
June Middleton and Vern Draffin at Fairfield Hospital.
Children at Hampton Convalescent Hospital.
Miss Davies, physiotherapist, with a polio patient.
Homemade frame for stretching muscles.
Heliotherapy on the balcony at Frankston Orthopaedic Hospital.
Fairfield staff with two patients in Thomas splints.
Fairfield Hospital ambulance.
Van for transporting patients to AFL games.
Reginald Webster in his pathology lab, Royal Children's Hospital.

I dedicate this work to the memory of my mother and father and my son,

to my husband Ed, to my family, Sam, Kylie, Owen and Emma,

and to all those who have felt, and continue to feel,

the tragedy of discrimination.

ACKNOWLEDGMENTS

Many people have helped this book come to fruition. I am grateful to the many librarians and archivists I met in Australia and overseas during the collation of the numerous primary sources used in this work: their knowledge and expertise helped me a great deal. Very special thanks go to my colleagues who offered wise counsel and listened to my endless musings on the life and times of Elizabeth Kenny and Jean Macnamara. I especially thank John Knott, Anthea Hyslop, Naomi Rogers, Kerry Neale and Barbara Rossall-Wynne, and the former patients of Fairfield Hospital in Melbourne who willingly shared their memories of surviving polio. I am indebted too to the members of Polio Australia who have written about their experiences.

I am forever grateful to my husband, Ed Highley, whose long experience as a professional editor has been invaluable. His support for this work, his willingness to read and comment on endless drafts and his ability to gently prod me into continuing when I got discouraged, have been essential. My thanks also go to Nathan Hollier, Joanne Mullins and other staff at Monash University Publishing for helping smooth the way to publication.

I have often thought about the privilege accorded to me to read and listen to other people's stories about having polio, and they proved to be a treasure trove in the writing of this book. Their stories are but a beginning, a scratching of the surface: there are many more yet to be told in the History of Medicine in Australia.

ABOUT THE AUTHOR

Kerry Highley grew up in the Sydney beachside suburb of Manly. Her first career was as a medical laboratory scientist, a profession in which she worked for many years before turning to History in 2000. In 2009 she received her PhD in the History of Medicine from the Australian National University for her thesis on the polio epidemics in Australia. While at the ANU, she tutored in Second World War studies and the History of Terrorism. Apart from polio, her research interests and writings have included aspects of the history of the Australian Army Medical Corps in the First World War.

PROLOGUE

A Wednesday morning in late summer. Manly beach, Sydney ... *Seven Miles from Sydney and a Thousand Miles from Care* ... declares the sign above the ferry terminal at Circular Quay. A breeze stirs the surface of the sand and out to sea a sole surfboard rider bobs around, waiting for the next wave. There are a few people swimming between the flags, but the mile-long beach is almost deserted, for it is on the weekend that great crowds of people overflow from the Manly Ferry to sweep up the Corso towards the beach.

Down near the water's edge sits a group of pale, thin children. Their legs are fastened inside steel bars with leather straps, and they poke straight out in front of their bodies like matchsticks. The brass buckles on the bands glitter in the sunlight. One or two try to wriggle on their bottoms towards the sparkling, foam-speckled water but a young woman, dressed in the uniform of a nurse, shoos them back to join the group.

A short distance from the group of children is a young mother with her daughter, who is playing with her toys in the sand. The child stands and begins to wander towards the group of children. As she does, her mother's voice pierces the still air ... 'Come back here at once, those kids have been very sick, and you might catch something'.

This was Australia in 1952, a time before Jonas Salk discovered a vaccine to prevent poliomyelitis. Across the vast land parents are frightened that their child could be the next to catch the deadly disease. No one, scientist nor doctor, could tell them what to do, or how to prevent it happening. What was poliomyelitis? Why were they so scared?

This book will tell you why, and how it could happen again.

Chapter 1

INTRODUCTION

Most Australians born before 1960 can remember the widespread vaccination campaigns that were initiated against polio with first the Salk, then the Sabin vaccines. The Salk immunisation program introduced into this country in 1956 was heralded as the beginning of the end of the 'war against polio', and populations in countries as geographically widespread as Australia, New Zealand, Canada, Sweden and the United States of America breathed a sigh of relief that science had finally, after years of painstaking research, discovered a vaccine against polio.[1] No longer would communities in Australia fear the unpredictable and puzzling epidemics that had visited the country with increasing frequency since the turn of the century, nor would parents fear that a child's sudden rise in temperature and aching limbs heralded a life-threatening attack of polio. For two generations in the twentieth century, polio's influence was profound, and it was the most feared disease of childhood and adolescence. Yet the polio epidemics in Australia have received scant attention from social historians.[2]

Polio generated panic and fear in families with young children. It arrived silently and suddenly, often with symptoms that could easily be attributed to a chill, or sunstroke, or eating tainted food, or a dozen or so seemingly trivial ailments. For the lucky ones, the encounter with the poliomyelitis virus did not give rise to full-blown symptoms of infantile paralysis and, within a few days, they recovered. For the unfortunate, exposure to the virus initiated paralysis, primarily affecting the legs. The poliovirus did not distinguish between rich and poor, or by race or creed, or between those who were physically robust and those who were not. The suddenness with which apparently healthy children succumbed to the virus meant that the disease was regarded with particular dread.[3]

In pre-Second World War Australia two women, Dr Jean Macnamara and Sister Elizabeth Kenny, symbolised the rift that existed between accepted medical treatment for the paralysed body, and an alternative treatment. This is an important thread to this story, a battle between establishment medicine and the threat posed by an outsider who questioned the orthodoxy of the day. Polio epidemics highlighted the difference between new and old medical theories and practices, and they stimulated a fierce debate in Australia and the United States of America about the role of treatment in the care of the paralysed body, and who was qualified to prescribe new therapies.

In Victoria, Dr Jean Macnamara followed the orthodox approach using splints, plaster casts and braces to protect and control the body before commencing therapeutic exercise — usually after a period of some months. In her clinic in Townsville, Sister Elizabeth Kenny endorsed and practised a method of treatment opposite to that endorsed by orthodox medicine and its foremost advocate, Jean Macnamara. Kenny believed in little or no form of constraint for the paralysed body, apart from sandbags and a foot board, endorsed gentle stretching of muscles in the early, acute stage of the disease, and used hot packs to relieve pain, spasm and tightness in muscles.

The anxiety that parents felt about polio in mid-century Australia was not misplaced. Polio was the only epidemic disease to record an increased incidence in Western countries in the twentieth century. As the century progressed, the intervals between epidemics in Australia became shorter, indicating that polio was becoming endemic. Some reports by researchers have suggested that the 1937–38 epidemic in south-eastern Australia was the severest,[4] but figures released by the World Health Organization (WHO) in 1954 did not support that conclusion. In Australia, the epidemics from 1951 to 1953 saw the median incidence of polio rise to double that in 1937–38 (see Annex Table 1).[5] Almost 31,000 cases of poliomyelitis were reported to Australian authorities from 1912 to 1963 (see Annex Table 2), and thousands of survivors worldwide are now experiencing late effects of having had polio.[6]

Polio is an infectious disease and, in Australia, it came within the jurisdiction of the Public Health departments in the various states. The disease is caused by an enterovirus, and it enters the body by way of the mouth, before multiplying first in the tonsil area and then in the intestinal lining. The virus is spread by faecal contamination of food and water. In young children it was most commonly spread at the age when they started to socialise with others from outside the family, and most often by minor contamination, usually from fingers placed in the mouth. In children with immunity, the exposure to the virus produced no ill effect apart from a general malaise. In the unfortunate few, the virus passed from the intestine into the blood. If it then reached the nervous system it produced effects ranging from a simple headache and fever with some changes in the spinal fluid — non-paralytic poliomyelitis — to paralytic disease which could rapidly become fatal.[7]

People with acute poliomyelitis were admitted to hospital, an institution that has changed from one that primarily provided shelter and care for the sick, the poor and orphans, to one that has become a symbol of medicine and its specialised knowledge. By the beginning of the twentieth century, most large cities in the Western world possessed private, public and specialist hospitals including those that admitted patients suffering from infectious diseases.[8] Because polio is highly contagious, survivors were separated from family and friends in isolation wards until the acute, infectious stage had passed. Feelings of rejection, sadness and grief at the loss of their former able-bodied self were common. Physicians were not able to assess how badly the virus had weakened or damaged the nerves supplying muscles until the acute phase had passed, and this evaluation took place in a rehabilitation ward. Weeks, months and sometimes years of arduous, often painful, physiotherapy to strengthen the affected muscles began. Long stays in hospital were common for polio survivors, the convalescent stage usually lasted around eighteen months, but some never went home.

By the early twentieth century, orthodox medicine[9] had consolidated its authority in the allied health professions of nursing, radiography, laboratory technology and physical therapy. Western societies turned to medicine and science as the foremost weapons against disease. Medicine embraced modernity and the advances in technology, diagnostic techniques, pharmaceuticals, and surgical and rehabilitation techniques learned during the First World War. The medical profession expected that medical knowledge should come only from within its accepted canon of scientific expertise and experimentation and, in particular, that erudition about anatomy and physiology had to be learned from its own texts and from cadavers in the dissection room. No other scholarship was acceptable or permitted. Specialisation in medicine became firmly entrenched, and specialists defended their areas of expertise. Specialists were acknowledged as experts not only by the general public, but also among their medical peers, and that gave them increased social and professional status.

Elizabeth Kenny risked a great deal when she challenged medical orthodoxy about the best way to treat the paralysed body and, because she did so, she made a significant difference to the lives of many polio survivors. Her ideas and techniques on treatment marked a turning point in physical therapy, but she would make powerful enemies in the medical world in achieving her goal of having her method accepted as a legitimate alternative to orthodox treatment. Unfortunately, most Australian survivors of polio were denied access to her treatment because of the dominance of allopathic medicine in Australia, and an unwillingness by medical practitioners to return to the medical pluralism that had flourished in pre-Federation Australia. The major player in alternative medicine in Australia had been homeopathy but, by 1930, homeopathy was no longer a provider of mainstream medical care. Its Melbourne hospital was renamed as Prince Henry's, and orthodox medical staff dominated those prescribing homeopathic remedies.[10] Unlike the situation in the United States of America in the 1930s, where 'nearly a quarter of American healers were Christian Scientists, osteopaths, or chiropractors of some stripe',[11] medical pluralism was suppressed in Australia, and alternative healing techniques like homeopathy, chiropractic and osteopathy were actively opposed. The medical profession in early twentieth century Australia was conservative and slow to change under the influence of social evolution. Nowhere was that more apparent than in Victoria, where the BMA forbade 'consultation with irregular practitioners'[12] and employed the same tactics as it had earlier done with the homeopaths to overwhelm and eliminate the Kenny method of treating polio from within the state, and ultimately from Australia.

The campaign directed by many Australian medical practitioners against Elizabeth Kenny and her clinics may have been motivated more by disdain for her non-medical status than for her methods of treatment. Doctors and nurses delineated and defined their 'occupational territories' in the treatment of polio in 1930s Australia within a hierarchical structure, with medical practitioners occupying the top position and directing subordinate nurses to carry out treatment decisions determined by them. Indeed, the real reason for the criticism of Kenny may have been that she represented a threat of non-medical interference into an area of medicine that practitioners considered to be their sole preserve.[13]

The battle for acceptance between these two major personalities in polio treatment in Australia began many years earlier with the unexpected and unexplained rise of the deadly disease. In the first two decades of the twentieth century, advances in public health and sanitation improved the morbidity and mortality rates of many common childhood diseases. Ironically, those advancements also provided optimal conditions for the re-emergence of an old foe, infantile paralysis or poliomyelitis.[14]

In the early part of the twentieth century, polio was viewed as a shameful disease, associated with dirt and poverty. Society and officialdom remained entrenched in their belief about traditional associations between dirt and

Introduction

disease as they struggled to explain the epidemic in New York in 1916.[15] There was confusion about the cause of the disease. Many Americans resorted to xenophobia, pointing to the influx of immigrants in the early twentieth century, alongside official and public attempts to link polio with those who lived in poorer, urban areas, while refuting any possible link between the disease and the middle class.

The more advanced a country in public health standards of hygiene, the more likely it was to experience epidemics of polio. From the second to the fifth decade of the twentieth century, epidemics were almost entirely confined to Scandinavia, the northern United States, Canada, Australia and New Zealand. In these countries, polio was relatively severe, and involved children aged from five to ten years. The disease showed an increasing tendency to produce severe paralysis in young adults. Polio was, and is, a different disease in infants and adults. This is probably due to the fact that because standards of hygiene in the general community had improved, the age at which children were being first exposed to the poliovirus was becoming progressively later and, if paralysis occurred, the effect was generally more severe. In infants under three months, exposure to the poliovirus produced either no outward symptoms or a mild, flu-like response. Higher average polio rates are consistently associated with lower average infant mortality rates and vice versa.[16] The contemporaneous notion in the northern hemisphere that polio was noticeably a disease of summer and autumn was found not to be true in Australia, when the severe epidemic of 1938 appeared in winter.[17]

The facts about the transmission of the poliovirus were unknown until the early 1950s, and various theories were expounded in Australia and globally about its aetiology and spread. Some experts suspected droplet infection from coughing, sneezing or spitting, while others — inspired by the success of research into diseases like malaria and the plague — concentrated their efforts on animal or insect vectors as transmission agents. In the nineteenth century the miasmic theory as the cause for illness was popular. Defenders of miasma disputed the germ theory, and specifically its claim that a relationship existed between a distinct micro-organism and disease. Large cities like Sydney, Melbourne, New York and London produced copious amounts of human and environmental waste, and there was widespread community apathy about cleanliness and sanitation. The stench from open drains in city streets that overflowed with dead animals, household waste and raw sewage, added weight to the argument of those who claimed that illness was caused by breathing in 'miasma' or foul-smelling air.[18] Proponents of miasma believed that if the air were foul-smelling from rotting vegetation and corpses, then disease would be even more likely to breed in the over-crowded tenements of city slums.[19] Public health reformers campaigned vigorously to get urban dwellers to open their homes to the benefits of the sunlight and fresh air that they believed would kill germs. The influence of miasma adherents like Florence Nightingale was seen in the mid-nineteenth century development of the 'pavilion plan' for hospital design; the underlying rationale being that the improved ventilation in the wards would help reduce the high mortality rate.[20] Miasma adherents continued to theorise about the relationship between noxious vapours and disease right up until the late 1930s, while others concentrated on epidemiological studies to try and unlock the secret of how polio spread from one human to another.[21]

The Australian public expected medical science to provide the answers to the conundrum posed by the epidemiology and treatment of polio, but the failure of doctors and scientists to explain how and why polio appeared in the population added to public fear and apprehension and, in the 1920s and 1930s, press coverage in Australia shaped the way that information about polio was dispersed within the community.[22]

Polio epidemics often began silently. A child complained of a slight cold or a headache or sometimes an upset stomach accompanied by vague, aching pains in the limbs, symptoms that were characteristic of many of the common childhood illnesses. Many parents ignored their child's grumbling, and sent them off to school or out to play with other neighbourhood children, or to finish some household or farmyard task. Because the symptoms often seemed innocuous and not a cause for concern, polio spread quickly through a vulnerable community via carriers as well as those who later became ill. Subsequent epidemiological studies suggested that fewer than five per cent of cases produced paralysis, but for those who were paralysed, the effect on their lives and of those closest to them, was profound. The human body can be black or white, tall or short, fat or thin, but the dichotomy that appears more exclusionary than any other is that of disabled and able-bodied. Stereotypic labelling of the disabled body in the early twentieth century often related physical deformity to mental illness. In post-Federation Australia, the language of eugenics was widespread, and many medical and scientific journals actively supported intervention in reproduction to bring about a better future for Australia. Eugenics, and the science of improving the quality of the human race by selective breeding and the forced sterilisation of the 'unfit', was a classification that often included the disabled, both physically and mentally. Polio survivors had to readjust to their changed body and new identity, a task made more difficult if they had

Introduction

previously harboured discriminatory feelings about the disabled body and its place in society.[23]

This book examines the lives of many who were afflicted by polio. It looks at many aspects of the patient experience in Australia and in the United States of America, and includes vignettes from the United Kingdom and New Zealand. My wish is to inform readers of how the experience of polio affected those who suffered from the disease, their families, and the broader community within a broader context of social, cultural and political influences both in Australia and internationally.

In bookshops, patient experiences of the illness vie for the attention of the reader alongside the social histories of the disease. In polio narratives, the survivor's voice gives witness to how the experience and pain of polio has been moulded over time by social, cultural and technological change. Many printed sources contained material about patient stories of experiencing polio.[24] As part of my research I travelled to the United States of America and Canada and examined many letters from patients and the parents of children with polio detailing how the experience of having polio had affected their lives and those of their family. The Elizabeth Kenny manuscript collection held at the Minnesota Historical Society was invaluable for providing insights into polio and its treatment in that country.[25] I found a remarkable international community in the large cross-section of recollections I examined, and this speaks of an authentic coalescence of personal fragments about experiencing polio in the twentieth century.

Personal narrative has a long history — we have spoken, listened and written stories for each other for thousands of years — but narratives about the polio experience span but a few. In the West, epidemic polio appeared and then disappeared within three generations. Over that period, the shifting voice of the narrator brought an understanding of living with a disability to a wider audience. Stories about how polio has affected lives have become more common, especially from the middle class; but, unfortunately, stories of how the poor and the marginalised coped with the disease are few, mainly because their stories lie submerged within case histories in our public hospitals and institutions, buried within statistical analyses of prognoses, treatment and outcomes.

The moving and poignant stories of polio survivors who were trying to make sense of what had happened to them, of how they coped with the pain, and of their struggle to come to terms with a different physical body revealed patterns in the experience. The polio epidemics were a cruel lesson for many who suddenly became different in a world that valued conformity. We all like to portray ourselves in a positive light, and memories are often selective, as well as notoriously unreliable. Naturally, memories recalled some years after the event are sometimes coloured by an individual's reflection on how the experience of having polio affected their later life.[26]

Many polio survivors have shared their story with others in support groups like Paraquad Victoria, and formalised their experience of polio by having it published on the worldwide web. Time and again, these and other interviewees were recalling events that occurred in their childhood, at a time when they had little understanding of what was happening to them and were offered little explanation. For children, hospitalisation was often a terrifying experience, and the memory remained with them for the rest of their life. Strong feelings of loneliness, bewilderment and abandonment were common in children, while resentment at losing their independence, and of being 'treated like a baby', surfaced frequently in adult accounts. And, of course, there was always the topic of hospital food.

Elizabeth Kenny shook the complacency of the medical establishment, which firmly believed that muscles affected by the poliovirus remained frail and vulnerable for a lengthy period, and that gentle movement of limbs in the early stages of paralysis was dangerous. That dictum became more and more entrenched in the 1930s and '40s, with the result that polio survivors were encased in plaster casts for many months. With its introduction of early, active treatment, the Kenny treatment discouraged attitudes of passivity in patients, and encouraged independence and acceptance of the disability. Keeping the affected limb or chest warm with hotpacks undoubtedly helped to relieve pain, and gentle passive movements helped keep joints mobile and prevented deformities. Kenny encouraged her patients to remain autonomous, to retain agency over their bodies, and to work with the Kenny therapist to bring about recovery. That relationship was far removed from accepted medical practice of the era where the active care-giver gave medical treatment to the passive care-receiver.

Writing the history of medicine has changed from a time when it was primarily concerned with the great discoveries and the celebrated men and women involved: now medical history also tells us about social, economic and political change. I reveal how some epidemiological and scientific beliefs about polio have been adopted, and others discarded or modified over the past fifty years.

There are many voices in the history of polio: previously the story was of great men and women and their great deeds, and not the people who

Introduction

felt the pain, or fought to breathe, struggled to stand unaided and learned how to walk again.[27] The disabled are no longer silent and invisible. Many are articulate, educated and determined to take control over their own bodies — and their numbers make them a powerful political, cultural and social force for good. This book is also about the medical practitioners, both sanctioned and censured, who struggled with each other for the right to treat the paralysed, and strived to mend their broken bodies. It was important to understand the relative positions of medical power and influence in Australia in relation to other countries in order to unravel the reasons why an alternative, successful, but unorthodox method of treating the paralysed body was largely denied to Australian survivors of polio in the middle of the twentieth century. In the end, both the advocates of new methods of polio treatment, and those who opposed them, conceded some ground. For the majority of Australians, that reconciliation came too late.

Chapter 2

I'M AFRAID IT'S POLIO …

After I was admitted to hospital I can remember the doctors in white coats, and the nurses and sisters giving me something to drink, and then nothing else. I was evidently unconscious for many days. When I eventually became aware of my surroundings, I was in a big ward with lots of other children. I knew I was in hospital, but I didn't know what had happened to me. My arms and legs felt heavy. I hurt all over, and every time anyone walked near my bed the vibration sent pain shooting through my body and tears would run down my face. I couldn't tell anyone because I couldn't speak, my vocal cords were temporarily paralysed.

There were all these boxes on the other side of the ward … I'd heard people talking about coffins but I had never seen one. I thought [the boxes] were coffins with dead children, but I couldn't understand why their heads were sticking out. I was terrified. I couldn't ask, and I thought they might put me in one.[28]

(Nita Lawes-Gilvear, Launceston Hospital, Tasmania, 1937)

Polio often began suddenly, and early symptoms in children were often vague, but sometimes dramatic. In Melbourne in 1913, Ilma Lever's mother didn't believe she was ill and, 'pulled my legs because she thought I was pretending not to be able to walk … she always blamed herself for my dislocated hips'.[29] Richard Owen, 'fell down in the yard, and couldn't get up',[30] while seven-year-old Gary Buchanan, 'felt sick and developed a bad headache … the next morning I tried to sit up but couldn't move … I felt agonizing pain'.[31] Quite a few children mentioned having a splitting headache. A few days after she went swimming Katherine Pappas 'couldn't walk … I kept falling over, but my mum thought I was fooling'.[32]

I'm Afraid It's Polio …

Pamela Solomon was six years old in 1956 and living in Coonabarabran, NSW, with her widowed mother when she developed

> a sore throat, then I couldn't talk, then I was paralysed all over. Mum would try to move me and I would scream with the pain — the doctors didn't know what was wrong with me and they told Mum I was spoilt. It took them three weeks to decide to send me to the Children's Hospital in Sydney.[33]

In Pennsylvania in 1956, seven-year-old Cindy Bernstein awoke to the sound of her mother calling her to get up and get ready for school. She remembered:

> being groggy, trying to climb down from what I thought was so high a bed, and falling as soon as I put my feet to the floor. I made my way to the top of the stairs and then I completely lost it. I don't remember exactly what happened then but I remember finding myself in a crumpled heap at the bottom of the stairs and Mom being rather hysterical.[34]

In New Zealand, a two-year-old was diagnosed and treated at home for 'gastric trouble', finally being admitted to hospital after she developed paralysis, but she died four days later. Another baby was treated with saltwater baths because the doctor 'did not know what else to do', while a young boy with polio 'was not diagnosed for eight and a half years'.[35]

In early twentieth-century Australia, death rates in childhood were dominated by a high incidence of infant mortality due to gastrointestinal disorders, followed in order by diphtheria, whooping cough and pneumonia. Infantile paralysis was relatively unknown, and it was therefore understandable that a doctor would first suspect gastroenteritis as a possible cause of a child's vomiting, pain and raised temperature.[36] In 1908, doctors at the Children's Hospital in Melbourne were treating '1000 babies a week for diarrhoea during the summer months'.[37]

For many adults, the first indication that they had contracted polio was the appearance of flu-like signs — fatigue, nausea, fleeting aches and pains. Symptoms deemed to be not severe enough to warrant taking time off work, or to visit the local doctor: 'Take an Aspro and have a cup of tea, it will soon pass', they told themselves. But for many the aspirin did not help as the hours passed and, as the mild fever started to worsen, and limbs started to feel weaker, doubts began to surface about exactly what was wrong. It became an effort to sit up in bed to sip the tea and increasingly difficult to walk to the bathroom. Then it became impossible, as previously strong and healthy legs collapsed, no longer able to bear the load. Pain in the lower back and limbs increased and, for some, it became difficult to breathe, all symptoms that indicated that the acute phase of poliomyelitis had begun, and the virus was circulating in the bloodstream after breaking through the mucosal cells lining the gut. This period was known as the 'viraemic phase' and lasted for a few days.

Others adults described similar experiences. One Melburnian was ill 'for about a week with a high fever and sore throat'[38] that seemed to subside, before coming back 'much worse', while another, a twenty-one-year-old woman, pregnant in 1949 with her second child, thought that the pains in her limbs were signs of impending childbirth.[39] Dulcie Black was admitted on a Friday evening to Fairfield. By the following Monday the staff, who had become 'worried that the baby's heartbeat was getting slower and slower', induced labour. White remembered that she 'couldn't push, so they moved me to the end of the bed and the doctor sat there with a bucket — it was a boy'. The baby developed polio a week later and was admitted to Mt Eliza Hospital.[40] It was rare for a newborn to develop polio from its mother as maternal antibodies passed across the placenta and protected the unborn child. Dulcie's baby was probably infected during birth from minor faecal contamination from his mother who, being in the early, acute stage of the disease, would not have had time to produce sufficient antibodies. She did not see her child again for twelve months. Geoff Golding had 'a hot lemon and an Aspro and got into bed'. Two days later, after falling over and being unable to get up, he was seen by his local doctor who 'tested his reflexes' and had him admitted to Fairfield the following morning. Within four days he was completely paralysed and had been 'put into the box'.[41] There were no laboratory tests to confirm or dismiss a diagnosis of polio until lumbar punctures were introduced in the 1930s. What is surprising is the fact that, fifty years later, cases continued to be wrongly diagnosed:

> The local GP didn't recognize my fever and stiff neck as polio ... he gave me M&B tablets[42] and cough mixture ... didn't think it was my place to tell the doc I had polio ... another doctor came a few days later ... just as much of a loss as the first ... my sister, a nurse came to see me ... she rang her own GP and a Dr Powell came to see me ... 'Into Fairfield you go', he said.[43]

In 1951, Hazel was a 'happy, healthy wife and mother of three young children' in the Riverina, 400 miles south-west of Sydney when she was 'struck with polio'. For six weeks her doctor tried to find a hospital bed for her, anywhere in New South Wales. Eventually, Royal North Shore in Sydney agreed to take her and she spent over five months in a ward flat on her back.

As John Smith describes in his chapter, 'Memories of Polio', approximately fifty per cent of polio survivors from the 1950s that he interviewed related how they were initially treated for another complaint. Smith concluded that 'while one would expect that during the 1950s anyone who presented with a febrile illness would be tested for the disease it was not so'.[44] For instance, in 1961 Ron Gillam was told, 'you are too old to have polio, it's arthritis'.[45] A physician from Western Australia who himself contracted polio agreed with John Smith's assessment:

> Although a lumbar puncture was done, there was no specific test[46] ... but mind you, the diagnosis was not, in general, exceedingly difficult to make providing one understood the characteristic features, and did some specific tests ... if I hadn't had medical knowledge there's no chance I would have survived ... I had to give instructions to my medical attendants.[47]

Some adult sufferers had difficulty convincing hospital staff they were ill — 'they reckoned I was putting on a bit of an act'[48] — while others were sent home with aspirin to relieve 'severe back pain' and told to 'come back tomorrow if the pain hadn't gone'.[49] Occasionally, hospital paramedical staff had reached well-founded conclusions about the diagnosis, but, mindful of the fact that it was the professional responsibility of the doctor to communicate prognoses, were unwilling to encroach on medical territory by offering an opinion. A radiographer in Perth remarked to her patient, 'you look like you've got infantile paralysis to me, but it's none of my business'.[50]

Gloria was six years old in 1955. She remembered waking up one morning and discovering that she 'could not move her arm', so her worried mother took her to the Boston City Hospital. After examining her, nursing staff told her mother she 'was constipated ... to take her home and give her an enema':

> The next day I couldn't move my whole left side, so she brought me back. They again told her I was constipated and I needed an enema. She told them, 'There's something wrong with my daughter and I'm not moving'. The doctor examined me and told my mom I had infantile paralysis ... I was in an iron lung for four years.[51]

Most parents felt responsible, and worried about what they had done wrong. A seemingly simple instruction to a child to ignore a headache or an aching limb — 'it's only growing pains'[52] — and to carry on as normal later magnified parental feelings of guilt and remorse at a perceived neglect of a critically ill son or daughter. Should they have been more careful in their supervision of their child? Should they have forbidden rather than allowed that visit to the beach, or the purchase of that ice-cream cone, or that trip on the tram to the picture theatre?

Some parents believed the illness to be retribution for some transgression they had committed. 'It's God's will', pronounced the pious baker in Noorat, the small Victorian town where young Alan Marshall went down with infantile paralysis like a 'pole-axed steer'.[53] Many parents tried folk remedies before sending for a doctor: 'in 1952 in rural Minnesota you didn't go to the doctor the minute you ran a fever … you waited until you were sure that something was wrong'.[54] Besides, for many families, the cost of sending for a doctor was prohibitive and viewed as a last resort. A number of narratives examined reveal a delay between the onset of symptoms and the correct diagnosis, for many physicians did not know what was wrong. One family doctor told a young boy's mother, 'you think it's polio, but it isn't. What you've got to do is make him do exercises and snap out of it.'[55] By the time paralysis became evident there remained no doubt about the diagnosis, but for some children it was then too late:

> My boy took sick and I called the doctor who diagnosed a cold when he had all the symptoms of polio. I took care of him for five days. He called another doctor who diagnosed it but it was too late, my baby was dying. It's hard to write this as my heart is broke [sic].[56]

Most parents sought reassurance from physicians that there was nothing they could have done to prevent the disease, for the majority of parents in the early- to mid-twentieth century still had great faith and trust in the ability of the medical profession. The association of the profession with science and the rise of specialisation had helped Western medicine gain an unassailable position over traditional methods of healing like folk medicine or homeopathy. More and more individuals came to the medical profession in the expectation that their illness would be identified and treated.

People relied on medical and scientific authorities for advice and directives on how to avoid disease and maintain good health, and because those authorities were unable to explain either how polio was transmitted from person to person, or what could be done to avoid catching the disease, the general public soon sensed the confusion and contradictions that existed within the professions and began to lose trust in their power to inform.

Myths and rumours often abounded. Popular theories in Victoria in 1937 about how polio was transmitted were varied — sometimes plausible, often bordering on the comical. Some Victorians believed sunstroke was the cause, others that it was the fault of domestic animals like dogs and cats, while some miasma adherents in Brighton 'blamed the foul Elster Creek for carrying and giving off the virus'.[57] Public health authorities worldwide exhorted housewives to be constant in their efforts to reduce dust because it was a 'germ carrier', and to install fly screens to keep 'filthy flies' out of the house because 'they carried polio'.[58] Tasmanians were nervous about the epidemic across the Bass Strait, and some refused to buy food that had been 'wrapped in Melbourne newspapers'.[59] There was a lot of superstition about. A story appeared in a newspaper of a pound note sent by mail from Melbourne to someone in Tasmania, 'but the person didn't know ... put the envelope inside the kitchen range to disinfect it ... the thing caught fire and it burnt ... a pound was worth a fair bit of money ... you didn't burn a pound note, no way.'[60]

Camphor bags worn 'around the neck' were believed by some to offer protection against the virus,[61] while others remained wary about 'handling money in the till' or 'speaking on a public telephone'.[62] Others believed that diet was to blame: popular targets included processed flour and sugar, preservatives in food and pasteurised milk. In the United States the most popular theory of causation blamed 'ice-cream, candy, soft drinks and summer fruits' while sharks, rubbish tips, insects, spiders, electricity, plant pollen, feather pillows, cemeteries, uncircumcised males and, inexplicably, tickling of children also had their adherents.[63] In 1937, the discovery of the virus in faeces[64] gave added impetus to the directive by health officials to avoid swimming pools during epidemics, and added to concern about contamination of water supplies. Twenty years later, bizarre theories about transmission of the virus still proliferated. For example, a Queensland mother was convinced that 'breast milk and cabbages' possessed vitamins that prevented polio, based on her observation that all the cases detected in her area had been 'bottle-fed'.[65] Sadly, she did not elaborate on her evidence for including cabbage in the diet.

The failure of doctors and scientists to explain how and why polio appeared in the population added to public fear and apprehension and, in the 1920s and '30s, press coverage in Australia shaped the way that information about polio was dispersed within the community. Newspapers published the latest statistics on polio notifications and deaths, and compared them with previous years' figures, and pictures of children and adolescents in iron lungs, or in braces or on crutches, confirmed to parents that their fears about the disease were justified.[66]

In crowded urban communities with rudimentary plumbing, where sanitary systems were primitive and polio was endemic, almost all children were exposed to various infections from an early age and, if they were fortunate, they survived and developed an immunity to further infections by the same agent. Improved sanitation, especially of the water supply, meant that common diseases like typhoid became less frequent, but those same advances in public health reduced exposure of infants to the poliovirus. Epidemics of polio increased with improved sanitation. The immunity that early exposure to the virus bestowed happened less frequently and, as a result, many children reached adolescence and adulthood without being introduced to the virus and developing antibodies. Without any natural immunity to polio, those susceptible members of the population were then at risk of becoming ill. Furthermore, the likelihood of an epidemic of polio occurring within a community rises as the general level of immunity drops and as contact occurs between the immune and the non-immune in a population. That was what occurred in Australia, New Zealand, Scandinavia, Canada and the United States of America in the early decades of the twentieth century. Large sections of the population lacked immunity to the poliovirus because of improvements in sanitation and, instead of being an endemic disease, polio became epidemic and infected many adults and young children who had escaped exposure in infancy.[67]

When parents realised their child was not getting better but worse, they often took matters into their own hands. Alan Marshall's father drove him the twenty miles to the small hospital in town on 'the brake, the longshafted, strongly built gig in which he broke the horses'[68] while another child was taken to hospital in a 'hearse, it doubled as an ambulance'.[69]

Before the 1930s, physicians relied on their clinical judgement to distinguish polio from similar diseases affecting the central nervous system, but the diagnosis was difficult because of the co-existence of epidemic meningitis, the symptoms of which were often indistinguishable from polio. Frequently, doctors were reluctant to deliver a verdict until they were absolutely sure it was polio, because they knew the traumatic effect their decision would have on families. No doctor wanted to make an incorrect diagnosis.

Margo Ashton was nine years old, and the only child of working-class parents in Port Melbourne when she contracted polio. She clearly recalled: 'the doctor sitting by my bed as we waited for the ambulance to come. The worried look on his face is still with me today, I know he was preparing my parents for the worst … the entire family was shocked … they wondered if I would live.'[70]

In his classic case study in Baltimore of parents of children diagnosed with polio Fred Davis argued that the 'doctor's unwillingness to make a firm diagnosis of polio seemed to serve several purposes'. First: 'it afforded the doctors some protection in the event that the tentative diagnosis was proved wrong'; second: 'it relieved the doctor to some extent of the unpleasant task of breaking the bad news to the parents'; and third, some felt that the diagnosis would be better handled by the family if there was a brief interval between seeing the patient and the delivery of bad news.[71]

Before the diagnosis was pronounced, some parents might have contemplated the possibility that their child had caught polio, but many did not want to think about the likelihood, or voice their concern to a doctor. It was almost as though until the symptoms were 'named', then the patient, the parents and to some extent the family doctor could deny the possibility of polio. Optimism one minute and pessimism the next was common in parents. However, once the diagnosis was confirmed, emotions intensified over the following days as families were catapulted from a state of relative security and confidence about the health of family members into one of fear and uncertainty. To see a child healthy and active one day, and next day to be confronted with the likelihood of death or permanent severe disability was traumatic, and difficult for parents to cope with.

When families were finally confronted with the truth of the situation, men and women alike 'wept and broke down … my grandmother told me years later that she had never seen my father cry except on that day'.[72] Some parents could not look at each other 'without bursting into tears … all we could think about was the twisted body of our beautiful boy'.[73] The adult Gary could still remember the look on his mother's face when she said to him, 'Don't move and I'll get help'.[74] Images of 'crippling, iron lungs, and death' dominated parental responses to the news and, for many, the diagnosis of polio challenged basic conceptions and fundamental beliefs about their role as devoted and caring parents.[75] For others, finally knowing what was wrong with their child was better than the uncertainty that had existed previously.

Many families felt ostracised by their community: 'parents and friends of my mother walked on the other side of the road and they were treated something terrible'.[76] After his small daughter was admitted to hospital with polio, Mr Parker recollected that 'we weren't allowed to go into the shops in the Victorian town of Sale or to walk through the general part of the hospital. We had to go around the side to the infectious diseases ward.'[77] Another father remembered that 'neighbours wouldn't walk near our front door, they would cross the street. We were a pest house, a plague house, no one visited.'[78]

Elsie Thomas was eleven years old when she contracted polio in the 1937 Melbourne epidemic, and her mother was so concerned that her dressmaking business would be 'ruined, if people saw the ambulance outside the shop and knew that someone had infantile paralysis' that she arranged for it 'to come to the back entrance'.[79] Such was the level of ignorance in the community about the transmission of the disease that, as late as the 1950s, many believed that rehabilitated patients were infectious: 'Once we got back to walking a bit we were allowed to walk around the block. [Outside the hospital.] But people would see us coming and they would all cross the street'.[80]

In contrast, some families were overwhelmed by the kindness of others: 'the whole neighbourhood pitched in, they would take turns cooking dinner so that every evening my mother did not have to worry about the next meal, or where it was coming from'.[81]

Some children believed that catching the disease was 'a terrible thing that happened to you if you disobeyed your parents' or 'if you didn't finish your meal'[82] or 'fought with your brothers and sisters', or if you went swimming: 'swimming was definitely the way to catch polio'.[83] When one young boy saw his mother for the first time since being admitted to the ward he yelled out, 'Momma, I'm sorry', because he felt responsible for catching the virus.[84] A four-year-old taken to Fairfield Hospital in Melbourne remembered feeling that she must have been 'very bad … and for my punishment I was taken away from my family and sent to this strange place that was full of fear'.[85] Another recalled: 'I didn't understand this world or why I had been taken there, but I learned to be good and quiet and do as I was told. I learned that I was all alone.'[86]

The young boy responded to his situation by becoming subdued and withdrawn, reflecting his despair at being separated from his parents. Hospital staff may have misinterpreted his reaction as a sign that he was settling into life on the ward, but it was more likely that he had suffered emotional damage from his hospitalisation.

One of the major reasons that people seek the help of a medical practitioner is for the relief of pain. The pain of polio was often excruciating, but until the Australian therapist Elizabeth Kenny made its relief a priority of her treatment regime, and showed how the lessening of pain could be used as a diagnostic tool, pain was often given token acknowledgement. In the acute phase of polio, skin became hypersensitive to the touch of others. Charlene Pugleasa recalled that when her brother 'touched my skin it hurt really bad … with a piercing pain'. When the doctor came he lifted her neck from the pillow causing her to 'scream with pain'.[87] Charles Mee felt 'relentless pain for days, like the pain of a tooth being drilled without novocaine, but all over my body'.[88] Painkillers were refused because medical staff feared that the medication might cause additional damage.[89] In Tasmania in 1937, Nita Lawes-Gilvear remembered hurting 'all over' when nursing staff walked near her bed: 'the vibration sent pains shooting through my whole body'.[90] In Kentucky in 1944, a thirteen-year-old boy lay on his parents' bed in the 'blast-furnace hot sun' while waves of 'muscular spasms and pains' swept over him 'repeatedly, unremittingly'.[91]

Polio patients retained full sensory awareness throughout the acute phase of their illness. Unlike patients who suffered spinal cord injury, polio sufferers could feel the pain in their limbs, and quantifying the extent of that pain to outside observers was fraught with misinterpretation. As Naomi Rogers observed, some physicians believed that 'pain was usually present only when movement is a factor, and was always relieved by immobilisation' of limbs; moreover, 'some physicians … admitted that they had frequently denied the significance of pain in polio, and it was a matter of reproach that we have so long evaded the questions raised by this striking symptom'.[92] From early in her career, Elizabeth Kenny recognised that pain was a significant factor in polio, and her first task was to try and lessen it with the use of moist heat packs on affected limbs.

Reading the first-hand accounts of experiencing polio were often heartbreaking. Some writers told of their childhood, of their fears when no one could explain what was wrong, and of being separated from family members; married couples told of their grief and feelings of loss at being separated from each other and from their children; and some parents wrote of the guilt they experienced when fundamental beliefs about themselves as devoted mothers and fathers were challenged by their child's sudden, life-threatening illness. Emily recalled that after she got polio: 'There was a big change in my relationship with my parents, and had a lot to do with that they really couldn't protect me anymore. That innocence stopped and I was really young for it to stop.'[93]

Because the majority of polio patients in the twentieth century were treated in an infectious-diseases ward and then later in a convalescent hospital, the experience of illness for the patient was transformed. No longer would it be lived out within the confines of the family home, but in an institutional setting. For those who were critically ill, the journey to the hospital signified the beginning of the separation process from family, as few parents or spouses were allowed inside the ambulance. 'My first memory ... pain, my mother and tears ... I was in an ambulance, alone ... and I was being taken away. I was sick and scared'.[94] Paradoxically, although the experience was frightening for many children, for others it was strangely exciting: 'I asked the man to turn the siren on ... that's the last thing I remember'.[95] For those in pain, the ambulance journey was almost unbearable, each jarring bump or pothole in the road increasing their suffering.

Families often felt some relief once the patient had been transferred to the ambulance, and hoped that they could move quickly to the next phase of doing something practical to help. This was a hope that rapidly faded once they were confronted with the strict and unyielding face of a hospital bureaucracy that removed participation by parents or family members in any decision-making, and insisted on total control over the body of the patient. They would soon discover that hospital staff disclosed little about progress and prognosis, primarily to avoid committing themselves to a deadline for recovery, but also to keep the decision-making process within the confines of the hospital. With people disabled by polio, that dependence, lack of autonomy and medicalisation of the body would extend beyond the hospital into the domain of after-care treatment.

Chapter 3

STAYING ALIVE: LIFE IN HOSPITAL

I don't know who 'Thomas' was, but he certainly thought up a cruel and frightening treatment. The splint was like a wire frame that I was tied into day and night so that I couldn't move. My arms were stretched out like on a cross and my legs were apart. I couldn't move my head. There was a hole in the frame below my bottom to go to the toilet. It was so embarrassing. I was cold all the time from the metal, but I wasn't allowed to complain. I spent a long time tied in this thing, staring at the ceiling and unable to move at all.[96]

Hospitals have changed over time from institutions that primarily provided shelter for the homeless, the sick and orphans to the specialised centres for training doctors and for conducting research that exist today. Traditionally, clinical medicine was the most difficult subject to teach and, because of the large numbers of patients, charitable or volunteer hospitals provided the main opportunity for students to study the effect of disease and trauma on the living body.[97] Thus, as Michel Foucault argued, through the development of that 'constant gaze upon the patient',[98] people admitted to hospital became a medical exhibit to be observed and studied by doctors, and their bodies transformed into an object that provided clinical training.[99] Charitable hospitals banned the admission of the chronically ill (including the disabled), the mentally ill, children, pregnant women and people with infectious diseases. Until the creation of specialist hospitals or isolation wards within existing institutions, hospitals refused to admit infectious cases for the simple reason that, because they could not be isolated from other patients, the risk of contagion and cross-infection was too great.[100]

Once admitted to hospital, patients were usually given a spinal tap or lumbar puncture to confirm the diagnosis,[101] a procedure that many thought was painful, while others barely noticed it. Those who did experience pain never forgot it. Neither did parents forget; many of them remarked on their anguish at hearing their child screaming from behind the closed doors of the examination room:

> A nurse came in with an enormous needle, and it was so terrifyingly long that I thought they had made a mistake, that surely it was a veterinarian's needle meant for horses. I was afraid it would go all the way up into my brain.[102]

> An ambulance took me to Fairfield Hospital and I was put into a bed. A nurse came in with an enormous needle. She told me it would not hurt. The lumbar puncture without any local anaesthetic made me nearly jump out of bed in agony.[103]

As is the case with any painful experience, the reaction varied with the individual and some practitioners were more skilful with the procedure than others. Robert thought it felt like someone was 'driving a wooden stake into my back'.[104] Geoff Golding remembered feeling the pressure 'of the needle going in, but it was not painful ... I was lucky, Dr Kett was marvellous ... don't remember any pain at all'.[105] Thomas Daniel was a senior medical student in Boston in 1954, and part of his duty roster at the local infectious diseases hospital was to admit suspected polio cases and do a spinal tap. On many occasions, the patient was a sick and frightened child. Through trial and error, he realised that the severe headache that often followed the procedure could be avoided if the patient remained flat for several hours, but recalled that many of the children were so 'agitated and upset, that telling them to lie flat was about as effective as telling an angry mule to stop kicking the walls'.[106]

Admission to hospital was followed by isolation in an infectious diseases ward, far away from the support of family and friends. Many young children remembered the emotional trauma of the separation. One boy recalled that when he was separated from his mother she 'cried hysterically' and told him, 'Don't say goodbye, that means I'll never see you again'.[107] Some children pleaded with their parents not to 'leave me here'.[108] Separation was recalled as 'absolutely horrendous ... and you were punished if you cried, and put in a cubicle because you upset the other children'.[109] Some children felt completely 'overwhelmed by the sight of so many sick and crying children, enclosed in row upon row of small, white cots'.[110] Many young children were filled with fear:

Staying Alive: Life in Hospital

> Things happened so quickly. My world turned upside down, things spun out of control. Mum and Dad disappeared and all these strangers took over and they took me away. I was put in a room with high ceilings. There were all these other children there and all sorts of terrible things were happening to them. Some were in boxes that hissed and wheezed while others were tied up in bed and couldn't move. I started to cry, I wanted my mother. But they were cross and told me to be quiet.[111]

Parents had to leave crying, often hysterical children in the care of nursing staff. Some children became quiet and withdrawn, traumatised by the separation: 'Several years ago my mother told me tearfully of her anguish at that time because when I came out of isolation I wouldn't look at or speak to either of my parents for quite a while, but just turned away from them and stared at the wall'.[112]

Many overworked nurses were upset because they did not have the time to comfort distraught children properly. One Melbourne child remembered, 'in the hospital ward every single kid was crying',[113] and in England six-year-old David 'cried myself to sleep. When you'd wake up there would be another little boy crying in the next cubicle. It was awful.'[114]

Sister Woodruff nursed at Caulfield Convalescent Hospital during the 1937 epidemic and recalled,

> There was only one nurse on duty at night in a ward of thirty children … our case load was so heavy. If you couldn't pacify one then you'd move it to another room … because one crying would wake up the others. It must have been terrifying for the kids … it gives me the horrors to think about it now. It was so cold in Melbourne and we couldn't keep them warm under the bed frames. I preferred working at Royal North Shore Hospital in Sydney where the Kenny treatment was used.[115]

All medical and nursing staff worked hard during the polio epidemics, and conditions did not vary greatly between one generation and the next, whether in Australia or in the United States. The first case of polio admitted to Fairfield Hospital in Melbourne in the 1937 epidemic was on 12 July.[116] By the end of August, four additional wards had been allocated to polio patients, nine respirators were in use, and the Medical Superintendent, Dr F.V. Scholes, had requested that 'all mild cases of diphtheria and scarlet fever be isolated at home',[117] so that beds could be re-allocated to the polio wards. Hospital authorities quickly realised they had an epidemic on their hands. By December, it had peaked. Nine hundred cases had been admitted, and forty-eight people had died. There were twenty-one respirators available, and thirty-four children were each being given a few hours inside an iron lung — Scholes remarked 'that's all they required'. Exhausted Fairfield Hospital staff tried as best they could to cope with a 'very heavy workload', and the Superintendent recalled how he had 'crawled over cases lined up in hospital corridors, to fall into bed'. His report to the Commonwealth Director General of Health, Dr J.H.L. Cumpston, painted a vivid picture of conditions at Fairfield in October 1937:

> The polio epidemic is going strong, the northern and western suburbs are being hit now, Footscray and Brunswick being the worst. Coburg, Preston, Northcote and other populous working class suburbs have so far been hardly touched, so we have a long way to go yet. We have now topped the 500 mark, and nearly 440 have been admitted to Fairfield. The place looks like a battlefield.[118]

Worried authorities in other states asked Scholes for permission to send medical and nursing staff from their hospitals to gain experience in nursing acute cases of polio, a request that he agreed to without hesitation.[119] With over 900 patients, and thirty-four of them sharing respirators, every spare pair of hands helped. Dr Scholes noted that a related but unexpected feature of the epidemic was a drop in reported cases of diphtheria and scarlet fever to the lowest for many years, which he attributed to the fact that 'children from Melbourne were not mixing freely'.[120] Obviously, many parents were keeping their children at home. By July of the following year the epidemic had disappeared almost as quickly as it had appeared. In all, 1277 cases had been admitted with polio; of these, seventy-six had died — a mortality rate of 5.95 per cent. Medical and nursing staff breathed a sigh of relief and focused their attention on a large number of new admissions suffering from measles.[121]

Across Bass Strait, nurses working in the Infectious Diseases Hospital in Launceston in 1937 'worked seventy-two hours' per week, with one medical officer remarking, 'we worked like blazes, on duty virtually twenty-four hours'.[122] No one had the time to sit with a frightened child, however much they wished to. Launceston Hospital had one of the few Kenny-trained nurses in Australia, Sister Alison Grueber, who worked in its respirator ward. In *The Great Scourge*, Anne Killalea painted a vivid picture of the frantic pace on Grueber's first day at work:

Arriving for work after a five-hour train journey, the Public Health nurse was met by a scene of 'pandemonium'. The wards — one entirely emptied in readiness for fresh cases — were very hot, children were crying, electricians and carpenters were noisily installing two new respirators, and rows of children on the verandahs, in four different stages of infection, were hot, dirty and uncomfortable ... Finding basins and towels by herself, Sister Grueber began sponging children ... found other patients in smaller rooms, and cleaned thirty-two children, most with fever. Finally off-duty about 9 pm to have a meal, unpack and undress, she was called to re-dress in her uniform and help lay out one of two patients who had died. No sooner was that done than a third expired. In bed at 4 am, Grueber managed two hours' sleep before her second day began at 6 am.[123]

Some children found that the Kenny 'Blue Sisters'[124] seemed to have more time to spend with them, were 'more affectionate, because they held you more, whereas in the ward the treatment was very distant and unpleasant'.[125] Seven-year-old Shirley, a patient in Hampton recalled

the warmth and loving care of the 'Blue Sisters'. The physical contact involved in the bathing, massage and passive exercise fulfilled a child's need for human contact. Funny how things have moved on — the hugs I received from those wonderful women would probably not be allowed now.[126]

Many children were bewildered and afraid they were going to die because no one would tell them what was wrong with them. 'I was put in a bed in a huge room with high ceilings. There were all these other children there, and all sorts of terrible things were happening to them. Some were in boxes that hissed and wheezed. Others were tied up in bed and couldn't move'.[127] One survivor of polio remembered, 'I used to think it was funny that nobody would come [to see me in hospital] ... and I had two nurses who used to come in all dressed in white with masks ... but nobody would say why'.[128] For eight-year-old Gary the relief at seeing his mother again was overwhelming: 'One day as I just lay there the ward sister came in with my mum, the nearest I had been to her for weeks ... I remember crying as I felt mum's hand on my arm'.[129] Older patients also felt the pain of separation, but could understand what a diagnosis of polio meant and the risk they posed to other family members.

It appears that little changed in the strategy of preparedness for polio epidemics over the following twenty years. Administrative, medical and nursing staffs were still caught unawares and unprepared for the rapid spread of the disease once it became established within a population. The Medical Superintendent of Fairfield Hospital was not the only one to use a military metaphor of a 'battlefield' in 1937 to describe working conditions during a polio epidemic; the doctor in charge of the epidemic in Tasmania was described as managing it with 'military precision'. In Launceston Hospital the pressure of work on medical staff, 'eventually took its toll':

> Dr Lewis, hurrying across to the ID (Infectious Diseases Ward) one night, slid to the bottom of a frosty path, and broke his leg. He slept for the next month or so in the ID where … the noise of the respirators was 'frightful'. While this same doctor managed the strain by occasionally throwing himself down on a patch of lawn for twenty minutes, another was invalided for ten days with exhaustion. Dr Fulton caught the disease he was treating.[130]

In Minnesota a young resident medical officer recounted how it was 'like being in combat, you had to be on the ball and ready to go all the time. We were tired, exhausted, and frightened at the same time. We didn't want to get polio ourselves … or bring it home.'[131] The death of a child was singularly traumatic for many of the medical staff: 'It really bothered me terribly for many weeks that I couldn't save that small child … the memory of that day and the child's name remains with me forever'.[132] In 1955, Dr Berenberg, a paediatrician at the Children's Hospital in Boston, described 'a busy night' during the epidemic:

> The hysteria in the city was beyond description. We'd get 150–200 people at the same time because families had to wait until Dad got home from work with the car. The police would keep them in an orderly line, and we used to do a lot of our preliminary screening in the automobile … if the kid looked ok they stayed in line … the ones who were obviously in respiratory distress or couldn't move an arm we would give them a card so they could move up to the head of the line. On the worst night that line went back more than half a mile. Another doctor and I spent the whole night just going back and forth.[133]

Those patients in respiratory distress from paralysed chest muscles were not only in severe pain, but also unable to breathe on their own. In most cases, that meant adapting to a new life in a respirator or iron lung, a machine that would encapsulate some of the most iconic images of the twentieth century. Rows of iron lungs lined up in hospital wards, the heads of patients protruding from the metal cylinders and looking in essence like the exemplification of an Orwellian dystopia or the stuff of nightmares. Iron lungs were in short supply in Australia in 1937; the American ones were extremely expensive to ship across the Pacific Ocean and had to be returned if they needed repair. Some respirators were 'jerry-built' by the Mount Lyell Company in Tasmania, while Professor Aubrey Burstall of the University of Melbourne invented the 'cuirass', a respirator that was attached to the abdomen and upper chest and operated like the iron lung on a negative-pressure principle. Initially, the cuirass was made from aluminium, but later designs were made from fibreglass, thus bringing greater mobility and independence to polio survivors. The portable, wooden respirator produced by Adelaide inventor Edward Both for around £100 was introduced in 1938. The 'Both' respirator, which unfortunately resembled a coffin, was subsequently modified and produced in England at the Morris Cowley car works by the philanthropist Lord Nuffield, who then distributed them free to hospitals in Britain and throughout the Commonwealth.[134] In the United States the development of the first respirator to treat polio victims was credited to Philip Drinker of the School of Public Health at Harvard University. Many polio survivors recalled their fear when they first glimpsed the respirator machines, and Tony Gould was one of those. He was an officer in a Gurkha regiment in Hong Kong when he contracted polio in 1959, and he remembered 'screaming with pain' when lifted from his stretcher to the bed in the isolation ward. For Gould, 'worse was to follow':

> They lay me down between the jaws of a yawning box that had appeared from nowhere. For a moment I thought they were going to operate on me without an anaesthetic and I swore at them ... I couldn't believe what was happening to me. Now my head was sinking backwards towards the floor. Suddenly it came to me that they had made a terrible mistake, that this was a coffin and that they were burying me alive. 'I'm not dead' I wanted to shout, but all I could do was pull my head away from their clutching hands.[135]

Gould was febrile and probably delirious, so his panic and confusion about his circumstances were understandable. Many children and adults found the placement in the respirator[136] a frightening experience, but for an equal number the relief from the effort to breathe was welcome. Geoff

Golding thought it 'felt bloody wonderful going into the tank ... it took hold of you like a lover's embrace, and took a great load off you because you didn't have to think about breathing ... besides, I felt too sick to be bloody scared'.[137] Chest muscles that had strained to draw breath started to relax: 'The weight, the unbearable weight on my chest continued for a few breaths; then, as the dials were regulated, it lifted as if death itself were lifting from my body and soul'.[138]

While many patients viewed the respirator as an 'Angel of Salvation', for others it was a prison, and they longed to be out of it and to be free again. One thought that although it was 'scary initially', once she 'got used to the rhythm of it, it was all right'.[139] Although the respirators were often described as 'noisy, like living in a tin can',[140] and 'uncomfortable ... I remember waking and thinking someone was trying to strangle me but it was [the collar on the] iron lung',[141] most realised that, although being in an iron lung 'was not a great place to be' that 'it kept you alive'.[142]

A Perth doctor who was a sufferer of polio in 1950 credited the respirator with saving his life. However, he believed it was due more to luck, rather than medical expertise, that he survived:

> Being treated in an iron lung is a fate almost worse than death ... there was no management of anything to do with respiration ... everything was based on clinical management ... once you were placed in an iron lung, it was miraculous if you ever came out of it and survived the experience.[143]

Most patients in the respirators had 'sandbags laid along each side'[144] of their body to keep them immobilised, but that immobility caused other problems. Nursing patients in a respirator was constant and painstaking work, and access to them was limited to portholes on the side of the tank. Throughout the day, nurses inserted and removed bedpans and urinals, made observations of temperature and blood pressure, suctioned airways, bathed bodies, cleaned teeth and attended to bedsores, but opening the portholes meant that the delicate balance of air pressure was upset, and often left a patient gasping for air. Those unfortunate enough to have bulbar polio had to contend with the added complication of not being able to swallow, thus placing them in real danger of drowning in their own secretions. Their plight was not helped by having to lie flat on their backs. To lessen the likelihood of choking, the head of the tank was lowered to help drain the chest through a tracheotomy but, as a result, the patient often slid up to the head of the tank. Occasionally that led to pressure on exposed skin, causing bedsores.

Hospitalised in Perth, a patient remembered that he had 'four bedsores, one on each shoulder and my elbows plus a carbuncle on my back. I think the thing that saved me from dying was the penicillin. I was given six hourly injections of penicillin in my bottom, which was pretty much skin and bone and that was pretty painful'.[145]

In the United States the situation was similar. Kathryn Black described the room where her mother lay:

> Wards of tank respirators looked something like the boiler rooms of giant ships, with the blur of gauges, tubes, latches, and dials. The six-foot metal cylinders that breathed for patients lay like coffins on stands that raised them to table height. Intravenous bottles hung from aluminium poles next to the respirators, and at one end of each lay a head. Polio had not left Mother lying prettily against fluffed white pillows, but palsied, in a torpor. A rubber collar separated her head from her body, her brown hair was matted from perspiration and fell back from her face, and her long, slender neck was marred by a raw, sunken hole, with a metal fixture holding a rubber tube.[146]

The respirators saved the lives of many who would otherwise have died, but some patients did die in the machines. Nursing staff did their best to spare others from the knowledge that a fellow sufferer had succumbed, but for those whose lives were dominated by the rhythmic thumping and wheezing of the respirator bellows, the signs of death were unmistakable — the rapid footsteps of nursing staff to the bedside, the swishing sound of curtains being drawn, the sudden silence, and then the squeaking of the mortuary trolley as it was wheeled into the ward. Occasionally, nursing staff turned the mirrors above the tanks away so that 'patients couldn't watch while a body was wheeled out in a now silent machine'.[147] Nita Lawes-Gilvear would sometimes 'wake up in the night and hear the trolley being wheeled in to take another girl away ... you didn't know if you might be next ... I just dreaded the sound of trolley wheels in the night'.[148] In New York, ten-year-old Edward remembered when 'a couple of kids died. We were told by the nurses, "Their mother came and picked them up during the night". Even at that age I wasn't buying it. We used to talk about that: "Do you think your mother would come here in the middle of the night?"'[149]

The sound of the iron lung whooshing and thumping was not the only distinctive sound in the acute care ward. Some of the patients who could not talk would summon the nurse's attention by 'clicking' with their tongues:

When an emergency occurred, like a machine malfunction or the power went down and a child began to smother, there was pandemonium. Feet came running, then more and more feet. The kids who were able to called for help, but most were so weak that their voices didn't carry, so they clicked for attention with their tongues. That mysterious sound was how they communicated. Sometimes the whole room clicked to get attention, and my own heart pounded, listening for the rescuing feet. Afterwards, if it was something really bad that happened, a mother could be heard crying in the hallway for the rest of the night.[150]

The realisation that their lives depended on the respirators brought added fears for patients. Most hated the feelings of imprisonment, helplessness and total dependency on nursing staff. Many men felt emasculated. Lorenzo Milam was 'incensed at the indignity of being forced to wear a diaper at the age of nineteen'.[151] Others deeply resented the loss of privacy:

People would capriciously and suddenly enter my most private spaces to do what was 'best' for me, they were like hostile invasions, and I felt violated[152] ... they would enter the most personal and private parts of me as they reached inside to move a leg or an arm, or insert a needle or a bedpan.[153]

As much as they despised the lack of independence and privacy, most feared what could happen when they were removed from the respirator. A process of weaning patients usually commenced when fever had subsided and the spread of paralysis had ceased. Initially for a few minutes, then building up to several hours a day, they were given the opportunity to see if they could breathe unaided: 'The weaning process was quite brutal. It was with a stopwatch, literally. It was perfect behavioural conditioning. They would give little prizes for each advance: "Three minutes, all right, you can have a football."'[154] A polio survivor in Perth detailed his battle to learn how to breathe outside the iron lung following severe paralysis in 1956:

with breathing excercises they used to open up the lid of the tank and say "breathe" and you would try and breathe. You might go for two or three minutes and that was it ... it took months and months to build up my breathing ... after four or five months I could breathe for an hour or so.[155]

Medical staff believed that gradual removal from the respirator would encourage previously paralysed chest muscles to work on their own and become stronger and, for most patients, that process took somewhere between three and five months. Some never left the tank. Another great fear for respirator patients was what would happen to them if a power failure occurred in the hospital, and that ever-present risk was another reason that medical staff encouraged patients to attempt to breathe on their own, albeit briefly. Every minute counted for those in the respirators as hospital personnel raced to operate the manual pumps:

> Members of the staff of the Fairfield Infectious Diseases Hospital today saved the life of a twelve-year-old girl in an iron lung by operating the respirator after storms had cut off the hospital's two sources of power … they worked in relays for over three hours to operate the hand pump.[156]

During the period of isolation, gowned and masked parents were sometimes allowed in to the bedside for a brief visit, but more often had to make do with a glimpse of their child through a window. Sometimes children were not told the reason their parents were not allowed to visit them in isolation: 'We weren't allowed to have visitors in hospital for months. Sometimes Mum and Dad came, but they weren't allowed in. No one told me they had been or that they weren't allowed to come in, and so I just assumed I had been rejected and abandoned'.[157] Another child 'wondered why everyone had deserted me, except for these strange people dressed in white'. One young boy remembered feeling 'like I had the plague … it was very scary'.[158]

Although it appeared that the initial acute phase of polio was not as traumatic for the adult sufferer because they could understand what was happening to them, the convalescent period seemed far worse for adults than for the children. On the whole, other family members did the best they could to take over the role of the sick parent and care for the rest of the family, but for those in hospital the enforced separation from their children was frightfully hard. One woman sadly recounted that, because she was 'in hospital for months on end, I never saw my babies … it nearly broke my heart … wondered if I'd ever see them again'. She cried for her children 'for months'.[159] When finally they were allowed to return home many recounted that, although they had 'survived' the experience of polio, they had paid a terrible price, for their children 'didn't know' them.[160]

Polio also imposed a financial burden on families, especially if the breadwinner contracted the disease. In some cases, the loss of income was only temporary, but for those who faced permanent disability, the future was bleak. In the United States, the National Foundation for Infantile Paralysis developed a program that was funded by the annual 'March of Dimes' drive to assist patients and their families with medical and hospital expenses. No such scheme operated in Australia. As Claudia Thame noted, 'only if the community at large was threatened by the ill-health of a person, was the disease of public interest', thereby justifying the need for additional public expenditure.[161] Diseases and health problems that were not perceived as being important for the health of the nation were judged to be the responsibility of the individual. Sufferers of tuberculosis frequently infected other members of their own family and the community, and many hid their condition for fear of social opprobrium, but it was not possible for polio sufferers to do the same because hospitalisation was generally necessary. It is a shameful fact that fifty years ago, the disability allowance for polio survivors in Australia was less than half that for tuberculosis.[162] That discrepancy was probably due to the fact that the convalescent tubercular patient was still infectious, and therefore a risk to the health of the nation. In 1951, representations were made to the Federal Minister of Health seeking an increase in the disability allowance for polio sufferers, but the acting minister H.L. Anthony refused, stating that while it was 'unfortunately true' that anxiety about financial loss was often part of chronic illness, polio could not be compared to tuberculosis. In the case of tuberculosis, it was of 'national importance that sufferers should restrain their natural inclination to work until all risk of recurrence had passed'.[163] Anthony added that he could see no valid reason why the disability payment for a polio survivor should be increased. But he was mistaken: virologists were already aware that individuals recovering from polio could be infectious for up to six weeks following the onset of the disease.[164] They were just as likely to infect others as were sufferers of tuberculosis. As a result of that decision on pension payments, more spouses were forced from the home to seek full-time work, causing increased physical and emotional stress for all concerned. Families had become increasingly aware of the financial burden if a child or breadwinner became ill with polio, and when commercial insurance against contracting the disease was introduced to the United States in 1949, the demand was unprecedented. The cost was US$10 for cover of US$5000 over two years: 'Customers lined up outside the insurer's offices from early morning and the police were often called in to keep the queue orderly. Applications flowed in at such a rate that the clerical staff could not process them quickly enough.'[165]

That same year, the New South Wales Government announced that it had set up a committee to investigate the polio epidemic, and people were advised they could take out insurance against polio for 24 shillings a year.

The premium would provide cover of £1000, paid at the rate of £10 per week for one year. If, at the end of the year, 'the person was not cured, then the balance of £480 would be paid out'.[166]

Hospitals during the mid-twentieth century had restricted visiting hours, a practice that D.J. Wilson argues was 'to facilitate control over the patient'.[167] The prevailing belief was that children were less likely to cooperate with hospital staff if parents visited frequently, but Fred Davis has argued that curtailed visiting hours were an attempt to loosen a child's 'ties with home', thus substituting parental authority with that of hospital staff, and immersing 'the child in the hospital's subculture of illness'.[168] No child under seventeen years of age was allowed to visit inside the hospital and, as a result of that policy, some young children 'hospitalised for years forgot they had brothers and sisters'.[169] Perhaps the saddest part about this attitude to children in hospital and their parents was that it was accepted as normal by almost all nursing and medical staff. But conditions in the wards were difficult for all concerned, and overworked and exhausted staff did their best. Wards were often chaotic after parents left, with children crying and refusing to eat or go to sleep: 'I always recall Sundays in hospital for the torrent of tears that followed the departure of parents, and the vomiting of jelly and custard afterwards'.[170]

Understandably, hospital administrators were worried about cross-infection between wards, and the risk of visitors carrying the virus back into the community; but, paradoxically, nursing, medical and ancillary staff moved freely between the hospital and the outside world, and had no restrictions placed upon their movements. Personal possessions of patients were confiscated, even clothing: 'if you dropped a book on the floor, it was never picked up … it was swept out and we lost them'.[171]

One young boy, whose parents had spent hard-earned money on purchasing him a 'new suit' to wear into hospital in Tasmania, 'had it taken from me, and when I asked for it they said, "It's got wogs on it and you can't have it. My mother was quite upset about that."'[172]

Administrators may not have been worried about the virus being carried outside hospital walls, but many people in the community were concerned, and they regarded hospital staff with trepidation: 'If the sisters and nurses wanted a seat on the bus they pinned their Fairfield Hospital badge to their lapels and the bloody bus emptied!'[173]

Many families felt ostracised by their community: 'parents and friends of my mother walked on the other side of the road and they were treated something terrible'.[174] In northern NSW, twelve-year-old Shirley had lived on a farm before she contracted polio. After she was hospitalised, 'no one was allowed to come near the farm for many months, the house had to be fumigated, and any food my parents ordered was left in the ice-cream box up the road.'[175] Twenty-six-year-old Margaret 'didn't have any visitors in the hospital, even my father didn't come, everyone was so fearful of polio'.[176] Some schools destroyed students' possessions:

> The school called to tell my parents that everything I had in my locker was gone. They had burned them. And they had burned my desk … and all my school books and they had fumigated my locker. My mother told me years later how awful that made her feel.[177]

As is the case in every profession, there was a marked variation in the standard of nursing care. Some nursing staff were viewed as being particularly harsh; terms like 'appalling' or 'abusive' or 'sadistic' were used by some patients to describe their experience in hospital. Simon Parritt remembered being 'put out in the sun and just left there. I ended up with severe sunburn.'[178] After Beatrice was put into bed, 'the nurse, a sadistic woman, arrived and pulled me down to the footboard, then she told me "we keep our feet on footboards here."'[179] Eileen Murray recalled that her first memory of Hampton Hospital[180] was when she was 'wheeled into a spare ward, and left there all day because I wet the bed, and of the nurse who slapped my face for doing it'.[181] Lynne Ellis was a patient in Prince Henry Hospital[182] in suburban Sydney in 1951. She recalled,

> one Sister who was a real martinet. She would not allow patients to have family photographs on their bedside lockers. All that she would permit was a bowl of fruit or possibly, but grudgingly, a bunch of flowers. We were not allowed to have screens around the bed when using a bedpan. It was 'too much work for the nurses' she would say. We weren't allowed to have baths either … quite often Sister would stand at the door of the ward and announce 'I hate polios' … she left us in no doubt that we were a dreadful nuisance.[183]

At variance with those memories there were many patients who remembered nursing staff as 'lovely and kind'.[184] Gloria Smothers particularly remembered one kind nurse who 'read books to me every day'.[185] Some young nurses empathised with other girls who were the same age, and in pain. Valda Heath remembered one nurse who 'would cry with me and rub my arms when I sobbed getting treatment'.[186] Marguerite Swann was a four-year-old patient in Fairfield Hospital in 1951, and retains vivid memories that are branded into my soul of the isolation and loneliness and the kind nurse who came and sat next to my bed and helped me to relax by getting me to watch the shadows of the leaves on the wall, and to see if I could see the fairies there. The next night I called out again, hoping that she would come. But a very grumpy nurse came and told me sharply to be quiet and go to sleep.[187]

The overwhelming number of complaints by Australian polio survivors was firstly about the food provided in hospitals, and secondly about alternatively freezing or sweating in a bed with only a thin, hard, coconut-fibre mattress between them and a fracture board. Many suffered from bedsores because of immobilisation in splints: 'They had these long prams like trolleys to wheel us about on, and we were picked up and put on them, frame [Thomas splint] and all. We were often taken outside but the people seemed to forget about us and left us there when it was raining, or too hot.'[188]

Hospital policy for long-term patients favoured verandah accommodation with canvas blinds that were rolled down at night, and back up when the day shift came on duty. Balconies or verandahs were a legacy of Victorian miasmic theories about the need for fresh air and sunlight in wards, but were subject to extremes of temperature. Pauline Bazley was in Bendigo Base Hospital, and her bed

> was on the verandah, hot in summer and freezing cold in winter ... the rain would come in under the canvas blinds ... I got pneumonia four or five times. There was little to compensate for being exposed to the elements ... our beds faced a brick wall ... the really scary thing was the big, black spiders that used to fall on our beds as we lay still on our backs.[189]

Conditions were the same at Fairfield Hospital. In winter, 'it was very cold on the verandah at Fairfield, I had seven blankets on my bed to keep me warm',[190] while in summer, 'ancillary staff did their best to lower the temperature on the verandahs ... I remember that the gardener used to come and hose down the tin roof in summer'.[191] In Tasmania, winters were even colder than on the mainland:

> There was no heating in the aftercare ward. We began to feel the cold, especially on the frosty nights because you could not put your hands under the bedclothes when they were in splints. The plate of metal that our feet were bandaged to was extremely cold. So groups of ladies started knitting woollen socks and covers for our hands. They made coloured rugs that were placed over our chest and tucked in round our

shoulders at night. They were a help but many nights we would wake up shivering with the cold and everyone seemed to be getting bad colds. Some got pneumonia and died.[192]

For Australians hospitalised during the epidemics, the food in hospital was usually appalling, tasteless and lacking any nutritional balance. Little in the way of fibre was given, no fresh fruit and just a few vegetables which, if offered at all, were more often in the guise of unpalatable slurry. In *The Great Scourge*, Anne Killalea gave an example of a typical hospital menu in Tasmania in 1937: 'Bread constituted breakfast, and bread and custard for tea. Lunchtime alternated between a choice of tripe or mince'.[193]

For some in-patients, doing something to avoid eating the unpalatable food provided some relief from the boredom of life on the polio wards. In Fairfield Hospital, young Brian Caulfield did not 'like hard-boiled eggs, so we'd wrap them up and lob them up into the ventilating shafts ... they are probably still there',[194] while Edna Thilby, who 'hated porridge' used her tin plate to 'fling it out onto the lawn, it must have been thick with porridge, ghastly, lumpy stuff. We had porridge seven days a week for breakfast, and that's all we got.'[195] Also in Fairfield, Marguerite remembered being given 'baby food through a bent glass straw before graduating to grated apple mixed in with almost liquid mashed vegetables'.[196] Another remembered jelly that was 'so rubbery' that we used to throw it at each other.[197] Some children were physically ill after being forced to eat food they did not like: 'I could not eat that milky hospital food. The nurses would feed me rhubarb and custard, one would stand one side and hold me, and the other would shove food into my mouth. Then I would vomit. I lost a lot of weight.'[198]

Ian Dury loathed the fact that he was a 'prisoner to hot milk — with this bloody little jug thing coming towards you. It looked like a teapot, but it was for pouring milk into people's mouths.'[199] Many parents and visitors were appalled by the quality of food, and brought in supplies from outside. Sometimes they had to smuggle these past a hawk-eyed Ward Sister: one woman remembered lowering down a rope 'so our husbands could send up meals we'd ordered'.[200] Grandparents were enlisted to help: one devoted couple came in to visit several times a week carrying 'a baking dish full of rice pudding', while other parents 'lobbed chocolates over the hospital walls'[201] for the more mobile to retrieve and share with others. More often than not, the junior nurses joined in the rebellion against hospital food and 'would take the hat around, and one would go to the corner shop and buy eggs and make us scrambled eggs'.[202] Sometimes bribery was used to cajole patients to eat: 'We were allowed to listen to the radio in the afternoon if we ate our supper. One day I didn't eat my green beans and the nurse wouldn't let me listen.'[203] Many patients hospitalised in Fairfield during the 1950s had trouble swallowing the food and were fed by nasal-gastric tubes for long periods. Noel Spurr recalled that the first food he 'could keep down was "Cheddarette" biscuits, and when I came home people said I was like something out of a concentration camp'.[204]

For all involved, challenging the power of the institution in small ways gave a feeling of empowerment, a means of regaining their image of themselves as a person and not merely a patient. Frequently, those who were in hospital regained some sense of independence by working out means of subverting the authority of the system, whether it was by working out how to wriggle out of a Thomas splint at night after staff had done their rounds — 'I very soon learned that by turning my hand around I could get my arms out. Dame Jean [Macnamara] supervised this treatment and I remembered her saying, "If we hadn't put you in a splint you would have ended up like a corkscrew."'[205] David recalled how he and his roomate adulterated their urine specimens by pouring fizzy root beer into the bedpans before using them, and of the gasp of horror from the nurse when she checked them.[206] Life on the wards was not all bad: a genuine camaraderie often developed amongst those in the 'tanks', and it was usually the young and inexperienced nurse who was the target for practical jokes:

> In those days the nurses were pretty scared too. They would send the girl into a room full of three iron lungs and of course they used to be scared out of their wits. They tried hard to be self-confident and sometimes we played a trick on them ... they were told that those lungs were keeping us breathing and that if they stopped, we'd stop breathing. So we would pretend to choke, or have a fit ... and the poor girl would put her head out the door and yell 'Nurse' ... but generally the nurses seemed to enjoy working with us.[207]

Some patients rejoiced in the idea that they were viewed as difficult by staff; it gave them a sense of autonomy, but sometimes it was at a price. Rewards were given for compliance with hospital rules, and those rewards could easily be withdrawn. Amy Fairchild argued that some polio patients were termed 'bad' by hospital authorities because they 'vied with medicine for power and authority over their bodies and the terms of their recovery'.[208]

Having polio in the mid-twentieth century usually meant an extended stay in hospital, generally around twelve months and sometimes as long as four or five years. Some, like June Middleton in Victoria, never went home.[209] Those who had made the successful transition from respirator to a rocking bed, or who had learned how to 'frog breathe',[210] then joined other patients in the convalescent ward and settled, willingly or unwillingly, into the routine of hospital life. Most hoped that the move would prove a significant step in the road to recovery, but some were disappointed to discover they were still paralysed after the fever and pain had disappeared. For all polio survivors, many months would be spent in exercising weakened muscles and, in Australia, treatment usually followed one of two methods that were as different and controversial as the two women who promoted them. In Australia in the 1930s, some adherents swore by the unorthodox method of treatment devised by Sister Elizabeth Kenny in Queensland, while those who advocated the conventional approach of orthopaedic medicine followed the treatment regime supported by Dr Jean Macnamara in Victoria. Kenny's treatment advocated early, passive treatment of muscles in the acute phase of the illness, the use of heat packs to alleviate pain and tightness, and no immobilisation and splinting of affected limbs. Macnamara followed the more accepted treatment method of using splints to prevent contractures and deformities in limbs and then physical therapy once the patient had entered the convalescent phase and pain had subsided. Orthodox treatment gave medical practitioners and therapists the active role in treatment, whereas the Kenny method encouraged patients to reject their passive role and to retain agency over their body by working with the therapist to facilitate recovery. Whichever method of rehabilitation was followed, the recovery period was long, arduous, often very painful and imposed further stress on families and patients traumatised by the polio experience.

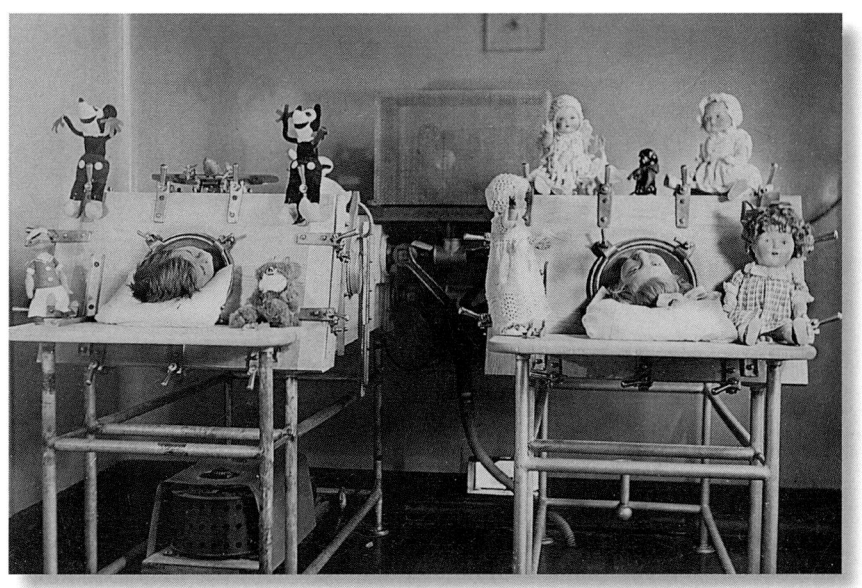

Children in gendered iron lungs in the Royal Children's Hospital, Melbourne.
Reproduced by permission of the RCH Archives

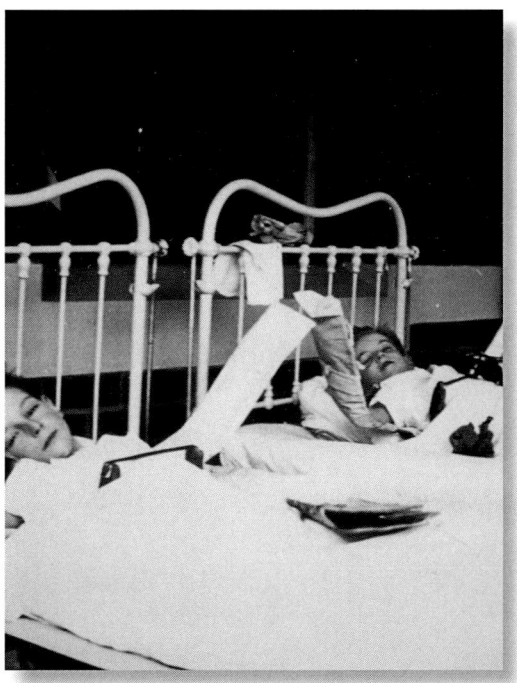

Children in Thomas splints on the balcony at Fairfield Hospital, circa 1938.
Reproduced with permission from the Fairfield Hospital archives.

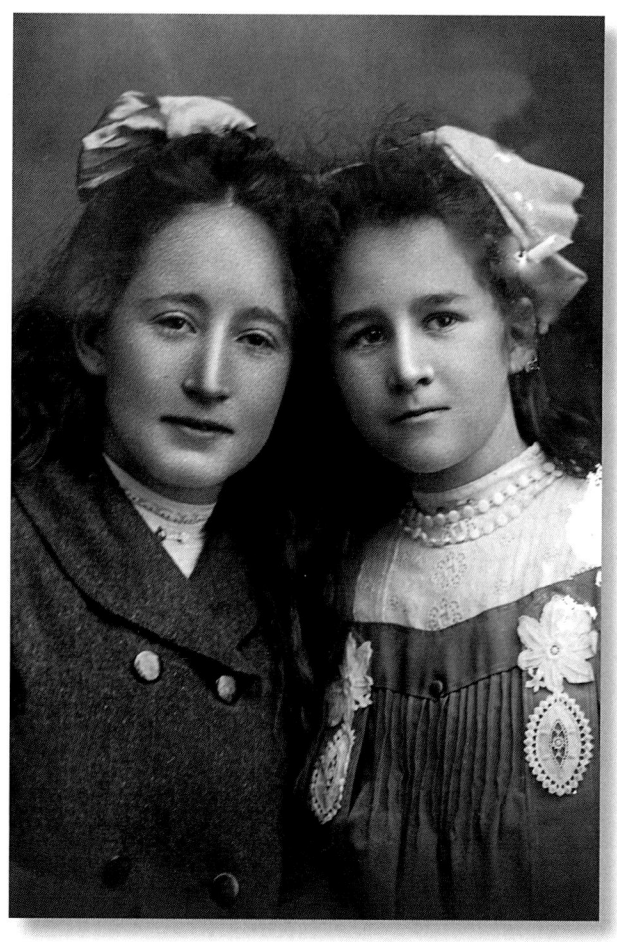

Molly and Jean Macnamara, circa 1909.
Reproduced with permission from the National Library of Australia

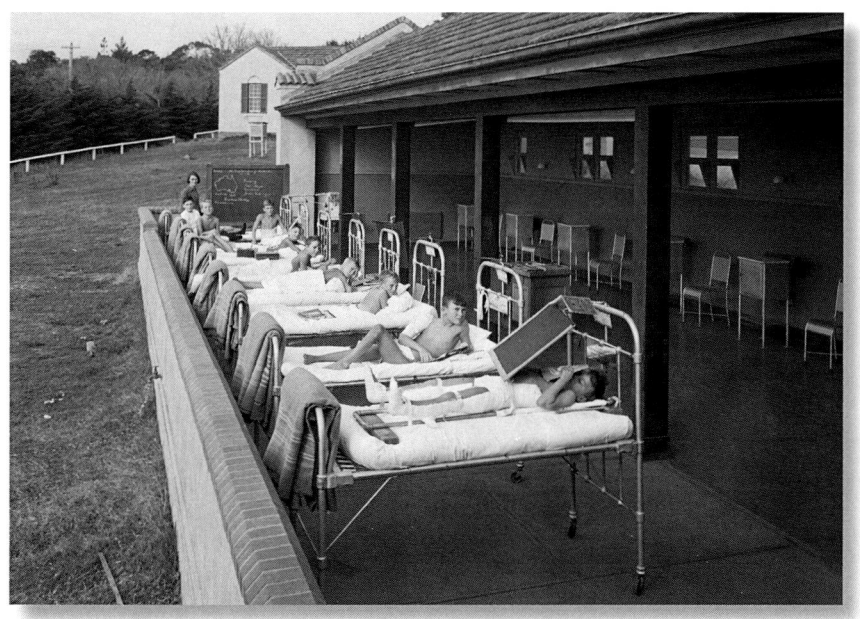

Children having heliotherapy at Frankston Convalescent Hospital, circa 1940.
Reproduced by permission of the State Library of Victoria (Harold Paynting Collection).

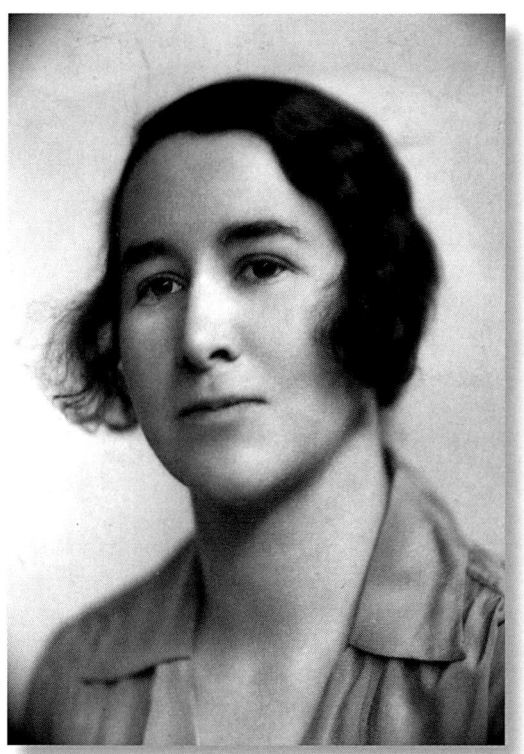

Jean Macnamara, circa 1931.
Reproduced with permission from the National Library of Australia

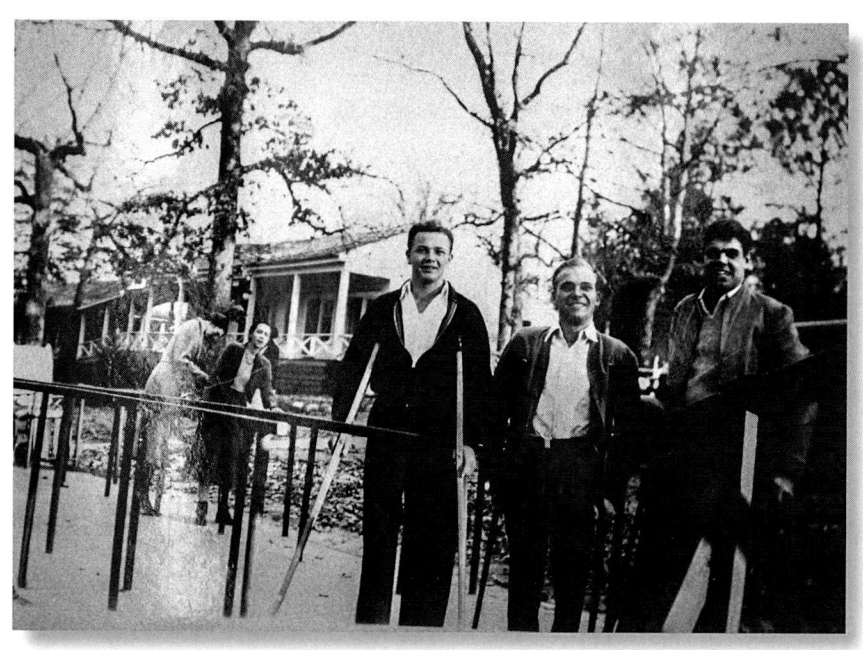

Polio patients, Warm Springs, 1933.
Reproduced with permission from the National Library of Australia

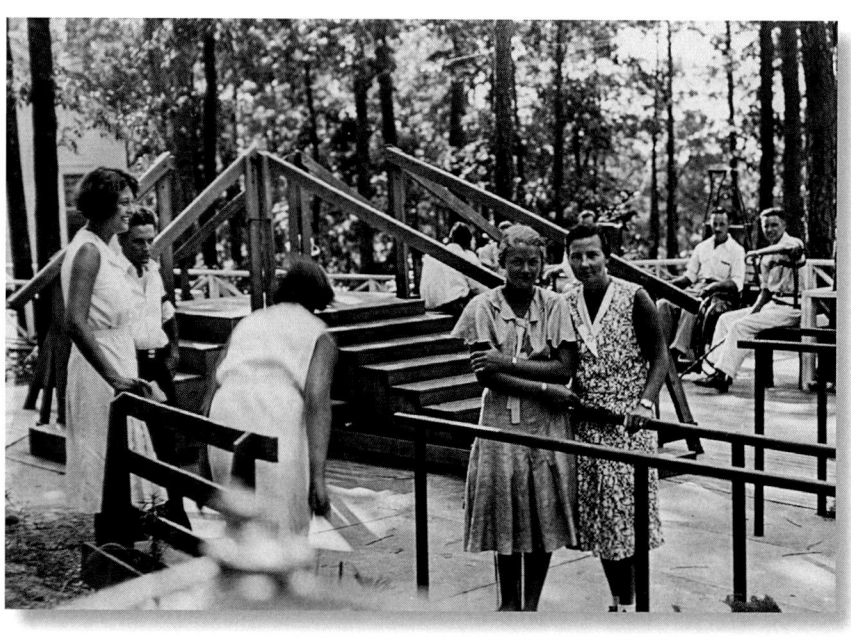

Polio patients, Warm Springs, 1933.
Reproduced with permission from the National Library of Australia

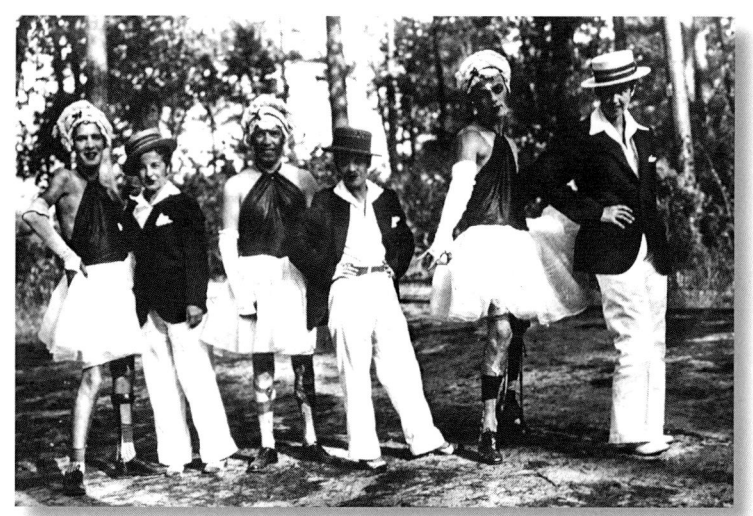

Concert given by polio patients, Warm Springs, 1933.
Reproduced with permission from the National Library of Australia

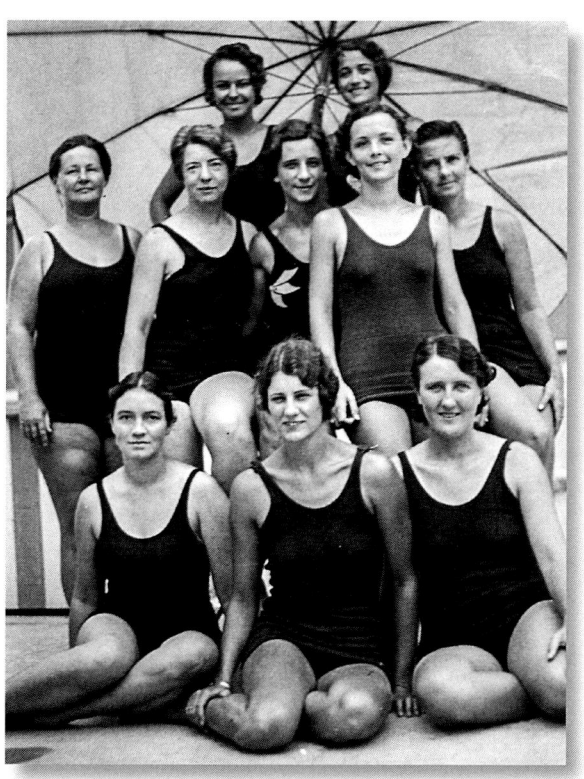

Physical therapists, Warm Springs, 1933.
Reproduced with permission from the National Library of Australia

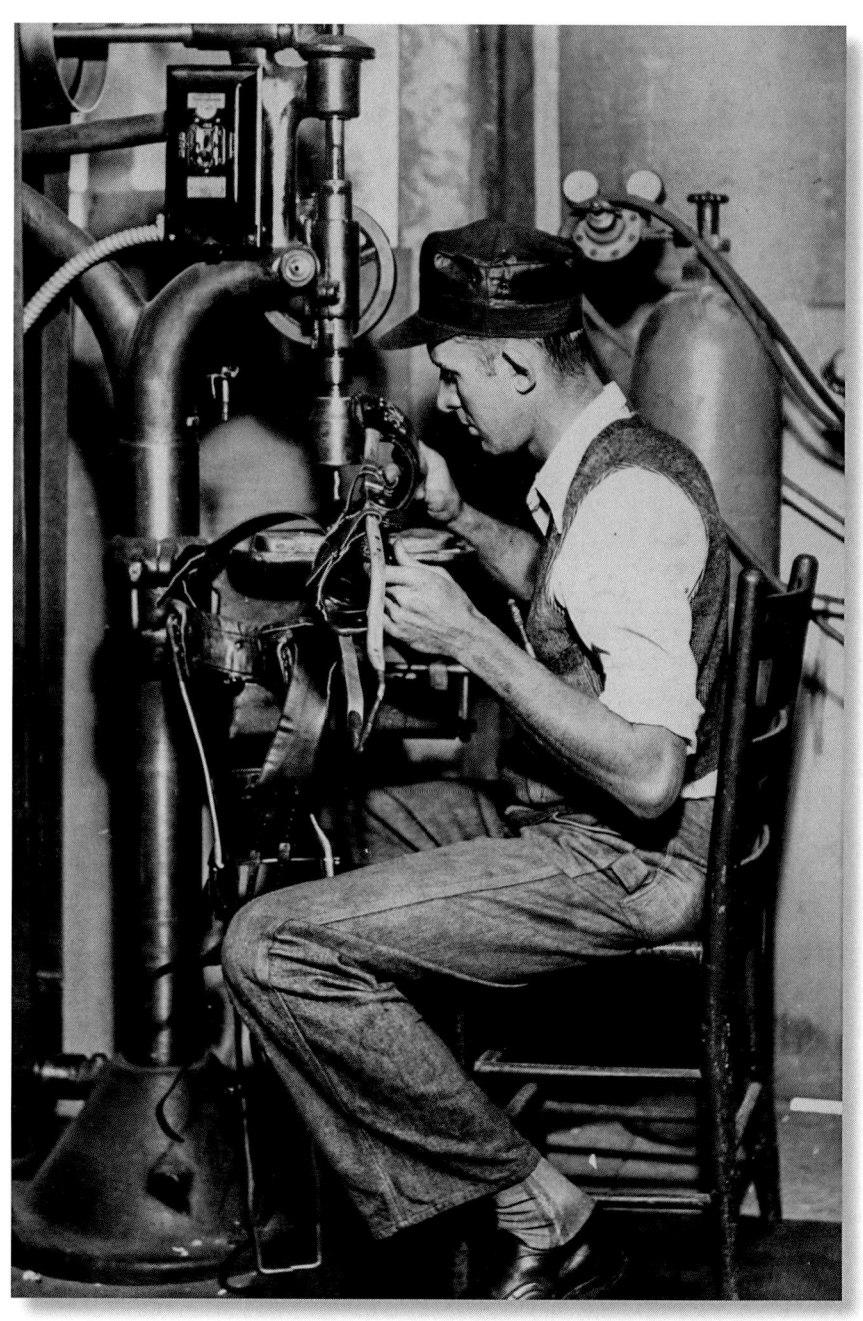

Splint workshop, Warm Springs, 1933.
Reproduced with permission from the National Library of Australia

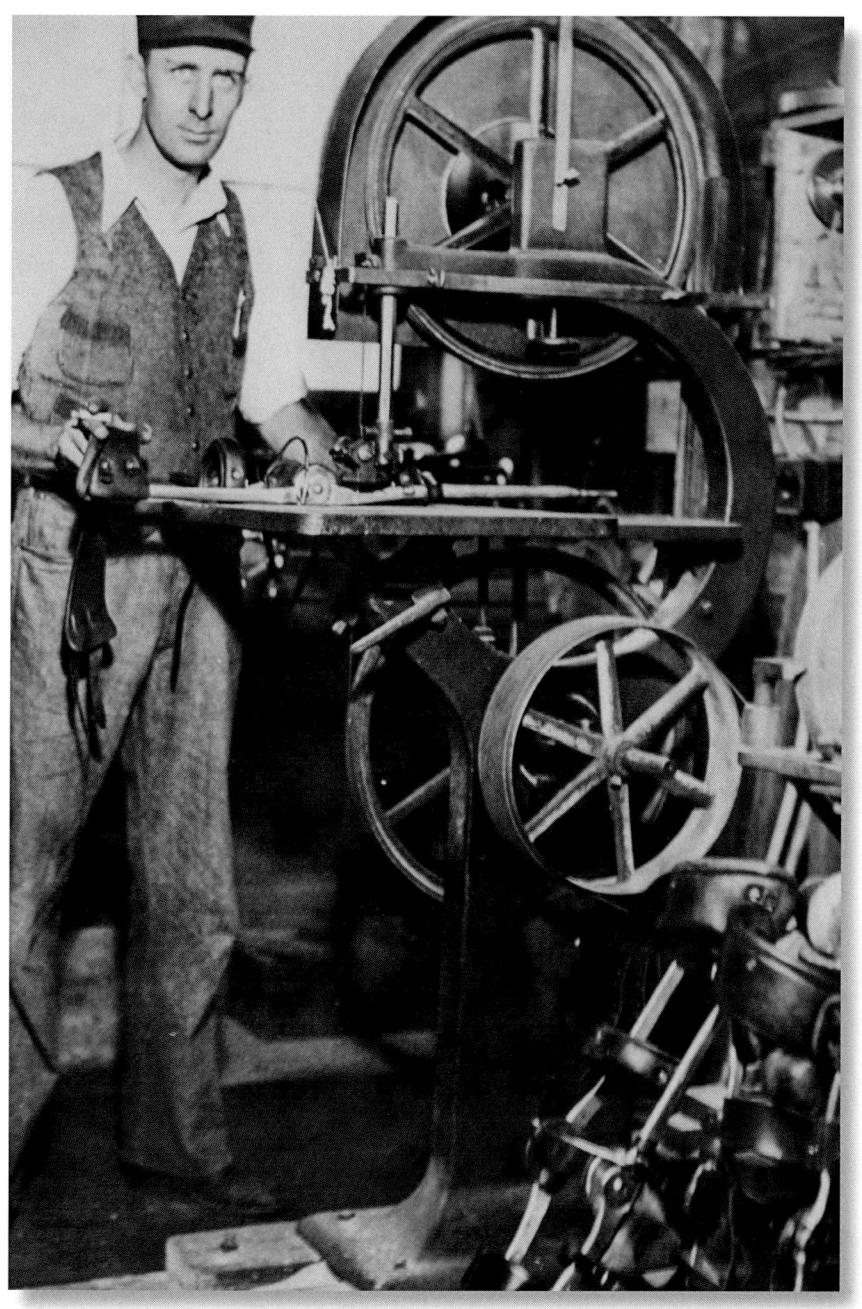

Splint workshop, Warm Springs, 1933.
Reproduced with permission from the National Library of Australia

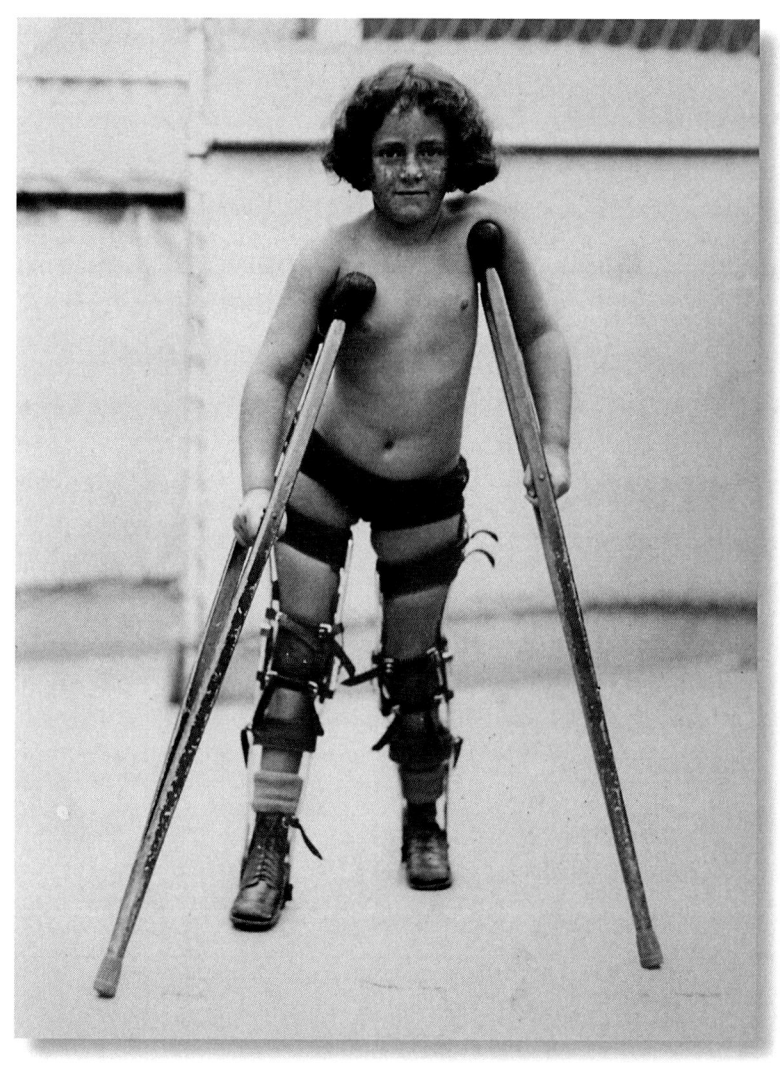

Child in splints, Warm Springs, 1933.
Reproduced with permission from the National Library of Australia

Chapter 4

SILENT TRAVELLER: POLIO IN AUSTRALIA

It is a major embarrassment for the Commonwealth Government that enlightenment about how polio spread and what control measures should be taken could not be clearly enunciated by health authorities. A definitive statement on the transmission of the virus and methods of controlling its spread is needed in order to shield government departments from misguided criticism and impatient agitation.[211]

Viruses and bacteria are everywhere; they are part of the normal dirt and grime of everyday life, and infants in 'cleaner' countries and communities were increasingly being reared in quasi-sterile environments that failed to stimulate immunity to normal endemic bacterial and viral flora.[212] Infectious diseases leave footprints in the form of serum antibodies in humans, and a rise in antibody level indicated that exposure to a specific disease had occurred. What distinguished polio from other infectious diseases of humans was the paradox that, as sanitation improved and other communicable diseases were conquered, the incidence of polio increased. Antibody levels to polio in many communities were found to be low or absent.[213]

Before 1880 there was no record of infantile paralysis or polio in Australia. Edward Ford's bibliography made no reference to either disease, but did quote one source by Charles Reeve in 1858 who wrote of the existence of 'diseases of the spinal cord and its membranes and the various forms of paralysis arising therefrom'.[214] Although the first official epidemic of polio in Australia was recorded in 1895 in the fishing port of Port Lincoln in South Australia,[215] some experts later came to the conclusion that 'sporadic cases of polio had probably been occurring for some considerable time'[216] and that polio was most likely endemic in Australia.[217] Polio is a notifiable disease and, as such, came within the jurisdiction of the Public Health departments in the various states.[218] Several of the early classifications are no longer recognised, for as diagnostic techniques evolved, many disease classifications changed. For example, until 1938 polio was also classified in some states as epidemic cerebro-spinal fever, meningitis, infantile paralysis or acute anterior poliomyelitis.

Notification became compulsory for polio[219] in New South Wales, Victoria and Tasmania in 1911, Western Australia in 1916, and South Australia in 1922. Once notification became binding, doctors were required to report their diagnosis to a central authority for collation of statistics and epidemiological analysis. Data were collected nationally from 1917, but before that year some states reported cases of infantile paralysis. Queensland and Tasmania reported five and three cases, respectively, in 1912 (see Annex Table 2). States had the power to inspect private dwellings and impose periods of isolation if the disease was present, and health officials also reported their findings on general household cleanliness and sanitary arrangements. The control of plague, tuberculosis and diphtheria had traditionally been the major problem for health authorities, and the outbreaks of plague in Sydney during the periods 1900–1909 and 1921–1922 did more than any other single event to bring about radical improvements to prevailing insanitary conditions.[220] However, public health control methods that had been successful in controlling other diseases did not appear to work against polio and, by 1915, the disease was beginning to cause concern.[221] At the end of 1917, cases of an illness that exhibited marked cerebral symptoms began to appear in some country towns in New South Wales, causing considerable alarm among residents. Local newspapers dubbed it 'The Mysterious Disease'.[222]

When a major epidemic of polio broke out in New York in 1916,[223] health officials instigated a vigorous campaign based on hygiene and quarantine. Patients and all contacts were quarantined for six weeks, and only the attending physician and nurse, health officer and representatives of the State Board of Health were permitted to enter or leave the infected building. A card warning that polio was present was fixed to an outside wall, and flyscreens were attached to windows. Family members over the age of sixteen could leave after being treated with disinfectant, and younger children could leave on the understanding that they would have no contact with other children for two weeks. Food was delivered to the quarantined house and left at the front door, mail was forbidden, and all books and toys burned. Dogs, cats and birds were treated and removed from the house and any animals found roaming in the vicinity of the quarantine area were destroyed. If the patient died, the funeral had to be kept private — family members were not permitted to gather together to offer sympathy and support. Schools were closed, and public meetings banned. Communities outside the affected area tried to prevent inhabitants from fleeing. Despite all the precautions, the epidemic continued to spread. Naomi Rogers has argued that the social response to the epidemic in New York was constructed within an atmosphere of fear — fear of dirt, of the poor and of the immigrant.[224] One of her key points is that before Franklin Delano Roosevelt contracted polio in the 1920s the image of polio was different: 'It was associated with the poorest, dirtiest children, not affluent adults in the prime of life, and with immigrants in slums, not Yankees from long established families'.[225]

Rogers showed how some health officials were unwilling to relinquish their historic assumptions concerning the link between dirt, morality and disease, and resorted to traditional methods of control — quarantine, fumigation and disinfection — to attempt to control the epidemic in New York in 1916, because they believed that the source of the disease lay within the crowded tenements of the inner-city slums. Clean up those areas and the disease would disappear, they reasoned. Officials identified flies as a target for their role in 'carrying the disease from working-class to middle-class' families, and implemented enthusiastic anti-fly campaigns that exhorted the housewife to be especially vigilant to keep 'filthy, polio carrying flies' from the house.[226] Rogers argued that it was not until Roosevelt became a survivor of the disease, and gave polio a new social meaning, that public and medical perception began to change about the association between dirt and disease, and to accept that the incidence of polio was not defined by class or race. When Australian officials studied the epidemiological findings published on the New York epidemic they realised they were dealing with a similar set of circumstances: the incidence of polio was greater in scattered country populations than in the crowded city slums, and public health control measures like quarantine that had been so successful in controlling other infectious diseases did not appear to work.[227]

The anxiety that parents felt about polio in Australia was not misplaced, and many viewed the prospect of a child becoming paralysed and suffering permanent disability as especially terrifying. Polio could transform the sufferer into the 'Other', and that 'Other' was seen as a contradiction to an ideal of a healthy childhood, followed by adolescence and successful adulthood. Epidemics in New South Wales and Queensland in 1904, and in Victoria in 1908, followed the outbreak of polio at Port Lincoln.[228]

That same year Alan Marshall had just started school in the small town of Noorat in south-western Victoria when he came down with the disease. Parents in neighbouring districts were worried when they heard the news about the young boy's illness, for many local people believed that sufferers of infantile paralysis were mentally as well as physically handicapped. Marshall recalled that 'Parents called their children in earlier, wrapped them more warmly and gazed at them anxiously when they coughed or sneezed', while many whispered anxiously to each other: 'Have you heard if his mind is affected?'[229] The origin of congenital defects was still shrouded in mystery and superstition, and there was no distinction made between an inherited or acquired disability. All were lumped under the one heading, and that was 'cripple'. In 1932, H.T. Parker gave a different reason for the apparently common correlation of physical with mental disability, rightly concluding that a lack of mental stimulation for the child was the problem, and not the disease itself:

> Without doubt, physical defects, whether inborn or the result of accident or disease, are not uncommonly correlated with mental disabilities ... physical defects could result in a lack of normal mental stimulus of the young child ... restricting intellectual development.[230]

There were epidemics of polio in the eastern states during the years of the First World War. Queensland suffered the most. In the epidemic at the end of 1915 the state reported the highest number of cases for the war period with a mortality rate of fourteen per cent. Whether the rate was as high for other states is not clear, because deaths from polio were not classified separately until 1922, unless a special report was produced, as was the case in Queensland.[231] In the 1937–38 epidemic, the death rate varied from six to ten per cent throughout the affected states.[232] Severe epidemics occurred in New South Wales in 1916 and Victoria in 1918. There was a moderate outbreak in Tasmania in 1930, and a mild one in South Australia in 1922.[233] Western Australia experienced a mild outbreak in 1925, and the first major epidemic occurred in 1948. Each epidemic brought a rise in notifications of the disease. The post-war years were the worst for all states except Tasmania,[234] and the decade between 1950 and 1960 also saw increased notifications of polio in the Australian Capital Territory and the Northern Territory.

In the summer of 1931–32, an extensive outbreak occurred in New South Wales and public health officials noted that the 'disease appears to be more feared by parents than any other' and that the press and public had made 'unusual demands for information about polio'.[235] Worse was to come. In the winter of 1937 an epidemic appeared in the bayside suburbs of Melbourne that proved devastating for the population of Victoria, and provoked panic on the eastern seaboard of Australia.[236] Hilda Bull realised almost immediately that the epidemic possessed several 'unusual and startling features'.[237] Cases were 'very severe', and the disease seemed to be extremely contagious. Great efforts were made by authorities to quarantine children in the area affected, but it spread quickly through residential areas into the city and the docklands. Parents became alarmed, and authorities tried to prevent them from sending their children to the country, but many did leave.[238] Streets where children usually played were deserted, 'picture shows and shops' were empty and, by the end of July 1937, all schools in Melbourne within a fifty-mile radius had been closed.[239] Worried parents flocked to the Children's Hospital, unwittingly exposing their children to a greater risk of catching the disease: 'There were apparently four "foci" in the city, chief of which was the outpatient department of the Children's Hospital'.[240]

Fear during the epidemic was intensified by ignorance of how the disease spread. In 1928, John Dale wrote of his apprehension about polio because he had 'little to guide him' about how best to combat an epidemic whose behaviour was 'so uncanny' and unpredictable.[241] Little changed over the ensuing ten years. However, by 1937 health authorities were aware that it was rare for hospital staff to become ill or for cross-infection to occur in wards — factors that suggested to them that the contagious period was short, and had passed before patients were admitted. The role of disseminating information on rapidly changing areas of quarantine, restrictions on travel and advice from public health authorities on transmission of the virus became the preserve of the media.[242] Parents were advised that children should not 'catch trams and buses unless absolutely necessary',[243] and popular myths about the transmission of the virus circulated. Theories ranged from sunbaking to animals as the culprit. As the panic about polio had spread in New York in 1916, 276,683 domestic cats and dogs were killed in the 'lethal chamber' of the Society for the Prevention of Cruelty to Animals.[244] Although a letter writer had suggested that 'cats transmitted the virus', it appears that Victoria's cats and dogs did not suffer a similar fate.[245]

Despite the rapid spread of the epidemic in Victoria, New South Wales remained comparatively free of the disease for some months, but health authorities were aware that social contact between the immune and susceptible members of the population had to be prevented. They approached the Commonwealth Government for help, but the Federal Minister of Health W.M. Hughes refused to nominate Victoria as an infected area, declaring that it was 'constitutionally and legally impossible'.[246] In response to Hughes, New South Wales officials acted quickly and amended the *Public Health Act* to impose restrictions on interstate travel. Tasmania and South Australia[247] did likewise. Up to twenty crossings into New South Wales were patrolled by police who were also stationed at railway stations, aerodromes and bridges over the Murray River. Cars and trucks were stopped and checked and, unless those in charge could prove that any child under sixteen travelling in the car had not had contact within the previous 21 days with any known source of the virus, or had not attended a school closed because of the epidemic, permission to cross the border was refused.[248] In Tasmania, family members of polio patients were isolated for three weeks, infected houses were fumigated, and travel permits introduced for internal journeys from north to south on the island. Epidemics in Queensland in 1924 and 1932 caused 'great alarm' in the population.[249] Officials noted that the disease spread along lines of communication throughout the state, and correctly deduced that it spread through personal contact. Public unease in 1937 to news that an epidemic of great violence had erupted in the South prompted the Minister to set up a committee to advise the Department of Public Health on how best to respond to the emergency. Queensland Health made the decision not to impose quarantine, concluding that 'although these measures were employed in several instances elsewhere at very great cost … nothing would keep the disease out'.[250] In the Northern Territory, the isolation period was extended to six weeks after a minor outbreak in the Aboriginal population at Alice Springs and Hermannsburg, but 'very little infection' occurred.[251] Two cases were reported at Alice Springs and one at Tennant Creek between 1937 and 1939. Health authorities were interested in the 'apparently low incidence of infantile paralysis' in the Aboriginal population and believed that it was due to either 'racial resistance' or 'early immunisation' and approached the Native Affairs Branch in Darwin for permission to 'collect blood' from 'natives of selected age, sex and habitat' following 'suitable inducement or incentives for the natives to subject themselves to the necessary blood-letting'.[252]

The results proved interesting, and added weight to the theory that Aboriginal children had been exposed to the virus at an early age and developed immunity. Over ninety per cent of Indigenous people in all age groups had antibodies to the Type II Lansing poliovirus.[253] Four years later another study was conducted against the two remaining types of poliovirus,[254] and showed that those two types were not endemic among Aboriginals in the Northern Territory. What the study also proved was that antibodies produced as a result of exposure to one type of poliovirus did not extend immunity to the others. In 1951 there was an epidemic among the white population in the Territory,[255] but no cases were reported amongst Aboriginals. Moreover, despite extensive travel throughout the Territory in 1955, the team from Adelaide managed to locate just one Indigenous person who showed signs of residual paralysis,[256] indicating that, although the disease was endemic, the paralytic form of the disease was rare.[257] Some historians have commented on the low incidence of polio in Australia during the war years, a fact that is borne out by consulting the official figures. However, in Queensland the figures for communicable diseases were 'affected by war conditions, especially the great increase within our State of populations not subject to the Laws of the Commonwealth or the State, which had contributed to rendering the maintenance of general sanitation and the control of infectious disease very difficult'.[258] As a consequence, no statistics were collected during that period.[259]

In 1940, Frank Macfarlane Burnet commented on the 'great change' that had taken place in the age incidence of polio since the early years of the century. In 1937–38, polio was no longer a disease of infants and young children; the peak incidence was occurring in the five to ten age group, with increasing numbers of teenagers and young adults affected. The ratio of cases between urban and country areas was no longer biased towards the rural. Previously, healthy carrier adults had arrived in country areas to spread polio from endemic urban areas. Now the disease was spread by contact between children, and the ratio of urban and rural cases reported was almost even.[260]

Several therapeutic methods were used in Australia during the 1920s and '30s. The favoured method in Australia was serum treatment, and its most forceful proponent was a graduate of the medical faculty of the University of Melbourne, Dr (Annie) Jean Macnamara.[261] She was born on 1 April 1899 to an Irish Catholic father and a diminutive, 'red-haired, freckle-faced' Scots Presbyterian mother in Beechworth, north-eastern Victoria.[262] John and Annie Macnamara, like so many of their fellow emigrants from Britain, had acclimatised to the harsher environment of their adopted country, but were nevertheless delighted when John was posted as Clerk of Courts to that prosperous town in the Victorian High Country. Plantings of European trees and shrubs had been transforming parts of south-eastern Australia into landscapes more reminiscent of Europe, especially during autumn and winter when deciduous trees turned vivid reds and yellows before shedding their leaves to receive an occasional blanket of snow. It was so unlike the behaviour of the native eucalypts, acacias and melaleucas of the Australian bush that remained green throughout the year, that Jean recalled her excitement at seeing a 'view of a snow-clad Mt Buffalo, and the Town Crier on a frosty night as he walked the streets proclaiming the news of upcoming meetings or flower shows'.²⁶³ Her childhood, and that of her elder sister, appeared idyllic, protected within the cosy, private world of a comfortable, middle-class family where both parents enjoyed the admiration and respect of the local community.²⁶⁴

In 1905, John Macnamara was appointed as Clerk of Courts at Camberwell in suburban Melbourne, and the family moved to Wattletree Road, Malvern, where Jean and her sister Mary (Molly) were enrolled in the Spring Road State School. Jean first won a scholarship to the Presbyterian Ladies College, and later one to Melbourne University to study medicine. In 1922, she received her degree in company with such luminaries as Frank Macfarlane Burnet, George Simpson, Kate Campbell and Reg Mackellar-Hall. In May, Macnamara was appointed along with Campbell and Kate Mackay as an RMO (Resident Medical Officer) at the Melbourne Hospital, a position that would give the women great clinical and surgical experience.²⁶⁵

The future for the girl from Beechworth looked bright. Jean Macnamara's career would evolve in a period that marked the consolidation of the prestige of the practice of medicine, reinforced by a general air of esotericism and deference. Following European settlement, medical care to the colony was provided by salaried surgeons working for the colonial government and, despite a guaranteed income, by 1820 there were only about three medical practitioners per 10,000 inhabitants in New South Wales. By the mid-nineteenth century, the number of doctors in New South Wales and Victoria had increased four-fold, with a high proportion of them working on the goldfields.²⁶⁶ Many medical customs and practices came to Australia from Britain and, as the association of the urban practitioner with the well-to-do in Australia opened up new social and political contacts, those linkages also increased their status within the profession, and in the general community. Successful physicians and surgeons became extremely wealthy and influential men. In 1846, a group of medical men in the Port Phillip District formed a medical association and, in 1855, combined with others to form the Medical Society of Victoria. The first issue of the *Australian Medical Journal* was published in 1856, and was seen as another step towards the goal of professional accreditation. A process of self-regulation began with the licensing of practitioners and registration with the Medical Board. However, that tightening of the rules did not prevent ordinary members of the public from practising medicine or surgery. Many simply erected a shingle to offer their services, placed a '"Dr" in front of their names' and went about the business of tending to the sick and infirm. Over seventy-five per cent of those who practised medicine in the colony in the nineteenth century were not qualified doctors or physicians, but chemists, dentists, midwives, homeopaths, herbalists and other alternative providers.[267]

The *Medical Act of 1908* and the associated legal framework established the market dominance of the medical profession. It also laid the foundation for the control that the British (later Australian) Medical Association[268] would exercise over other health professionals, in particular, nurses and physiotherapists. Tony Pensabene's study outlined how the previous guidelines governing supply and demand for medical services changed in Victoria when the profession gained control over the new knowledge of scientific medicine, and over the supply and working conditions of doctors. He argued that the beginning of the twentieth century was when the medical profession in Australia attained true respectability, mainly as a result of the strength of its professional organisation — one dubbed by J.A. Gillespie as 'the most powerful trade union in the British Empire'.[269] Evan Willis adopted a more Marxist view in his analysis of the rise of the medical profession in Australia, and argued that political and social issues played the dominant role in the rise of medical dominance, and that the possession of complex knowledge was also important, but played a lesser role. Willis believed that the profession achieved its dominance in Australia in the early 1930s.[270]

By the late nineteenth century, Melbourne had become a complex and sophisticated city of some 500,000 residents. It was a metropolis that mirrored British social order, with pockets of great wealth, juxtaposed with slums and poverty. However, despite the claims of being modern and civilised, Melbourne was an unhealthy city.[271] Health authorities soon came to realise that the city's hospital system could not cope with increased rates of infectious disease, and that a specialist hospital would have to be constructed. The question was, how was it to be funded? Most of the financial support for Melbourne hospitals came from voluntary contributions and charitable donations, and this did not allow for large capital expenditure like the construction of new buildings. In 1922, Frank Apperly, lecturer in Pathology at Melbourne University wrote to the Rockefeller Foundation asking for financial support to construct a new hospital and medical school at Parkville. He was seeking funds from the Foundation so that the endowment would not become 'the plaything of political parties' like the then current situation in Victoria. According to him, 'this important university has struggled along for 70 years always in a state of poverty' with almost non-existent facilities and despite the fact that Australia can produce the brains, the university had become a 'degree shop' with its best graduates going overseas to do research work. Stressing that his letter had been written out of love for his university, he hoped that his appeal to them would not be in vain. However, the Foundation later rejected his request stating they did not grant endowments for building construction.[272]

Both the Melbourne Hospital and the Children's Hospital had earlier adopted a policy of not admitting anyone with an infectious disease, notification of which had become compulsory in the early years of Federation:

> Diphtheria is nursed only now and then in the Children's Hospital, there being no department for the general treatment of disease. Children suffering from any contagious complaint have to be turned away ... their condition being more pitiable since there is no other children's hospital in the colony.[273]

Despite the ruling that 'children suffering from infectious diseases were no longer to be admitted', diphtheria and scarlet fever were common in the wards, probably because many children were asymptomatic when admitted for other reasons, and later developed full-blown symptoms of those infectious diseases.[274] In 1880 the Children's Hospital[275] erected a separate pavilion to isolate infectious children.[276] In her book first published in 1891, Grace Carmichael observed that: 'No communication was permitted with the main hospital except at a very respectful distance ... now and then one of the maids would take watch for an hour [over the patient] allowing me a few turns in the sunny garden; but this was rarely'.[277]

When the Melbourne Hospital began erecting tents in the grounds to quarantine infectious cases, the Central Board of Health took a dim view of that practice, and urged Melburnians to dig deep and raise funds for the building of a 'fever hospital' as soon as possible.[278] In 1904, The Queen's Memorial Fund Hospital, or Fairfield Hospital for Infectious Diseases as it became known, was opened. It was funded by a pro-rata levy on municipal councils, thus illustrating a new focus on infectious disease as a public health problem, and not the responsibility of the individual.[279] During 1937 all cases of polio from the metropolitan and central country areas of Victoria were admitted to Fairfield.[280]

The Children's Hospital in Melbourne had been sympathetic to the idea of appointing women resident medical officers to the staff, but official policy following the end of the First World War dictated that preference be given to male doctors returning from active service. However, in May 1923 that attitude towards the appointment of women 'softened'[281] and one of the two resident clinical assistants accepted was Jean Macnamara. By the time she arrived on the wards, Victoria had experienced three particularly severe epidemics of polio. Treatment of paralysis at that time was mainly supportive: prolonged rest and the splinting of affected limbs was the accepted method of treatment, a regime that would persist unchallenged for over ten years.[282]

Treatment of polio paralysis fell within the jurisdiction of orthopaedic medicine, a field that had emerged in the middle of the eighteenth century as a medical specialty dealing with crippling diseases of childhood. By the end of the nineteenth century, it had expanded to include fractures and other injuries caused by trauma to the human body. In 1889, the French surgeon Lucas-Champonnière had posited that immobilisation led to stiff joints and deformity, and that gentle massage and passive exercise would relieve pain, reduce swelling and help bone to heal.[283] Despite that, most surgeons and physicians believed that it was best to allow nature to perform its healing work by prolonged rest and immobilisation. No movement or massage was allowed and splints were devised to restrain the affected limb.

The First World War accelerated the growth of orthopaedics as a specialty within medicine, for the conflict provided an abundance of casualties needing surgery and rehabilitative treatment. Bodies mangled by the new technologies of mechanised violence returned to Australia to begin the arduous process of learning new ways of living with a body changed by war, and those bodies were highly visible on the streets of Australia's cities and towns. The use of explosives and heavy guns resulted in missing limbs, shattered bones, torn muscles, damaged nerves and paralysis. Joanna Bourke's study of the impact of the Great War on the male body detailed how:

> orthopaedic teams, consisting of doctors, nurses and voluntary workers, were established to provide for the treatment and aftercare of the disabled ... thus, the wartime economy created an army of people whose livelihood was dependent on maintaining a supply of cripples.[284]

The medical infrastructure that had evolved to care for the crippled child was strengthened by 'extraordinary therapeutic, rehabilitative, and surgical technologies for all cripples — male and female, adult and child, soldier and civilian'.[285] Hospitals cared for children and adults who had been admitted with polio, and those institutions were training centres for physicians, surgeons and, to a lesser extent, nurses and physiotherapists. Hence, the polio patient was transformed into an object that provided medical training or, as Foucault expressed it, the sick and the disabled became a medical exhibit.[286] With polio patients, this dependence, lack of autonomy and medicalisation of the body continued beyond the realm of hospital-based treatment. When the economic climate of the 1930s intervened and disabled patients were moved from hospitals, control over the individual body was transferred to outpatient clinics and convalescent homes. In 1930, an editorial in the *Medical Journal of Australia* was strongly critical of the formation of the Australian Orthopaedic Association. It regretted what it viewed as the 'formation of another extramural association' and the consequent removal of orthopaedic practice from the auspices of the BMA in Australia. In the *Journal*'s view, surgeons were more than capable of dealing with demands for orthopaedic surgery and no special organisation was, in their view, needed. What seems clear from that statement is that the BMA resented any interference with its authority, even from within its own ranks.[287]

Sir Neville Howse, Director General of the Australian Medical Services in the First World War, recognised that significant numbers of returning servicemen would require orthopaedic treatment, and arranged for a number of medical officers to attend a special course given by Sir Robert Jones at the University of Liverpool before they returned to Australia.[288] By 1920, there were around five specialist orthopaedic surgeons in Australia and one of them was Colin MacKenzie of Victoria. He advocated lengthy rest and immobilisation by splinting or plaster casts as treatment for polio paralysis and believed that treatment in the acute or febrile phase would increase the severity and likelihood of ongoing paralysis.[289] MacKenzie believed that recovery from polio could take years.[290] In addition, he coined the term 'muscle re-education',[291] the orthodox treatment recommended by orthopaedic specialists and carried out by massage therapists.[292] In 1928, a paper by Jean Macnamara on the early treatment of polio was published in the *Medical Journal of Australia*:

> Patients should be nursed on a hard bed with a firm mattress and a cradle to support the weight of bed clothes, and encased in a plaster bed or boots that extended above the knee with the feet at right angles. Immediate splinting should be started in the acute phase and morphia given if backache is severe.[293]

Thus, the standard pattern of treatment for Australian patients was to isolate and immobilise them in an infectious diseases hospital or isolation ward of a general hospital for two or three weeks until the acute, or febrile phase of the disease had passed. Warm saline baths were then given daily, and re-education of muscles with graduated exercises commenced. Treatment of polio was then, as today, aimed at treating the effects of the virus, and not the virus itself.

Some hospitals, like the Children's Hospital in Melbourne,[294] introduced heliotherapy or exposure to sunlight as another form of therapy. Polio survivors were given access to the 'simple magic of sunlight and clean, clean air', and nurses 'slathered them with coconut oil'[295] as their bodies were 'burned to various artistic shades of brown'.[296] Clearly, the dangers of skin cancer had not yet been recognised.

Dr MacKenzie was a supporter of massage as a therapy, and lectured the therapists as part of their training. In Britain, the revival of massage or medical 'rubbing' had been attributed to an influx of men and women from Sweden in the mid-nineteenth century.[297] However, a scandal had erupted in the 1890s when the popular 'penny press' ran a salacious exposé of some 'houses of ill-fame' that advertised their services under the name of 'Massage Establishments'. To the horror of the legitimate masseurs, in 1893 the *British Medical Journal* saw fit to warn readers against the use of massage on account of the number of 'unscrupulous persons practising it'.[298] The members decided that an accredited association was the only way to fight the smear campaign against their profession. In Australia, the massage therapists were more concerned with the threat to their professional standing by untrained operators who were free to advertise their services because there were no regulations in place to prevent them.[299] Dr Jean Macnamara gave her support to the therapists in 1934 when they made a formal protest to their Registration Board against Sister Elizabeth Kenny, 'an untrained, unauthorised person who was practising what she called "re-education of muscles."'[300] Macnamara's support for the therapists gave them professional respectability because of her position as a leading member of the medical establishment and an acknowledged spokesperson on matters relating to poliomyelitis. Although the polio epidemics presented an enormous challenge to the fledgling profession of physiotherapy, they also created an opportunity for wider recognition of its expertise in the treatment of paralysis.

Physicians and scientists were subjected to pressure by the public and anxious parents to do something to either prevent or lessen the effect of the poliovirus on the body. Developments in cell and germ theory during the latter part of the nineteenth century and in the early twentieth century had led to many advances in therapeutic ways of treating bacterial disease, and vaccines against smallpox and typhoid had raised the hopes of many scientists about the prospects for prophylactic medicine. In Berlin, two assistants of bacteriologist Robert Koch[301] developed an animal serum that worked against the toxins produced by the diphtheria bacillus and, although the mechanism of passive immunity was not fully understood until the work of Frank Macfarlane Burnet and other immunologists in the 1950s and 1960s,[302] the use of serum therapy in that pre-antibiotic era proved very popular. In Paris in 1915, Professor Arnold Netter was the first scientist to use serum collected from patients recovering from polio in an attempt to prevent paralysis developing in new cases. He based his theory on a belief that convalescent serum contained viricidal properties that could be harvested and re-used.[303] Across the Atlantic, scientists at the Rockefeller Institute in New York were also hard at work developing various sera for therapeutic purposes, and when Simon Flexner reported in 1917 that his laboratory work using monkeys to develop and test a serum against polio had proved very promising,[304] other researchers throughout the world decided to investigate the therapeutic use of serum in the prevention of polio paralysis.

The use of serum as a method of preventing polio paralysis rose to prominence in Victoria in 1925 following the outbreak of another polio epidemic. Wilfrid Selwyn Kent Hughes, member for Kew in the Victorian Parliament, persuaded the Melbourne City Council to set up a Joint State and Municipal Campaign against Poliomyelitis,[305] and proposed that funding for the campaign be met equally by the State Government of Victoria and by pro-rata contributing councils.[306] The views of Kent Hughes on unemployment relief and support for the concept of 'work for sustenance' were well known, as was his support for 'benevolent cases', including the 'physically decrepit', to be transferred from government responsibility to the charities. Those views probably ensured his sympathy and support for any campaign that was likely to reduce the numbers of the disabled in the community who, in his opinion, were 'not entitled to the same rights as someone who had laboured for twenty or thirty years in the service of the State'.[307] Some other conservative members of parliament held similar views about the pension rights of the disabled, and voiced the opinion that it was simply 'bad luck if Providence had sent a man into the world with a frail constitution' and, as a consequence, the 'State owed him nothing'.[308]

Acting on the advice of his father, Hughes appointed Jean Macnamara MD as Medical Officer to the Committee advising the campaign.[309] She was twenty-six years old and, through experience gained at the Children's Hospital, was already acknowledged within medical circles as having a special knowledge of the clinical and laboratory methods of diagnosing polio. It was a feather in her cap to secure a position that would prove to be professionally, as well as financially, rewarding.[310] Macnamara was concerned about the aftercare treatment of paralysed children, but by 1924 had decided to concentrate her efforts on investigating and implementing a preventive approach to paralysis using a vaccine or serum treatment. Physicians then, as now, usually chose either a research career based at the bench or a clinical career divided between consulting room and hospital ward.

As Medical Officer for the Committee, Jean Macnamara was responsible for serum supplies and for their distribution within Victoria and interstate. New South Wales set up a similar scheme in 1926, and Queensland in 1931, but few medical practitioners applied for serum.[311] Collecting serum for therapeutic purposes had been attempted during the polio epidemic in Melbourne in 1918, when the pathologist at the Children's Hospital, Dr Reginald Webster, sent out a circular letter to the parents of thirty-five previous polio patients asking for blood to be donated. However, the response was poor.[312] Seven replies were received from mothers of the children, but only four agreed to come in. When Webster attempted to remove blood from the four small children, each became so distressed that he abandoned the idea, and instead decided to test his theory about the efficacy of serum treatment on monkeys. His experiments, aimed at proving that human serum collected from polio sufferers would provide protection against the virus, were non-conclusive, but Webster was more concerned that the procedure of administering serum intrathecally[313] could prove counter-productive, even fatal to the patient, if the delicate tissues surrounding the spine were damaged. Injection of the serum required considerable expertise, and Webster believed that inexperienced doctors could cause increased trauma to the spinal cord, thus making it 'easier for the poliovirus to travel to the brain'.[314] His view was that violating the spinal column was not a procedure to be taken lightly, as the risks for the patient were very high. It was accepted that the procedure should be performed by an experienced practitioner, hence the appointment of Jean Macnamara in Victoria.

If a general practitioner suspected polio they contacted the Committee, and it was Macnamara's duty to travel to the patient's home with her instruments for lumbar puncture, and a microscope to either confirm, or reject, the tentative diagnosis. If the test was positive, and paralysis had not yet occurred, the patient was admitted to hospital and given warmed serum very slowly, either intrathecally or intravenously. In August 1925, a nine-year-old boy received serum at the Children's and recovered, adding further weight to claims about its efficacy.[315] However, later results were mixed: some cases responded, others did not, and some patients went into shock after being given serum because of the introduction to their body of a foreign protein:

Joan W, a female aged 2 years [was] admitted to the hospital on 12 January. She had been ill for five days previously with fever and vomiting, and after two days became drowsy, irritable and feverish, falling over repeatedly. The Spine Sign [patient asked to bend the head to the knees without pain occurring] was marked. Given 26cc of serum intrathecally and 44cc intravenously. She developed paralysis of right quadriceps, which recovered with rest in a splint and re-education over two to three months.

Dorothy D, aged 4 years was admitted to another hospital on 8 January 1929 after 36 hours of illness. She complained of headache and pain in the back of her neck. Twelve hours elapsed before serum was given, 25cc intrathecally, 45cc intravenously and 20cc intramuscularly. On 10 January widespread paralysis of all four limbs developed. She was splinted in a splint of Double Thomas pattern with foot pieces, head piece and malleable arm pieces. A corset was applied to prevent stretching of abdominal muscles, and moulded hand splints to keep the thumbs in opposition.[316]

The problem with basing a diagnosis on lumbar puncture was that polio was not the only disease that gave a raised leucocyte (white cell) count, and it is probable that patients suffering from other diseases like meningitis or Guillain-Barré syndrome[317] were mistakenly given serum. In 1918, Dr Douglas Stephen had concluded that an increase in leucocytes in the cerebrospinal fluid occurred before the onset of paralysis, but the following year Dr Reginald Webster was equally convinced that it was impossible to distinguish between meningitis and polio by examining spinal fluid.[318] However, Jean Macnamara agreed with Dr Stephen and, for several years, based her diagnosis of polio on the results of the lumbar puncture. By using her microscope at the bedside of the patient, Macnamara reinforced the belief that the new relationship between science and medicine as a 'source of social, moral, and technical betterment', would be a partnership that would bring great benefit to both physician and patient, because of the evidence science provided to reinforce a medical diagnosis. Bringing the laboratory into the home was an example of 'how science — as an ideal and as a body of knowledge — entered the physician's workaday world'.[319] Additionally, the diagnosis made possible by the use of the microscope was often an irrevocable step in altering a person's view of themselves. As Charles Rosenberg has argued:

From the patient's perspective, diagnostic events are never static. They always imply consequences for the future and often reflect on the past. They constitute a structuring element in an ongoing narrative, an individual's particular trajectory of health and sickness, recovery or death.[320]

The influence of newspapers and magazines in bringing the use of serum therapy to the attention of the public was such that many physicians were viewed as failing in their duty of care if they did not use serum once the diagnosis of polio had been made.

By April 1926, notifications of polio in Victoria had dropped and, although it was decided to abandon the campaign for the time being, the work of collecting serum from donors continued. To guarantee a constant supply of volunteers, Macnamara included those who had contracted polio some years previously as well as recent convalescents. Small children were not spared: parents were approached for donations and, as a further inducement, donors were offered £5 per pint plus travelling expenses. However, despite the lure of receiving a sum for donating their blood that exceeded the average weekly wage, many refused. One young woman from Geelong wrote to Macnamara and agreed to donate blood on the proviso that 'she could be done at home' because she had to help her mother 'to make up for some of the expense' incurred by her family during her stay in hospital, and could not afford the time to travel to Melbourne. Another family considered that the trauma involved for one of their children 'was not worth it' because their daughter Nellie cried 'hard when we ask her, so we will not go against her will on any account'. Furthermore, the parents believed that it was unfair to ask their other daughter Margaret because she had already 'done her share'. Although they were sorry 'to disappoint you [Macnamara] again' the family believed 'it wasn't any good forcing' their daughters to donate blood. Some donors were fearful of a procedure they viewed as painful. One wrote that she 'really suffered last time … thought I would lose my arm', and another, obviously alerted by another outbreak of polio and to the possibility of another appeal for blood, pre-empted Macnamara by writing to say that he 'hoped for the good of everyone concerned that there will be no more need of my life blood this year'. Mrs Finch of Richmond flatly refused to let her son Arthur give 'any more blood', bluntly stating that he 'was not yet walking, and is very thin'.[321]

In Victoria, the selection of donors was based on other criteria besides recent exposure to polio: suitable subjects were those with 'a good family history', or the 'right type' of person.[322] Scientists and the public have long known about hereditary diseases of blood,[323] and the threat from being exposed to contaminated blood through transfusion.[324] Blood has always occupied a very special place in the human psyche; it is essential to maintain life and has deep cultural significance. A problem with one's blood, be it from disease or loss, is a problem with life.

At the University of Melbourne, Jean Macnamara had studied under, and worked as an anatomy demonstrator for Professor R.J.A. Berry, a committed supporter of eugenics and the campaign for segregation and state intervention to limit reproduction by 'unfit' members of the population.[325] There is no doubt that she was influenced by hereditary determinism. After visiting a home for disabled children on Rhode Island in 1932, she wrote back to Australia that 'it was lavishly endowed, [but] some of the children were epileptic and spastic, and would be better knocked on the head than being treated like millionaires'.[326]

In 1931, Isobel Hodge was appointed as almoner to the Children's Hospital and, as well as duties that involved following up on the welfare of discharged patients and encouraging parents to bring their child to outpatient clinics for therapy, she also compiled reports for Jean Macnamara on suitable blood donors, and noted the family background and circumstances of the convalescent children. Hodge worked from '4pm to 9pm',[327] a time when most parents would be home from work, and her reports gave detailed descriptions about the family:

> Wooden house ... clean and well kept ... in a good locality ... single-fronted semi-detached brick house ... wooden house in factory locality ... neat wooden house in a good locality, father is a carpenter ... very respectable family ... newly painted ... a good home, father refused permission for child to be a donor ... neat house, large closed car ... house untidy at 4 pm ... mother busy vacuuming ... the patient did not make a good impression, but gave his consent.[328]

Obviously, Jean Macnamara was concerned with the suitability or otherwise of potential blood donors, and children from respectable working-class families or the middle class were those she deemed suitable.

Fewer and fewer former polio sufferers were agreeing to donate blood, and the scarcity prompted Jean Macnamara to begin research with Burnet at the Walter and Eliza Hall Institute to see if serum could be safely stored for longer periods.[329] In January 1929, she wrote to Simon Flexner in New York asking for reprints of Rockefeller University findings on the use of serum therapy as a prophylactic to prevent paralysis in polio.[330] While lamenting the fact that Australia's 'isolation' denied her 'the stimulus' of conversation with other researchers in the field, Macnamara sought Flexner's advice on applying for a Rockefeller scholarship[331] to study polio in the United States and Flexner advised her to contact Dr Richard Pearce of the Department of Medical Education. The Rockefeller Foundation was established and endowed by John D. Rockefeller in 1913 and launched its philanthrophic work in the field of public health medicine. The International Health Division was the main operating arm and conducted worldwide campaigns against various diseases including malaria, yellow fever and hookworm. Queensland was a major beneficiary of funds for hookworm research in the early part of the century. As well as medicine, the Foundation created a Division of Humanities and a Fellowship program to give researchers from foreign countries the opportunity to increase skills or gain research experience in the United States. By the end of 1952, the Foundation had expended over US$28 million on various Fellowships.[332]

In the Pacific region, epidemics of polio were not confined to Australia and New Zealand. An outbreak of polio in New Guinea in August 1929 graphically illustrated the havoc the virus could wreak on a population with little or no natural immunity.[333] During the four months to December, 600 New Guineans contracted polio, and twenty-eight per cent of them died.[334] In those who survived, the incidence and severity of paralysis was highest in the young adult population. Two Europeans also fell ill, but recovered. Macnamara was disappointed that she was not notified of the outbreak early enough by the Commonwealth Department of Health, and regretted that 'such a unique opportunity for studying the effect of serum therapy with controls in human patients' had been missed.[335] Her idea was to give one group of 'villagers' human serum, and to use another untreated group as a control. Shortly afterwards she wrote to Flexner to inquire if the Rockefeller Institute would fund a similar experiment if another outbreak of polio occurred in a 'native population' in any of 'Australia's mandated Territories'.[336] If the Institute agreed to her proposal, she would 'stir up the Commonwealth Government' and make sure she was notified promptly of an outbreak. That opportunity never eventuated. Macnamara continued her experiments at the Walter and Eliza Hall Institute with Burnet, although they were unable for 'financial reasons' to purchase enough monkeys for their research.[337] Macnamara corresponded regularly with Simon Flexner, and in 1930 she was awarded a visiting Fellowship to investigate 'the living organism at a molecular level' at the Institute of Physico-Chemical

Biology in Paris. That same year, the *Medical Journal of Australia* threw its considerable influence behind the 'admirable success' of the serum treatment advocated by Macnamara. According to the *MJA*, serum treatment would 'reduce mortality' and 'prevent paralysis altogether' if given early enough. Furthermore, the 'whole medical profession acknowledged her achievement' and her 'mastery over a disease that still plays havoc with young lives'.[338]

In June 1931, Jean Macnamara addressed members of the Tasmanian Parliament on the benefits of serum, and it was probably around that time that she became friendly with Enid Lyons, wife of the Labor MP Joseph Lyons.[339] She was already part of a Melbourne social elite that included former Prime Minister Stanley Melbourne Bruce and Lady Somers, wife of the Governor of Victoria.[340] Her position on the benefits of serum therapy was clear: if serum was administered 'the illness was of short duration' and, if it was not, splinting for 'as long as six years' was necessary. According to her, serum offered sufferers of polio the hope that they would not become 'hopeless, distorted cripples'. Instead, the majority could, 'by careful patient treatment', avoid paralysis and the prospect of prolonged treatment and, of even greater importance to the Commonwealth, this would mean a large reduction in pension payments.[341] Macnamara believed that any cost to the state for the supply of serum was based on sound economics, and as serum was the only safe weapon against polio, she noted how pleased she was to see the 'gratitude of young adults in Hobart' after they had been given it, and their willingness to donate their own blood to add to the stock of serum.[342]

However, criticism of the use of serum treatment for preventing polio paralysis was beginning to gain worldwide momentum. In New York in 1932, Maurice Brodie published results showing there was no difference between normal and convalescent serum,[343] and in 1935 concluded that serum therapy held 'little value' because 'increasingly large amounts' were needed. Moreover, Brodie doubted that the 'antibody could ever reach the virus'.[344] In 1932, the New York Academy of Medicine released the results of an experiment to test the efficacy of serum treatment in polio and concluded that 'it was no use at all'.[345] The same year, Dr W.H. Park judged that 'patients treated with serum did no better than those not treated'.[346] By mid-1933, some medical practitioners in Australia were also expressing doubts about serum therapy. In New South Wales, Dr Karen Helms determined that 'it was not possible to conclude that the recovery rate in people treated with serum was due to that alone'.[347] Not long after her report appeared in the *Medical Journal of Australia*,[348] both New South Wales and Queensland ceased the use of serum treatment. Despite this, Jean Macnamara remained convinced that serum therapy was an effective therapeutic tool for the prevention of paralysis, and cited Webster's research as well as that carried out by Flexner in New York to promote its use. The Poliomyelitis Committee in Victoria decided to continue collecting blood and dispensing serum in spite of mounting evidence against its use from colleagues such as Mostyn Powell[349] and Robert Southby, who concluded in 1935 that 'serum had no effect on either paralysis or recovery',[350] and from M. Brodie in New York and F.M. Walshe in London.[351] In 1937 the Committee appointed Frank Macfarlane Burnet to advise them on the use of serum. Some members were upset that Jean Macnamara was 'obtaining serum for her own private use' and expressed the view that the 'collection of serum was for the general use of the public and not for the benefit of an individual'.[352] Burnet's recommendation was unequivocal. In his opinion the use of serum was based originally on a wrong interpretation of experimental work in monkeys, and later experiments in Australia and overseas had revealed that it was of no therapeutic value. Furthermore, Burnet believed that if a medical practitioner wanted to use 'something for which there is no scientific basis' then 'he should be prepared to pay for it'. He doubted whether any 'municipal or government body was justified in spending public money to provide serum'. The Committee then resolved that no further serum would be collected from the public and, in May 1939, the Commonwealth Serum Laboratory (CSL) purchased the remaining stock.[353]

Some of Macnamara's supporters used serum on the basis that it 'did no harm', and instead brought comfort to patients and their families that *something* was being done to fight the disease. There is no doubt that there was a rapid transition from experiments with serum treatment in monkeys to human trials, a progression that would be unthinkable by today's experimental standards but, in the early twentieth century, researchers and clinicians were encouraged by the efficacy of serum as an antimicrobial therapy, and believed that it would be equally effective as a therapeutic agent against polio. As new scientific knowledge evolved in the 1930s — particularly that dealing with virology and immunology — the difficulties associated with serum therapy for polio became more clearly understood. Nevertheless, Jean Macnamara remained convinced about its efficacy, and persisted with the use of serum therapy, both publicly and in her private practice, until 1938.

In 1971, Dr John Paul noted:

> The demise of serum therapy after so many years of crude trials on which claims of its value had been made by so many physicians, a

number of whom were acknowledged authorities and occupied high places in the medical hierarchy, must have been a bitter pill to swallow, if such a metaphor is appropriate.[354]

Serum therapy was not the only form of prophylaxis used against the poliovirus. Frank Macfarlane Burnet reflected in 1968 that it had been 'active dogma in the 1930s' that the virus entered the body through nerves in the nasal cavity, and spread from there throughout the body[355] and, because of research that supported that view, a campaign was launched both in this country and in the United States, where 'thousands and thousands of children' had their 'high nasal passages' sprayed with a solution containing zinc sulphate and picric acid. The scheme was a failure, not only because researchers had concluded that the only way to effectively apply the spray was to 'turn a child upside down',[356] thus provoking loud screams and physical resistance from the children, but also because the chemical used in the spray 'caused burns and terrible headaches'.[357] Some children permanently lost their sense of smell from the injury caused to their nasal cavity.[358] During the Melbourne winter of 1937, a public health official observed that 'strikingly few' children admitted to hospital with polio showed 'any signs of a cold', and proposed that if a child had a blocked nose then perhaps the virus could not gain entry. A 'chance remark' from Burnet to a colleague – that 'a simple way of testing that theory' was to invent a nose clip – inspired the scientist to construct one. But when his children were shown the clip, they 'flatly refused to appear in public wearing such things'. And that, wrote Burnet, was the end of that exercise.[359] Nasal sprays were used in Hindmarsh, South Australia, until February 1938, when health authorities finally warned the public against buying 'worthless preparations' and declared nasal sprays as a prophylaxis against polio 'useless'.[360] In Queensland, the Department of Health declared that the spray was 'ineffectual and impracticable'.[361]

Jean Macnamara left Australia in mid-August 1931 to take up her Rockefeller scholarship and, while mindful of the fact that the BMA had told her it 'did not wish to have anything to do with the aftercare of polio cases', she decided that she would report to them on schemes operating overseas.[362] Although she found Paris 'dreary and dirty' and the people 'awful ... noisy and chattery ... the women had sallow complexions and long varnished fingernails ... and the children look sick',[363] she knew she was there to work, and her first task was to meet with Dr Daniel O'Brien at Rockefeller Foundation headquarters situated on the Left Bank. O'Brien soon realised that, because her 'interests lay more in the practical side and less along investigative lines', there was no point in her remaining at the scientific research laboratory in Paris. He was adamant that she should leave at once for the United States where a 'huge epidemic of polio' was happening with several thousand cases alone in New York. In his opinion, it was a 'crazy idea' for Macnamara 'to potter about in Europe while the war was in America' and he made arrangements with New York for her 'to proceed immediately'.[364] She persuaded O'Brien to 'let her have a few days leave in England' at her own expense and he agreed, provided she boarded the *Lafayette* at Southampton on 25 September.[365] In England, fate in the form of a grumbling appendix intervened and she sought confirmation of her self-diagnosis from a London surgeon who advised her not to travel to New York on any account, 'because none of us would want to risk an appendectomy on a French ship'.[366] That doctors make bad patients is a truism — perhaps doctors know only too well the uncertainties associated with a correct diagnosis, hence their reluctance to submit to doubtful and sometimes painful procedures. Macnamara informed O'Brien of her illness and he agreed to her taking ten days rest in the country before a decision was made on her future.[367] She remained unwilling to leave for the United States and that 'ten days rest' extended to eight months, much to the chagrin of Daniel O'Brien in Paris.

Macnamara spent her time in Britain visiting several orthopaedic hospitals where she soon realised that Australian knowledge of aftercare treatment was far in advance of that in Britain. She was not impressed with the work being done for the aftercare of children at Great Ormond Street, London's largest children's hospital. Apart from 'two Australians working there',[368] the treatment for crippled children was 'medieval', and hospital policy was to 'let the children become deformed' before 'operating on their crippled limbs'. No one in England knew 'how to treat polios as well as we do in Australia', and some of the 'old boys, whose word she had taken as gospel' were very 'so-so' when she spoke with them in detail about aftercare. She was 'furious' that she had paid '30 and 40 shillings for their books' as they were 'dithering fools'.[369] Macnamara was shifting her focus from scientific research to orthopaedic medicine, and it was understandable that O'Brien was annoyed; he had agreed to her leaving Paris in order to travel to the United States, and her Fellowship had been awarded on the basis that she investigate the virus 'at a molecular level' and not research orthopaedics.[370]

Macnamara finally sailed for New York at the end of April 1932 where she met Dr Carter at the Rockefeller Institute. He tried to persuade her to return to researching the poliovirus, but she refused, adamant that her interest was now in orthopaedic medicine.[371] In March 1933, she visited Warm Springs in Georgia where, in her opinion, the 'treatment of paralysis was not taken seriously'. The staff were 'poorly trained' and the Director of Physiotherapy 'did not know how to care for paralysed muscles'. Supervision of patients at Warm Springs was 'lax' and splints were worn only if they 'did not interfere with social activities'. However, she believed that the work by 'Dr Michael Hoke on the surgical treatment of paralysed feet was probably the best in the world'.[372] Jean Macnamara returned to Australia in September 1933 unsure about the future.[373] She found it very frustrating that parents did not appreciate how important it was for their children to grow up healthy and straight, so they could become part of a healthy work force and contribute to the economic productivity of the nation. While she lamented the fact that many in society had not yet realised that a 'man's worth should not be measured by his shape', she maintained that it was a 'good thing' that an 'instinctive horror of deformity' should be present in Australia. Because a large section of the population in Great Britain suffered from rickets or tuberculosis of the bone, Macnamara believed that people's sensitivities had been dulled, as they no longer reacted with 'shock and revulsion' to deformity:[374]

> The incentive to achieve recovery of muscle power is greater in Great Britain where the incidence of rickets, surgical tuberculosis, war injuries through the centuries have accustomed people to the cripple population. In Victoria these epidemics shocked a population unaccustomed to crippling, sensitive to deviation from the normal shape, and a condition which threatened to add 100 to 300 persons annually to the list of those eligible for invalid pensions.[375]

When asked in 1938 if she thought that mild cases of deformity were being splinted unnecessarily, she responded by saying it was the only treatment to prevent deformities from developing; moreover, if any child showed 'any weakness' when asked to hop on one leg, or walking on 'tip-toe', then it was 'safer to splint than not to'.[376]

In 1935, Jean Macnamara was informed that the King had proposed that she become a Dame Commander of the British Empire in recognition of her work with 'poliomyelitis cases and other crippled children'. A longtime admirer of Britain, Jean and her husband were both delighted and she accepted the honour. Macnamara became a passionate advocate for correct posture in children: a dedication that was reflected by her two daughters who wore 'high lace-up boots that supported their ankles even when they were almost in their teens'.³⁷⁷ That conviction informed much of her attitude to correcting perceived deformities, whether they occurred naturally, like knock-knees, or resulted from polio paralysis. She was not backward in giving advice to parents about drooping shoulders, or a curved spine. She examined country children while they were at the Lord Mayor's Camp at Portsea and sent off letters to parents chastising them for their laxness:

> We suggest that you, his parents should look at him in bathing trunks and consider his shape critically as you would examine that of a building you have built or a young horse you think of buying. You will notice that he does not stand tall with chin and tummy in, but is inclined to slump so that his chest is flat, his tummy protrudes, his back is hollow. If he continues to slump it is likely his posture will be bad in adult life. Do everything you can to encourage a pride in his carriage.³⁷⁸

Five years after she returned from overseas, Victoria experienced its worst epidemic of polio. Jean Macnamara supervised the care of patients at both the Fairfield Infectious Diseases Hospital and the Children's Hospital using orthodox treatment — bed rest, and immobilisation of affected limbs in a neutral position in order to avoid the over-stretching of weak and damaged muscle tissue. Her admirers were many and, to some, her knowledge of aftercare treatment exemplary and justifiably 'recognised throughout the world'.³⁷⁹ However, her views on treatment were not universally accepted, especially outside Victoria. Jean Macnamara followed orthodox medicine, a heroic approach that gave medical practitioners the active role in managing and treating polio paralysis. In 1946 she declared that 'pool therapy did more harm than good' and that 'drooping adolescents' were proof that the 'Red Indian had the wisest plan' and that their 'papoose board should be the standard sleeping crib for babies from two months to two years, and that children with knock knees should be splinted'.³⁸⁰ In 1954, Dr Peter Colville addressed the Third International Poliomyelitis Conference where he said:

> There is a wide divergence of opinion on the orthopaedic management of paralytic cases. This almost certainly reflects a general dissatisfaction with results obtained from all forms of treatment and an inability to obtain a rational assessment of results using different techniques. At present, no solution is offered to this problem, although it probably represents a great source of anxiety to patients.³⁸¹

The polio epidemics in Australia focused attention on, and highlighted the difference between, new and old ways to treat the body disabled by polio, and Jean Macnamara's influence on maintaining the dominance of orthodox treatment for polio paralysis in Australia until well into the 1950s was profound. Elaine Riska argues that the medical profession can be internally divided into an administrative or politically active elite, a knowledge elite and ordinary practitioners.[382] In her early years, Jean Macnamara was keen to be part of the scientific, knowledge-rich stratum, but by her thirties she had become more of a lobbyist for change. Her energies were widely spread in her later years, and one of her passions was to promote the use of myxomatosis in Australia in order to combat rabbits, whose numbers had reached plague levels since their introduction into Victoria in 1859, and were causing enormous environmental and financial damage in rural Australia. She was not one to back down from a conflict, and her colleague Dr Stanley Williams described her as 'vigorous to the point of ruthlessness in dealing with colleagues or other responsible people, including politicians'.[383] Her passionate support for the use of the myxoma virus brought her into confrontation with Francis Ratcliffe of the Council for Scientific and Industrial Research (now CSIRO) who maintained that the devastation to Australia's delicate topsoil had occurred before rabbits arrived, and who was not convinced that the virus would spread in the rabbit population. Also against her was 'the rabbit lobby' of exporters, trappers and furriers who battled hard to maintain their livelihood.[384] Dame Jean[385] relished a chance to prove that she was correct in her thinking on subjects as wide-ranging as milk as a possible carrier of the poliovirus, soil conservation, the benefits of composting and myxomatosis. However, she was strangely reticent when it came to expressing either a public or personal opinion about another woman who was to become a significant player in the field of polio treatment. That woman was Sister Elizabeth Kenny, and it was in rural Australia that accepted medical authority on the treatment of polio paralysis was first called into question.

Chapter 5

PUSHING THE BOUNDARIES: POLIO TREATMENT AND ELIZABETH KENNY

In the early 1930s in rural Queensland and northern New South Wales, a nurse by the name of Elizabeth Kenny was moving around the countryside tracking down and treating crippled[386] children. In so doing, she set herself on a path to challenge medical orthodoxy about the treatment of the paralysed body and, as a consequence, she also challenged the axiom about a nurse's role within the medical hierarchy. Medical practitioners occupied the top position and the responsible and dominant physician directed subordinate nurses to carry out treatment decisions determined by him.

Nursing in the nineteenth and much of the twentieth century was dominated by the Victorian attitudes of Florence Nightingale, an approach that demanded dedication, discipline and a willingness to work long, often physically exhausting hours in hospital wards.[387] Many doctors of that era doubted whether nursing could even be regarded as a profession, and considered the women as subordinates — 'assistants' in carrying out the therapeutic regimes they had devised for patients.[388] The traditional, wise woman healer was replaced by the scientific doctor, and Victorian nursing emphasised the character of the nurse and not her skills or knowledge. As the twentieth century progressed, those assumptions would collapse.

As a nurse, Elizabeth Kenny was expected to confine herself to the physical and practical aspects of patient care as dictated by her superiors, and not, on any account, to involve herself in the diagnostic or the scientific. Kenny's treatment for paralysed bodies divided communities within Australia, Britain and the United States. She gained support from a handful of doctors in Australia and from many in the United States, as well as sweeping condemnation in this country and overseas. Some medical practitioners eagerly embraced her therapy, while others were vehemently opposed to a treatment that contradicted conventional wisdom. As in all medical practice, opinions varied. However, broadly speaking, the orthodox treatment of polio could be summarised by the following:

> Absolute bed rest, immobilization for protection of weak and paralysed muscles by splints and plaster casts, and the gradual introduction of muscle training or 're-education' after the acute phase and muscle spasm had abated. Surgery to correct deformities was generally performed and, in the case of children was initiated in late adolescence.[389]

In 1953, Dr John Pohl recalled how children had previously been taken to the operating theatre to have paralysed limbs 'straightened out under anaesthetic' before plaster casts were applied, and of how the children 'screamed with pain when they regained consciousness': 'Well, as doctors, we knew that if we didn't force them into plaster casts they would end up crippled, twisted and deformed. The whole idea was to prevent that happening and that was the accepted and universal treatment.'[390]

Elizabeth Kenny advocated early intervention of treatment, as soon as possible after the initial diagnosis. Her priority was to try and alleviate the pain from spasm in affected muscles by applying hot packs for up to twelve hours a day.[391] When spasm ceased, muscle re-education was introduced to develop a mental awareness of 'alienated' muscles and to re-establish co-ordination. At no time were splints or braces used and patients were allowed to remain in a 'natural rest position' in bed supported by sandbags. Kenny opposed any form of surgical intervention to correct deformities.

Other writers have argued that the campaign directed by many in the Australian medical profession against Elizabeth Kenny and her clinics was motivated more by a disdain for her non-medical status than it was for the methods of treatment she used,[392] and that Kenny represented 'the threat of non-medical interference' in an area of medicine that practitioners considered to be their sole preserve.[393] Medical practitioners are not only powerful because of their specialised knowledge, but also because they occupy positions of privilege within class structures in society. Nursing in the twentieth century was seen as an excellent example both of patriarchal subordination and as an ideologically driven exploitation that equated nursing with nurture and mothering, the natural preserve of women. As a nurse, Kenny was expected to devote herself to the physical and practical aspects of patient care, and not to involve herself in diagnosis or science.

Following her death on 30 November 1952, *The Sydney Telegraph* reported that Elizabeth Kenny was 'one of few Australians to gain an international reputation'.[394] Yet she failed to achieve any lasting success in her own country. Why was this?[395] In 1943, a paper published in the influential *Journal of Bone and Joint Surgery* concluded:

> Patients receiving the Kenny treatment are more comfortable, have better general health and nutrition, are more receptive to muscle training, have a superior morale, require a shorter period of bed rest and hospital care, and seem to have less residual paralysis and deformity than patients treated by older conventional methods. The Kenny treatment is the method of choice for the acute stage of infantile paralysis.[396]

Despite Kenny's efforts to establish her method of treatment in Australia before she left for America, she was largely unsuccessful.[397] By 1942, there were a few Kenny clinics left in Queensland, and a handful of Kenny trained nurses. In most parts of Australia, treatment reverted to that recommended by Dr Jean Macnamara and other orthopaedic specialists, and most polio patients in Australia continued to be 'strapped and bandaged in a full body splint', for as long as 'two years, unable to sit up to eat, drink or use the toilet'. Some patients were discharged from hospital in 'a brace with steel bars and calipers', and with legs so weakened from inactivity that 'if I let go of the crutches, I'd fall over',[398] while others made a complete recovery without any treatment. Such was the effect of exposure to the poliovirus, no one could determine what the outcome would be.

In contrast to the situation in Australia, across the Tasman in New Zealand 'almost all hospitalized patients in the 1950s were treated by the Kenny method'[399] using a combination of hot packs and passive movement of limbs during the acute stage. In 1954, The Third International Conference on Poliomyelitis concluded that

> The idea that paralysed muscles should be fixed in a position of relaxation is now quite untenable. Furthermore, it has been fully established that frequent passive movements improve the condition of all paralysed muscles.[400]

Why were most polio patients in Australia in the 1940s and 1950s denied a treatment that had become widespread throughout the world?[401]

Apart from many papers in scientific journals discussing her method of treatment, very little has been written about the life of Elizabeth Kenny apart from a few biographies,[402] and a co-authored autobiography, *And They Shall Walk*. Her work captured the imagination of many in the 1950s and '60s; nonetheless, the majority of the books on library shelves focused on the juvenile market.[403] During her lifetime, several venerable institutions including the Neurological Institute in Brussels, Harvard University and Johns Hopkins University in Maryland acknowledged Elizabeth Kenny's theories on polio treatment. She was awarded three honorary doctorates from American universities: a Master of Science from Rochester, a Doctorate of Science from Rutgers, and a Doctorate of Humane Letters from New York. Why was it, then, that Elizabeth Kenny, voted in 1952 as America's most admired woman, was humiliated and ignored by the medical profession in her own country?

The seeds of mistrust and suspicion displayed towards Kenny as she battled bureaucracy and the medical profession to have her radical treatment acknowledged were sown in the years between 1915 and 1930. Despite the fact that she claimed she had been a matron of a country hospital before enlisting in the First World War, two of the trained nurses who knew her well and worked with her as a nurse overseas were convinced that she was not a qualified nurse, based on their belief that her knowledge in certain areas of practical nursing was 'very limited' and that she 'did not know things she should have'.[404]

The root cause for the differing response between Australia and America to Elizabeth Kenny's treatment method rests with the influence exercised by the two governing medical associations, namely the British (later Australian) Medical Association (BMA) and the American Medical Association (AMA). In the early twentieth century the AMA did not control the practice of medicine to the same extent that the BMA did in Australia. In Victoria, the influence of the BMA was stronger than in any other state. Unlike the situation in Queensland, where the government had weakened the power of the BMA by barring medical representation on hospital boards, in Victoria the BMA had full representation on boards and was hostile to the introduction of a national health scheme or indeed any interference by the state in patient care. In the United States, one quarter of American medical practitioners in the 1930s were not regular physicians, and osteopaths, homeopaths and Christian Scientists monopolised the Health Insurance industry.[405] In 1925 the United States granted homeopaths, osteopaths and chiropractors in certain states the legal right to practise. The situation in Australia was the opposite. Unconventional practitioners were often viewed as 'quacks'[406] and the code of ethics of the BMA forbade 'consultation with irregular practitioners'.[407] Elizabeth Kenny steadfastly refused to be associated with alternative medicine, and always insisted that her treatment be carried out in hospitals under the supervision of a medical practitioner.

Tom Aikens recounted a meeting in 1938 between Kenny, himself and some friends at the Kenny clinic at Royal North Shore Hospital in Sydney. One woman (a fan of astrology) made a chance remark to Kenny asking if she was a Sagittarian. Aikens recalled that Kenny 'looked like thunder' and, before hurriedly leaving the room, said 'in an icy voice ... "Goodbye Mr Aikens, I'll see you this evening, and don't bring your friends."' Kenny suspected that the woman had tried to trap her into an admission that she worked by the stars or some other occult process in her treatment and cures, '... and I couldn't have things like that said about me. How the doctors would pounce on it to destroy me.' Some supporters of Kenny freely admitted that her attitude towards the BMA bordered on paranoia, that she saw 'an agent or a spy of the BMA behind every rose bush'.[408] Lack of openness and minimal communication between the parties concerned bred mistrust on both sides.

So, who was this woman who challenged medical orthodoxy on the treatment of polio in the twentieth century? Who was Elizabeth Kenny?

She was born on 20 September 1880 at Kellys Gully, a small railway terminus five kilometres south of the town of Warialda in the New England district of New South Wales,[409] where Michael Kenny was working as an overseer on the building of a bridge. Elizabeth was the fifth child and fourth daughter of Michael and Mary Kenny, and they named her after Mary's maternal grandmother, Elizabeth Pearson, who had married James Moore from Northern Ireland just before the family left County Donegal to sail to Australia in 1841. James and his brother Richard became successful graziers, and farmed cattle and bred horses on their large property, Moore Park, near Armidale in New South Wales.

The Moore brothers eventually owned large tracts of land in New England, enjoyed high status within the farming community and competed at local agricultural shows where they won many trophies and ribbons for their stud horses and brood mares. All the Moore offspring, including Elizabeth's mother Mary, were born at the estate. Michael Kenny was twenty-seven years old when he emigrated to Australia in 1861 from County Kilkenny to try his luck in the goldfields of New South Wales and Victoria. Like thousands of other young Irishmen before him, disillusionment soon set in and he abandoned his search for gold and moved on in search of work. When tall, redheaded Michael Kenny appeared in the Armidale district, there was an instant attraction between the educated but 'dreamy' Kenny and the equally statuesque and attractive Mary Moore.[410] There were a few murmurings within the Protestant Moore family about Michael's Catholic faith but nothing that stood in the way of the intended union, and the pair married in Inverell on 30 May 1872. The difference in their faith appears not to have troubled Michael and Mary Kenny, for each respected the other's belief, and a spirit of religious tolerance prevailed within the household.[411] All the Kenny children would be brought up as Protestants, with Elizabeth christened in the Anglican Church in Warialda.

When Elizabeth was around six years old, the family left Warialda and moved to land owned by the Moore family at Falconer, five miles outside Guyra, a small township where in the mid-1880s the railway had just arrived. Their home was a bark hut,[412] a popular first dwelling for rural Australians that required no specialised tools for construction. Saplings were used for the frame and tree bark covered the walls and roof. Bark huts were surprisingly comfortable, made warm in winter by an indoor fireplace, and airy enough in summer to catch the evening breeze. Although Mary Kenny was renowned for having a talent 'for always making everything very comfortable', the simple bark hut was certainly not the beautiful home described in Kenny's autobiography, *And They Shall Walk*. A family member later remarked 'that bit was all rot ... a load of rubbish'.[413] Elizabeth's cousins Mary and Minnie Moore also lived in the small township and the following year another cousin, Millicent Moore, moved from Moore Park to Guyra. Although she remembered her home was better than the Kenny's because 'we always had a maid, and someone to help, and an iron roof with seven or eight rooms', Millie did not believe her family was 'any better off ... it's just the way things were in those days'. She remembered her cousin Liza Kenny as a 'big, sturdy, well grown girl, an ordinary child, not one to get up to mischief ... always looking out for her younger sisters'.[414]

From 1860 until 1912 it was compulsory for a child in New South Wales to attend a state primary school from the age of six until twelve. High schools, as we now know them, began in 1912, and if parents wished a child to go beyond grade six in the earliest years of the twentieth century, they had to attend grammar school. As was the case in many small towns in Australia, the Guyra community had raised funds to build their own school and, in 1884, the two-roomed building opened its doors for sixty pupils. The school had classes from first to sixth grade. According to her cousin, Elizabeth was a good pupil: 'very quick, with a wonderful memory ... always reciting poetry like her mother did'.[415]

Throughout the 1890s, southern Australia remained in the grip of a protracted drought. In the punishing winter of 1895, no rain fell in the New England district from 'May to October, and hard frosts' destroyed any remaining pasture that had survived the drought. The land the Kennys farmed in Guyra did not belong to them and, with no financial ties to bind them to the district, Mary and Michael left to seek a better life in Queensland. Elizabeth's family moved around the countryside a great deal during her childhood, a custom that was common amongst working families in rural Australia, when men roamed freely over large distances seeking labouring or agricultural work. A network of family ties and a tradition of bush hospitality made the journey easier but the constant upheaval adversely affected the education of the children. In the spring of 1893, the family collected their belongings, said farewell to the Moores and boarded a train for Gowrie Junction, the small railway station near Toowoomba.[416] In Gowrie Junction there was a small public primary school in nearby Wetalla that Elizabeth may have attended, but she was now thirteen years old and sixth class was the highest grade. One of her classmates remembered her as 'reserved, a quiet and gentle girl, who walked in a stately manner even then'.[417]

The following year, Michael Kenny moved his family from Gowrie Junction to take up a position caring for the teams of plough horses at Headington Hill, the large estate owned by Davenport and Fisher on the Darling Downs. The period from 1898 until 1905 was a time of stability for the family. Both of Elizabeth's parents possessed a deep sense of reverence for education; her mother tutored in the Scots tradition of a love of words, literature and poetry, and her father was educated in Ireland in 'Latin and mathematics'.[418] At some point between 1905 and 1907, the family moved again to Spring Creek and from there to sixty acres at Rockfield, between Headington Hill and Nobby where Mary Kenny planted a large orchard with apple, quince, pear and mulberry trees, traces of which remained till the early 1960s.[419] When quizzed on her education in later years, Kenny insisted that she had been privately educated and had graduated from St Ursula's College in 1902 (when she was twenty-two years old). That was unlikely, for although the Ursuline nuns operated a number of schools in Australia, including St Ursula's College in Armidale, the Kenny family was living in south-east Queensland in 1902, and it was doubtful that they would have been able to afford to send their daughter to boarding school. St Ursula's College in Toowoomba did not open until 1911 when Kenny was aged thirty-one. Elizabeth Kenny's narration of her own history was often a pastiche of fact and fiction.

How did the young Elizabeth Kenny learn about anatomy and muscle structure? Throughout her life, she maintained that it was her involvement in teaching the calisthenics prescribed by Dr Aeneas McDonnell of

Toowoomba for her eleven-year-old brother Willie, described by her as a 'thin, weak boy'.[420] Bodybuilding, or physical education, had emerged in the late nineteenth century as part of a wider movement towards health and fitness and was based on the idea that outward physical robustness mirrored interior moral vigour. Kenny's sisters, Julia and Mary,[421] remembered the excitement in the household when the long-awaited book by Eugene Sandow arrived in the post.[422] Sandow believed that everyone could benefit from his program, even the bedridden. It is interesting, considering Kenny's later method of muscle 're-education', that Sandow endorsed passive exercise 'assisted by a nurse' and believed in the power of the will to bring about improvement: 'One of the essential points of my system is the cultivation of the willpower. The mind of the patient is concentrated upon the muscles and parts of the body brought into play by the movements made.'[423]

A few years later, another book in this field was published in Boston, USA, by Wilhelmine Wright, who had been treating paralysed children for ten years with a method similar to Sandow's. Wright believed, 'there exists in many paralysed limbs a possible amount of muscular power that is not suspected, and will not be available unless cultivated and developed'.[424]

In later years, many medical practitioners based their criticism of Sister Kenny and her method on the accusation that she 'stole' the work of others. That criticism is unjustified. Building and refining a method based on previous findings, and the sharing of ideas is, after all, common in scientific endeavour. Moreover, Wilhelmine Wright maintained that 'braces and plaster jackets' were the only way to prevent deformities in limbs, an approach condemned by Kenny, and did not advocate the commencement of treatment until three to six weeks after paralysis occurred. In contrast, Kenny advocated early intervention of treatment, gentle stretching of muscles, no restraining splints, and the use of 'hot packs' to reduce pain and muscle spasm in affected limbs.

In January 1907, word reached Mary Kenny that her mother Elizabeth was in failing health,[425] and her daughter made the journey south to Guyra to help care for her grandmother. After arriving at Granny Moore's she taught Sunday school at the Presbyterian Union church and, when her grandmother's health improved, she moved in with her cousin Minnie[426] and her husband James. The Bells owned the local bakery,[427] and the popular Elizabeth, 'a very handsome girl, tall with black, curly hair … quiet and dignified', helped behind the counter. Several of the customers asked her if she knew where they could sell their farm produce, and Elizabeth saw her chance: 'that's how she got into selling potatoes … but then she always had big ideas'. As Kenny remarked to her cousin, 'Min ... it's better to be a lion for a day, than a sheep for all your life'.[428]

Guyra was famous for its potato crops, Guyra Blues, Satisfactions and Manhattans, and Kenny became a commission agent for a local auctioneer, Tom Sole,[429] who sold at the Brisbane market. She would ride with James Bell in his baker's cart to outlying farms to buy the new crop from the farmers and, although there were three other competing agents in Guyra and an oversupply of potatoes in the market, Kenny 'wiped the floor with them ... she made some good money'. Reg McAllister noted that, during that period, potatoes sometimes sold 'for as low as thirty bob a ton'.[430] No witnesses from her time in Guyra made any mention of Kenny practising as a nurse, but a few added she did help quite a few new mothers, including her cousin Millicent following the birth of her son in 1911. That same year, a Nurse Sutherland arrived in Guyra to offer her services.[431]

When she visited town while working as a governess at the Avery homestead at Ben Lomond, Elizabeth Kenny became friendly with Margaret Sutherland. Kenny approached Sutherland at the Scotia hospital to ask for work. However, Sutherland's daughter was quite adamant that Kenny did not do any nursing, but had instead 'helped out in the kitchen'.[432]

The question of whether Kenny received formal nursing education in Australia has been debated elsewhere.[433] My research indicates that she did receive some training, but not in an acknowledged hospital or nurse training scheme, and that conclusion rests on studies conducted of the *Guyra Argus* during the time that Kenny lived there with Granny Moore. Throughout 1911 regular advertisements appeared for the Sydney Norland Institute,[434] an establishment that began in 1908 to meet the 'increasing demand for trained ladies as Children's Nurses'. Norland believed that it was 'eminently suited to women who had a natural sympathy with young children ... and who wished to receive scientific and practical training in nursery nursing'.[435] The year's training cost forty-five pounds.[436] There were four intakes of students per year, and it was likely that Elizabeth Kenny joined either the February or May enrolment in 1911.[437] When she was at Norland she met Eleanor Mackinnon, who proved to be a loyal friend and staunch supporter of Kenny and her work until Mackinnon's death in 1936.[438]

Three of the twelve months' training at Norland was spent in Sydney Hospital or the Benevolent Institution, and is probably when Kenny gained her midwifery and surgical experience before being awarded a general efficiency certificate.[439] Kenny returned to Guyra in 1912 to see the ailing Granny Moore and, while she was there, she commissioned Mr King, the local tailor, to make her 'two nurse's capes, a red nightingale and a long one'.⁴⁴⁰ Thus kitted out, she boarded a train for Clifton in Queensland, to set herself up in charge of her own private hospital, a task that was neither difficult nor uncommon for an enterprising woman of modest means.⁴⁴¹ Once the negotiations were complete with the seller of the property and the rooms furnished with beds, linen and household furniture, most nurses simply placed an advertisement in the local newspaper, and sat back and waited for the first patient to arrive on the doorstep.⁴⁴²

There seems little doubt that Kenny did not receive the general nursing training in Australia that would have made her eligible for registration with the Australasian Trained Nurses' Association (ATNA), despite the fact that Kenny's nephew recalled that his aunt claimed 'she had been apprenticed to a lay midwife called Sutherland at Guyra'.⁴⁴³ That date and the memories of various witnesses including Sutherland's daughter do not add up; neither does her claim to have been a bush nurse during the period from early 1911, a period widely quoted as when she encountered her first case of infantile paralysis.⁴⁴⁴ She arrived in Clifton from Guyra in 1912, and soon established her hospital that she called 'St Canice',⁴⁴⁵ but the locals referred to the large, cream-painted wooden house near the Clifton racecourse as 'Nurse Kenny's Hospital'. Patients were mostly maternity cases but, in an emergency, she took in general cases.⁴⁴⁶ Dr Hammond was the local GP, and an eligible bachelor. Whether Kenny entertained ideas of matrimony towards him was not known, but she set out to make a good impression on him before his morning round, 'togging herself out in her nurse's uniform … stiff apron over a white frock, cuffs and collar and a nice veil' before 'standing at the front door to wait for his arrival before taking him in to see the mothers and babies' and, as soon as Hammond left, 'off would come the uniform, and she would put on a plain frock'.⁴⁴⁷ However, her efforts proved fruitless, for Hammond married his housekeeper on the eve of his departure from Australia with the Australian Imperial Force. He died in France in 1916. There appeared no doubt that her hospital in Clifton was well patronised. Dr Aeneas McDonnell referred his patients to her because of his 'high regard for her natural ability as a nurse' and believed that she was a 'fine woman who was doing a great deal of good'.⁴⁴⁸

Whether Elizabeth Kenny was qualified to conduct her hospital at Clifton is a point worthy of investigation. When the Queensland Government introduced the *Health Act Amendment Act (1911)*,⁴⁴⁹ one of the clauses stated that only registered nurses⁴⁵⁰ were allowed to conduct a private hospital.⁴⁵¹ However, several loopholes existed that may have given Kenny a chance to register: one clause that stipulated that nurses without formal training would have one year's grace to register[452] after paying a fee of one pound to the Queensland Nurses' Registration Board, and another that, 'Nurses would be registered who could show three years spent in the bona fide practice of nursing with the production of two certificates from qualified medical practitioners'.[453]

As no evidence has come to light that she was practising as a nurse before 1912, she would not have been eligible to take advantage of that clause and it is my belief that she never registered with the QNRB because the Sydney Norland Institute would not have qualified as an accredited hospital. In September 1917, the ATNA published a full list of its members and Kenny was not one of them. She was not alone. In Queensland during 1913–1914, approximately seventy per cent of practising midwives were unregistered, and in the Rockhampton area there remained a sizable contingent of 'untrained nursing staff' as late as the early twentieth century.[454] That is not to say that many of those untrained women were not skilful and knowledgeable in their standard of nursing care, as the medical practitioners who worked with them acknowledged.

In 1912, Mr Beeby, the Health Minister in New South Wales, acted to ensure that 'the reputable woman without full qualifications must not be deprived of her means of livelihood', by insisting on the right to intervene and override the clause.[455] But nurses knew that the only way to raise the standard of the profession and gain recognition was by introducing a common standard of training throughout Australia.

The question of whether Elizabeth Kenny was justified in calling herself 'Sister Kenny' is somewhat easier to evaluate, despite the fact that some of the details about her enlistment and service as a nurse in the Australian Imperial Force (AIF) remain confusing.[456] When Britain declared war on Germany in 1914, the Dominions rallied to the defence of the mother country, and many members of Elizabeth Kenny's family enlisted for service. By the outbreak of war, Bill Kenny was a member of the Militia and the Queensland Police Force, and no longer a skinny and frail boy. The calisthenics had worked, and he had developed into a man of 'six feet, one and a quarter inches' with a reputation as a 'fine weight thrower … and a crack rifle shot'.[457] When he enlisted in the 2nd Light Horse Regiment in August 1914, Elizabeth wanted to sign up as well, but she knew that the newly formed Australian Army Nursing Service (AANS) would not accept her application, for she had no accredited hospital training, no certificate of general nursing or midwifery, and was not registered with ATNA. However, she was not prepared to let such a small matter as a piece of paper stand in the way of realising her ambition, so she put St Canice up for sale,[458] and made plans to leave for England.

Trained nurses in Australia were outraged when, in 1915, the Joint War Committee in the United Kingdom declared that nurses whose qualifications had been previously rejected as not up to standard, would now be accepted for home service in the Red Cross and in the Anglo-French hospitals in France.[459] The idea that partly-trained women would be on an equal footing, receive the same wages and perform the same duties as their fully certificated sisters prompted letters of protest to nursing journals in Britain and Australia. Nurses in Britain feared that the Voluntary Aid Detachment (VAD) workers would flood the market after the War 'posing as trained nurses' and compete for jobs with those better qualified, and while they acknowledged that many VAD were good workers, they maintained that to be a good nurse they had to start at the bottom and learn their work thoroughly, for in the past much of the work by the VAD had been 'shoddy, ignorant and emotional'.[460]

Several sources believe that Dr Aeneas McDonnell helped pave the way for Kenny to be accepted into the Australian Army when she arrived in London in 1915.[461] As a medical examiner for the Nurses Registration Board in Toowoomba, Honorary Captain in the Australian Army Medical Corps (AAMC), a member of the State Medical Board and the ATNA Queensland Council, McDonnell was a man of considerable influence. Recognised as a fine surgeon, he was also a great friend to nurses and had helped secure better pay and conditions for them. A letter of introduction and recommendation from Aeneas McDonnell about Kenny's prowess as a nurse would have carried great weight with military authorities.

Some sources on the life of Elizabeth Kenny have written that she enlisted in 1915, and was wounded in the battle of Ypres while serving in France.[462] However, at the time she was supposed to be overseas, Kenny was nowhere near the Western Front. She was still living in Clifton, Queensland, and according to an inaccurate newspaper report 'had been accepted for the Front' and was due to leave Clifton on 19 June 1915,[463] possibly to board the P&O liner *Orsova*, due to sail from Brisbane for Plymouth on 7 July with a contingent of nurses for the Front. But Kenny was not present in the list of nurses who sailed, nor was she in the group photograph taken on board. Kenny caught a train for Sydney to join RMS *Medina*, scheduled to sail for Britain on 26 June. With her on board were Dr Katie Ardill and two nurses from South Sydney Women's Hospital, who were travelling to

London to 'offer their services to military authorities'.[464] It was not unusual for a woman to travel overseas alone during that period since '23 percent of passengers travelling from Melbourne to London or other British ports were women'.[465] Alice Perrott recalled that Kenny 'travelled as a civilian' on the *Medina*, and showed her a letter of recommendation from Dr Aeneas McDonnell of Toowoomba, one that testified to her skills as a nurse and her suitability as a recruit for the AIF.[466] The *Medina* arrived at Marseilles on 2 August and by midway through that month Kenny's photo had appeared in a Queensland newspaper above a caption advising readers that the 'well-known' Nurse Kenny was 'nursing wounded Australian soldiers' at the 3rd Western General Hospital in Manchester.[467]

Doctors and nurses were in very short supply in Britain, and in 1915 the War Office had started a scheme allowing a limited number of females with 'first-aid and home nursing certificates' to be accepted into military hospitals for a month on probation. Whether this was the means by which Kenny entered the military or whether she joined the Territorial Force Nursing Service after arriving in London has never been established, but one record showed that she was a member of the Army Auxiliary Nursing Service.[468] Despite the fact that Kenny wrote home in November 1915 stating she had been nursing in France, evidence to date does not support that statement.[469] She did not arrive in Britain until mid-August 1915, and visited her Irish relatives for three or four days the following month.[470] It was conceivable that she was interviewed by the French Flag Nursing Corps[471] while in London for duty in one of their hospitals in France, but the minimum period for service abroad was six months. What is certain was that Nurse Elizabeth Kenny was on the list of medical personnel employed to nurse wounded Australian soldiers on HMAT *Suevic*, which sailed from London on 8 October 1915.

By mid-December Kenny was back in Nobby 'spending a fortnight with her mother before returning to duty',[472] and entertaining the local population with stories of nursing in Britain, France and Belgium, most of which were probably fictitious. The first entry on her official service record lists her as embarking from Melbourne on the *Orontes* on 19 December 1916.[473] Sister Ella Morphett was also on board the *Orontes*, and she and Kenny became friends. They visited Ireland together in 1917, and shared seven trips on the transports to and from Australia during the war years. Between sea voyages, Kenny nursed at the Australian Auxiliary Hospitals (AAH) at Southall, Dartford and Harefield, where she nursed badly wounded and gassed Australians — 'very undisciplined soldiers but good patients'.[474] Masseurs had travelled with the first contingent of the AIF in November 1914 and, at first, most of them were employed in British Military hospitals in England where the treatment was viewed as 'very beneficial for wounded soldiers'.[475] Following the establishment of the AAH, small numbers of masseurs and masseuses were sent from Australia and the majority were stationed at Harefield Hospital. The Australian Army Massage service was the 'only one of the Australian army medical, nursing or related services' to accept both men and women.[476] Elizabeth Kenny would have had ample opportunity to observe the masseurs at work on the transports or in the wards, for in all more than fifty thousand patients were treated at Harefield during the war.[477] Kenny was classified as a Staff Nurse until October 1918, when all staff nurses with two years' service within the AIF were promoted to Sister, and she was given the right to wear two stars on each shoulder of her nurse's cape.[478] Thus, despite claims to the contrary that were levelled against her, Elizabeth Kenny was perfectly entitled to use the designation 'Sister Kenny' throughout her lifetime.

Her final voyage home to Australia was on board the *Marathon* in November 1918, and she was discharged in January 1919 with a war pension for 'Varicose Veins and Myocarditis'.[479] Elizabeth Kenny often told her supporters that she had 'a weak heart' and 'was not in robust health … could never have an anaesthetic because of her heart', but a physician who examined her in the 1940s said she 'had a heart like an ox' and that the reports of her having a weak heart on her discharge from the AIF were probably caused by a severe infection like influenza or pneumonia which could involve the heart muscle and cause a temporary heart murmur. Dr Jay Davis said that when he told her 'there was nothing wrong with her heart, she didn't like it, but went ahead and had the anaesthetic for her broken arm'.[480] Davis commented that many army doctors in 1918 discharged thousands of soldiers with an annotation on their notes of a systolic murmur. In fact their heart was normal because doctors then did not know how to differentiate between the different types of murmur. He thought it probable that Sister Kenny had been ill with either influenza or pneumonia during her war service. Her record noted she was hospitalised during 1916.

During the 1920s, Elizabeth Kenny lived with her widowed mother Mary at Nobby, nursed the sick and delivered babies in her local neighbourhood. It was during this period that she adopted a nine-year-old girl from Brisbane, Lucy Lily Stewart, to be a companion and aide to her mother and, for reasons that are not entirely clear, she also changed the child's name to Mary Kenny. There were outbreaks of infantile paralysis in Queensland in 1919, and in

New South Wales in 1920 and 1921. During that period she attended some cases,[481] and provided treatment for crippled children. She often travelled over the rough dirt roads with Stanley Kuhn, who remembered 'the faster I went, the more she enjoyed it'.[482] Her association with the Kuhn family led to her development of the Sylvia Stretcher, an event that has been fully covered in other works on Kenny.[483] One knowledgeable source insisted that she 'made a fair amount of money from that stretcher … an annual payment of between £150 and £200 from the Sydney manufacturers'.[484] That stipend, in addition to her war pension of four guineas per week would have ensured her financial independence and funded further trips overseas to promote her stretcher.

In 1916, Daphne Cregan was sixteen months old and a normal, healthy toddler when she contracted what was probably cerebral meningitis while her family was living at Ben Lomond in New South Wales.[485] Her father insisted it was not polio — 'we'd never heard of polio then' — and doctors were unsure how to treat the child's subsequent paralysis for, as her father remarked, 'no two of them had the same opinion'.[486] The family had taken the advice of a Sydney specialist to try massage, but 'that made no difference whatsoever',[487] and when they heard that Kenny had returned from overseas and was now nursing in Queensland they sought her help. Amelia Cregan was 'at her wits end' from the strain of caring for her disabled daughter and Kenny agreed to help. She went first to the family home to treat Daphne before taking the girl with her back to Nobby. When she first started to treat the seven-year-old in 1921, Daphne 'couldn't even feed herself',[488] and Kenny began exercising her hands by giving her piano lessons at the Good Samaritan Convent in Clifton. She worked with Daphne until 1925, giving her salt and sulphur baths, and massaged her arms and legs with goanna salve and olive oil before splinting them using 'bark splints'. Clearly, Kenny had not yet formulated her opinion on the benefits or disadvantages of splinting. For the four years she cared for Daphne, she was paid between £7 and £10 per week, money that Daphne's father insisted was 'worth every penny'. In 1929, Daphne's parents took her to see a Dr Royle at Lewisham Private Hospital in Sydney, who advised surgery. It was not successful, and according to her father, 'made her worse than she was'.[489] When Kenny started her re-education clinic in Townsville, Daphne Cregan was one of her first patients. It was when she began treating Daphne in 1921 that Elizabeth Kenny first began to explore her system of muscle re-education and treatment, and not in 1911 as often claimed.

By the mid- to late 1920s, Kenny was moving over great distances as far north as the Gulf Country and then south into northern New South Wales, and it would not have taken her very long to become aware of the plight of the crippled child in Australia. Treatment and care were almost non-existent.

Anecdotal evidence about Kenny and her skill with nursing crippled children had begun to spread throughout eastern Australia, and she realised that she could better serve the interests of the children by getting them to come to her, rather than travelling to remote towns and farms to treat them.[490] In 1930, she had outlined a scheme to Charles Chuter[491] to provide better health care facilities for those in the bush.[492] He supported her, and provided her with a 'station to station' pass, one that was later upgraded to an open pass for travel on Queensland railways.[493] By 1931, she was also treating patients in New South Wales.[494]

A stocky, balding figure with a reputation for being a hard worker and articulate negotiator, Chuter first met Elizabeth Kenny in connection with her invention of the Sylvia Stretcher and, although he remained a loyal and influential supporter for the remainder of his life, he was also known to 'get mad at Kenny and tell her off … to stop rushing at a thing like a bull at a gate'.[495] Kenny treated the young daughter of Chuter when the child became paralysed after contracting meningitis,[496] and one source believed that it may have been what Chuter perceived as the bungled treatment of his child that prompted him to question the motives of some medical practitioners who placed their 'private practice' before the needs of hospital patients.[497]

In 1915, a Labor Government had been elected in Queensland and the Home Secretary's Office became increasingly involved in the administration of public hospitals formerly within the auspices and control of voluntary contributors. Labor's view was that the voluntary system was not only unreliable, but was patronising as well in its discriminatory attitude towards the poor. In 1917 the Home Office assumed responsibility for the Brisbane Hospital when, following the redirection of a significant proportion of voluntary contributions to fund the war effort, the hospital was in danger of financial collapse. However, that danger was averted when the Government took over the Golden Casket lottery[498] in 1920 to fund Queensland's hospitals and, by 1927, over two million pounds had been raised. Many hoped that hospital admission would no longer be governed by an individual's ability to pay fees, and that hospital treatment would become available for all. Charles Chuter was appointed to the inaugural board in 1924,[499] and he soon set about implementing his conviction that only those who funded hospitals should sit on boards, and that members of the medical profession, if they were not benefactors, should be excluded. When Chuter went further and detailed a plan to abolish the honorary system in hospitals and replace those medical practitioners with full-time medical staff, the BMA in Australia realised that its power base in hospitals was about to be eroded, and bitterness developed between now Chairman Chuter and the Honorary Medical Officers (HMOs). After a showdown, the BMA prevailed and maintained its right to appoint honorary staff in hospitals, but medical practitioners remained excluded from the Brisbane Hospital board until a change of government in 1957.[500]

In 1929, Queensland voters elected the Country and Progressive National Party to office, but the inexperienced government was swept from power in 1932 when Labor was re-elected,[501] with William Forgan Smith installed as Premier. As was the case with previous Labor governments, medical reform was a key issue, especially reform of the hospital system and public health administration. Both the Premier and his Home Secretary, E.M. Hanlon,[502] believed that revamping health policy was vital for the economic and social wellbeing of Queensland and, soon after Labor took office, Hanlon amended the *Hospitals Act* to insist that any bequest to a hospital had to be 'paid into a special fund instead of being credited to the local authority'.[503]

In Townsville in 1933, Elizabeth Kenny set herself on a path to challenge medical orthodoxy about the treatment of the paralysed body and, as a consequence, she also challenged that dictum about the nurse's role in medical care. In May she began treating paralysed children, including three from Nobby,[504] in 'bathtubs and on tables' set up in the courtyard of Queen's Hotel near the waterfront in Townsville. The Queensland Government began to take note of her voluntary work when three doctors, Dungan, O'Neill, and the Government Medical Officer H.J. Taylor, requested that Kenny treat their patients. She had no staff at that time and was teaching mothers how to care for their children using her labour-intensive method. Kenny worked on the bodies of the children every two hours. With her 'hot packs' she found she was able to relieve muscle pain. She then used her fingers to feel the children's arms and legs for any sign of muscle movement or response. She recognised insertion points and how certain muscle groups worked in opposition to others. Slowly at first, then gradually increasing, she passively exercised paralysed limbs. Kenny was vehemently opposed to the splinting and immobilisation that orthodox medicine advocated for the treatment of polio paralysis, for she believed that it made the pain worse, and prevented the gentle stretching treatment she advocated.

That same year, Charles Chuter set about his task of bringing Elizabeth Kenny and her work to the attention of his superior E.M. Hanlon and through him, to the man at the top, Premier Forgan Smith who, along with Hanlon and Chuter, recognised his chance to gain further control over the access and organisation of medical care for the population by installing a government-run clinic. However, by supporting Elizabeth Kenny the Queensland Government would fuel the resentment directed towards her by the BMA in Australia. Many medical practitioners would come to view her clinics as an example of socialised medicine, a concept to which they were vehemently opposed.

During her time in Townsville, Kenny's work at the Queen's Hotel was supported by a legacy from the Estate of James Simpson Love,[505] a horse breeder, philanthropist and pastoralist of Townsville. Love had been a partner in the hotel and spent his final years there before his death in November 1933, and in his will he stipulated that none of his estate[506] was to go to the 'Roman Catholic Church or any Catholic Body'. Because of her adherence to the Protestant faith, Kenny and her clinic were eligible for inclusion.

No account of Elizabeth Kenny and her Townsville clinic can be complete without including a man described by Kenny's family as 'her greatest enemy'[507] — Dr Raphael West Cilento. According to his biographer, Cilento had begun a 'love affair with the tropics'[508] while serving as a medical practitioner with occupying forces in the former German New Guinea in 1919, and he was appointed as Director of the Australian Institute of Tropical Medicine (AITM) in Townsville in 1923.[509] Cilento was enthusiastic about the position because he enjoyed life in a tropical climate, but he had another, more personal reason for accepting the post. Cilento had for some time seen Queensland's public health as an 'administrative empire ripe for takeover'. The Townsville position was the first step in his plan to establish his empire.[510] Cilento managed to balance his commitment to the BMA with his ambition to head a public service department, two seemingly incompatible goals, socialised medicine versus private enterprise. In May 1933,[511] Cilento set out from Brisbane on a tour of quarantine stations in North Queensland and, because word about Kenny's work with crippled children was becoming known in medical and government circles, he called in to Townsville to meet Elizabeth Kenny.

It was a 'pleasant, unofficial meeting'; Cilento listened to Kenny's claims and watched her work with the children, but was determined to reserve his judgement until her methods could be tested.[512] The following month, following an invitation by Dr Harold Crawford, President of the Australian Massage Association, Kenny presented a demonstration of her methods at the Brisbane Hospital. Raphael Cilento attended the trial, which he felt was less than fair to Kenny and conducted in an atmosphere of hostility and disbelief, a mood not so much directed towards her treatment, but because she could not explain her method in medical terms, and used phrases like 'spasm' and 'alienation' to describe the symptoms. Harold Crawford believed that Kenny was at best a faith healer, and at worst a crank, and that she posed a very real risk to patients and their parents.

Following that demonstration, Raphael Cilento recommended to Hanlon that no decision be reached on the effectiveness of Kenny's treatment unless patients under her care could be observed for a minimum of six months. That advice placed the Minister in a quandary. The public were clamouring to have Kenny's method made freely available, but Hanlon was worried about freely sanctioning a method to which the influential BMA was vehemently opposed. While he was keen to exercise the Government's mandate to pursue its platform of socialised medicine, he also realised the need for an authoritative and respected medical figure to conduct the investigation into the effectiveness of Kenny's method; Raphael Cilento fitted the bill. When Premier Forgan Smith asked Cumpston to second Cilento to Brisbane to investigate Kenny, Cilento jumped at the chance to leave that 'dreary, detached, public service mortuary chapel called Canberra'.[513]

In February 1934, the Queensland Government set up the 'Experimental Muscle Re-Education Clinic' in Townsville with Sister Kenny in charge. The clinic was established for the primary purpose of testing whether her method of treatment could be taught to others over a period of four months;[514] the success or not of her treatment method was not then in question. The clinic had expected that seventeen patients were to be admitted but almost sixty turned up at the door, including some who had suffered with various types of paralysis for many years. Kenny refused to send them away. That humane decision was typical of Kenny's approach to her patients, and contributed to her very public falling out with Cilento and the medical profession.

In 1933, Sisters Annie Steele and Leila Cooper were working at the Lady Chelmsford Hospital in Bundaberg, but both women were keen to work with children, particularly in the area of child welfare. The Queensland Government had approached Matron Barron of the Child Welfare Training Centre in Brisbane for advice on suitable staff for the Townsville clinic, and Barron had recommended both Steele and Cooper for the positions. The nurses were keen, but were equally concerned to make sure that their reputation as nurses would not be adversely affected by working with Kenny. In a letter to Sister Steele, Raphael Cilento congratulated her on her appointment to Townsville, and sought to allay her fears by reassuring her that the Queensland Government would appoint them and not Sister Kenny. Cilento added, 'In the unlikely event of Sister Kenny's work being proved utterly worthless, your professional status would not be in any way impaired'.[515]

Leila Cooper travelled north from Bundaberg to Townsville in late February 1934 to take up her new position working at the Kenny clinic and, for a few months Cooper and the rest of the staff enjoyed their work and were happy. Cooper noted that 'Sister Kenny is just wonderful with the children and they just love her'.[516] The same cannot be said for Evelyn Swan, who was a trained massage therapist. Almost from the beginning, Kenny and Swan clashed both personally and professionally. Kenny accused Swan of trying to wrest control of the clinic from her, of criticising her method publicly and of upsetting the other two trainees.[517]

When Raphael Cilento returned to Townsville in June 1934 to report on the activities of the Kenny Clinic, he was to find a deeply unhappy Annie Steele, Leila Cooper and Evelyn Swan.[518] The nurses were worried about what they termed as 'reckless expenditure of money at the clinic',[519] and confided to Cilento that Kenny was a very difficult woman to work for, one who was subject to extreme mood swings, almost verging on paranoia. Steele was adamant that she tried to be loyal and obedient, but could not be a 'blind puppet, obeying her every crazy whim and wish'. In her opinion, Kenny had to be 'slightly mental, otherwise it is wicked for her to say the things she does'.[520] Cilento advised them 'to stick it out' because he felt that they would eventually be advised to leave the clinic by the Queensland Government. To the dismay of the two women, their confidential remarks to Cilento were relayed to Kenny. Both denounced him as a 'traitor'.[521] To Kenny, Cilento was 'despicable', and the two nurses had been 'mad to put their faith in any man'. Staff morale at the Kenny clinic had reached rock bottom, and mistrust was rife. Annie Steele confided to Matron Barron that she would be 'ready for Goodna if she couldn't get away from this place'.[522] However, both nurses believed that excellent work was being done with the children and that Kenny was getting better results than anyone else. On Saturday 30 June, Charles Chuter advised Kenny to replace Sister Swan because the 'government was of the opinion that married women should not be taken on as trainees'.[523] Kenny acted swiftly. Swan was immediately dismissed, but inexplicably reinstated the following Monday.

According to his biographer, Cilento was predisposed to view Kenny's treatment method 'in a favourable light',[524] but his subsequent report did not give Kenny an official endorsement of her methods and the seal of approval she needed to be able to open more clinics. Cilento selected seventeen of the most intractable cases of paralysis from the sixty patients available to form the basis for his judgement. Annie Steele thought the report 'an honest representation of all the available facts', but knew that it would not 'please Miss Kenny and, I suspect the Home Department'.[525] When Cilento's report was presented, he and Kenny disagreed loudly and publicly over the guidelines laid down in the initial agreement. Kenny then accused her staff of being 'disloyal and indiscreet enough to talk to Cilento', and 'took to her bed for ten days' with a 'bad pain around her heart'.[526] Both Leila Cooper and Annie Steele were convinced there was nothing wrong with Kenny except extreme petulance, along with a desire to elicit sympathy from her supporters. Kenny had been discharged from the Army with a heart murmur and she quite often brought up the subject of her ill-health. She once told Charles Chuter that she had 'an incurable heart condition' and that she knew that 'her life would be short'.[527]

Cilento insisted that the Townsville clinic was initiated to test the treatment method, while Kenny was equally adamant that the issue under investigation was whether her method could be taught to others. He claimed that one of the terms of reference for setting up the clinic — to see if the patients could 'be restored permanently to health'[528] — was untrue, and had never been agreed to by Kenny or the Government. Cilento refused to comment formally on any patient aside from his selected seventeen, despite the fact that he had examined a recent paralysis case, a child from Townsville who had been admitted to the clinic in March unable to walk. Within twelve weeks of the Kenny treatment the girl was walking and, although Cilento had informed her mother she ought to be pleased that Sister Kenny 'had cured her',[529] he refused to include the child's progress in his report.

Cilento noted that all the cases he reviewed had made some general improvement, but believed progress was more likely due to the general measures employed at the clinic, such as improved hygiene, exercise, housing and nutrition, and a sympathetic attitude, rather than any specific treatment. In his opinion, the object of the exercise had been to save the country from the burden of providing a pension by restoring the individual to a point where he could earn his own living. Because none of the patients had been 'completely cured', Cilento doubted whether it was worthwhile to either patient or the public to transform a 'physically low-grade potential pensioner into a physically high-grade pensioner, none the less dependent'.[530] Kenny was furious,[531] but perhaps the relationship between them could have been repaired if she had not publicly attacked him. Tom Aikens, the independent member for South Townsville in the Queensland Legislative Assembly knew Kenny well, and referred to the relationship between her and Cilento as: 'Like a dog and a goanna, both warily watching each other, waiting for another chance to pounce and fight'.[532] The recently knighted Raphael Cilento was deeply affronted by Kenny's criticism, for he regarded himself as her social and intellectual superior.[533] To Cilento, it was unthinkable that any nurse would dare challenge a decision made by a medical practitioner.

Kenny persuaded the Queensland Government to seek another medical opinion on the Townsville clinic, and they appointed Dr James Guinane, the son of the proprietress of the Townsville Hotel. Despite Cilento's urgings to 'just write a couple of sheets of paper',[534] Guinane submitted an extensive report that advised that four recent cases of paralysis had all recovered after the Kenny treatment. He recommended the adoption of her treatment, and stated that while Cilento was an expert on tropical diseases, in his opinion Cilento had no knowledge of infantile paralysis.[535] Cilento refused to comment publicly, and wrote to Minister Hanlon to advise him to 'exercise caution' when reading Guinane's report. As a consequence of this intervention, Guinane's detailed evidence on patient evaluation was removed from his report, and only the recommendations circulated.

Over the following six months the feud between Kenny and Cilento escalated, and he was forced to go public when increasing public support for another Kenny clinic in Brisbane meant he could no longer remain silent. Cilento issued a statement saying that neither he nor the Queensland Government approved or disapproved of the Kenny method. Furthermore, Cilento believed that public and scientific opinion would support his conviction that the money set aside for Sister Kenny's 'spectacular endeavour' would be better served if 'directed towards improving existing massage departments and orthodox treatment in our great public hospitals', a service that was being provided 'quietly and without publicity' by orthopaedic specialists.[536]

The battle lines were drawn. Elizabeth Kenny retorted that seeing the 'poor, little afflicted children doing so well' made her even more determined to overcome all the obstacles put in her way and she would, within a few weeks, take her treatment south into New South Wales and Canberra, where she gained the support of someone of even greater power and influence than Sir Raphael Cilento. In March 1935, William Morris Hughes[537] invited Kenny to Canberra to give 'a demonstration of her methods' to himself and Dr Earle Page. The meeting was instigated following a letter from

Eleanor Mackinnon, who told Hughes 'by getting behind this work you will gain more renown than during the war'.[538] Mackinnon also wrote to Prime Minister Lyons, describing Kenny as 'a modest gentlewoman who has worked for this great result and received a gift that is Christlike in its operations'.[539] Another supporter of Kenny was Dr J.H.L. Cumpston,[540] who had long been concerned about the plight of the crippled child in Australia, and had requested each state to nominate or set up a central body to coordinate activities for the care of cripples: 'The medical profession is, by nature, very conservative and has in the past, not given much attention to this tedious, disappointing and unremunerative work. Sister Kenny has enthusiasm and originality and has taken up with vigour a neglected field.'[541]

As a consequence of Cumpston's directive, the states decided that the Societies for Crippled Children would carry out the task and, in order to coordinate planning and find out what knowledge had been gained, the Commonwealth Department of Health[542] arranged a conference in Canberra for the following year. In 1935, some prominent orthopaedic surgeons[543] in Victoria were prepared to give the Kenny treatment a trial. While not 'prepared to give Sister Kenny's methods either unqualified praise or unqualified criticism', Dr Douglas Galbraith was 'definitely interested in her methods', and advised Hughes that he was 'prepared to strongly advise the Committee to place facilities at Sister Kenny's disposal in the Children's Hospital'.[544] Both Galbraith and John Whitaker[545] believed

> orthodox treatment in the large city hospitals has shown tremendous progress in the last decade, and we would suggest that the area where Sister Kenny has been working has not enjoyed such a high standard of orthopaedic work. Her results have thus stood out in marked contrast to existing methods of treatment, we don't believe this would be the case if she had been working in a capital city.[546]

In May, the New South Wales Government announced that it had decided to establish a clinic at the Royal North Shore Hospital[547] for treatment of patients by the Kenny method.[548] All seemed to bode well for the future of the Kenny clinics, but she suddenly announced that she was not opening the Brisbane clinic because she 'was not satisfied by the conditions offered by Queensland' and was affronted by 'Dr Cilento's refusal to endorse my method'.[549] Minister Hanlon declared himself 'amazed' at Kenny's decision, and declared that one of the Townsville nurses would run the clinic in her stead. Privately, Hanlon was incensed with Kenny, and instructed Charles Chuter to 'sack her', which he did:

I have the honour, by direction, to inform you that the cabinet has decided to conduct the Crippled Children's Clinic as a Government activity, and your services as Honorary Superintendent of that Institution will therefore no longer be required. I am instructed by the Minister to convey to you his thanks for the excellent honorary service which you have given to the community.[550]

Circling in the background was Cilento, a man who publicly criticised Kenny and her treatment, but who subsequently submitted a memorandum to Hanlon proposing that he should be 'established as administrator as well as advisory officer' of all the Kenny clinics in Queensland.[551]

How Kenny was persuaded to rethink her stand on Brisbane is not clear, but within a few days she was reported as describing the whole incident as a 'misunderstanding between her and the Queensland Government', and three weeks later the Brisbane clinic opened for business.[552] However, the situation in Victoria was not resolved for three years,[553] despite a vigorous campaign by several Melbourne newspapers[554] to have the Kenny treatment made available. It seems that the strength of the opposition towards her in that state was formidable and difficult to overcome. In October 1935, a Royal Commission was convened 'to enquire into modern methods for the treatment of infantile paralysis and particularly the Elizabeth Kenny method …'[555] Initially, Kenny supported the formation of the Commission, until she was made aware that she would not be able to give evidence on her behalf, and that the hearings would take place 'in camera'.

At the conference in Canberra in 1936, fourteen papers were presented over three days. Among them was one by Jean Macnamara[556] and one by Elizabeth Kenny,[557] who was described by one of the delegates as 'a rather isolated figure … grimly reticent in a heavy, severely tailored black suit with a hard, forbidding-looking black hat. She expected hostility, and at the conclusion of her paper she got it.'[558]

When Kenny had finished her paper, Dr Harold Crawford[559] of Queensland attacked Kenny, and strongly objected to 'children passing out of the hands of the properly trained specialists in the orthopaedic realm' to be treated by 'nurses who are inexperienced'. Furthermore, Crawford said that he knew of children treated by Sister Kenny 'who have developed deformities'.[560]

When the meeting broke up, Reg McKellar Hall, an orthopaedic surgeon from Perth, persuaded Kenny to have a 'cuppa' with him. He found her 'aloof' at first, but she warmed to him when he revealed that he was interested in what she was doing for the children, and wanted to learn about her method. They made arrangements to meet at the Kenny clinic in Sydney the following week.[561] Hall was impressed by what he later observed: to him her method demonstrated a great deal of common sense, particularly the removal of splints to allow patients 'to feel as though they had arms and legs'. He phased in the Kenny method at the Children's Hospital in Perth when he returned, and thus incurred the 'displeasure of Dame Jean Macnamara',[562] his former colleague from his days as an RMO at the Melbourne Hospital, who would accuse him of 'operating a cripple factory' when she visited Perth in 1948.

Kenny returned to Brisbane upset with the reception she had received in Canberra, but heartened by the news that the Queensland Government had extended its support of her by opening new clinics in Cairns, Rockhampton and Toowoomba to supplement those already operating in Townsville and Brisbane.

The year 1937 would prove to be critical for Elizabeth Kenny. The Queensland Royal Commission into her treatment method was due to bring down its findings, support for her work in Britain was juxtaposed with increasing attacks from the medical fraternity in Victoria and, in May, the *Medical Journal of Australia* had published a scathing review of her book.[563] Polio epidemics were raging on the east coast of Australia, and the public was searching for answers from public health officials, science and medicine. Scientists debated openly and amongst themselves about the epidemics, and frustration in the population increased as authorities failed in their efforts to define what polio was, or how it was transmitted or, more importantly, how to avoid catching it. The public turned to the media for information and advice, and when Victorian newspapers took up the cause of Elizabeth Kenny, the people rallied behind her. Some parents asked for their child to be treated by her methods in hospital, while others approached Kenny directly for help and paid her expenses to come to Melbourne.[564]

Kenny's work was beginning to gain attention overseas, and she was invited to speak at a health conference in London in June 1937. Mention was made of the possibility of providing a ward and patients for her to test her method and Kenny was elated. She was tired of fighting with the Victorian BMA and 'weary' of refusing applications from Victorian parents for treatment. 'It wasn't fair', she wrote to Dr Rae Dungan, 'for Victoria to neglect their own cripples especially when Victoria had refused the offer of a Kenny clinic of their own'. There were 320 patients attending the Brisbane Clinic and, with a further seventy-three on the waiting list they had no room for interstate admissions. Furthermore, her clinic at the Royal North

Shore hospital in Sydney was 'half-full of patients from Victoria' with 500 on the waiting list for admission.[565] Minister Billy Hughes told the Lyons Cabinet that because the clinic was so popular, he believed that it was likely to remain open permanently. However, Hughes was unwilling to commit Commonwealth funds to reduce waiting lists because that would create a 'precedent'.[566]

Once in Britain, Kenny found an influential supporter in Sir Frederick Menzies,[567] who took a great interest in her and arranged for two wards at Queen Mary's Hospital, Carshalton, to be made available in early July for her to test her methods. The major breakthrough for Kenny was that she would finally be able to treat acutely ill patients in the early stages of the disease.[568] The treatment was to be supervised by the British Orthopaedic Association, which was scheduled to present preliminary findings at the end of three months.[569] Although some nursing and medical staff at Carshalton had initially been dubious about her method, and 'thought she was mad at first', most became enthusiastic.[570] By September, Kenny sensed that the treatment was being well received, and she wrote to Charles Chuter to say she had asked that the London report be sent directly to the Royal Commission for evaluation before their findings were published. Several therapists had confided to her that the treatment was 'superior to any other method', while a member of the medical staff wrote to the Ministry:

> I inspected the ward and saw most of the children, many of whom were pathetic and pitiful examples of this dread infection — infantile paralysis. However, the whole atmosphere of the ward in regard to the nursing staff, the children etc., was bright and cheerful, and I detected an optimism amongst the nurses which encouraged me to think they were fully satisfied with the results so far achieved. This impression was emphasized as a result of personal enquiries and questions put to several of the nurses who had previously been treating cases by old methods.[571]

However, formidable forces were marshalling against Kenny in Australia. Some nurses employed at the Brisbane clinic wanted to leave, citing reasons that the treatment was 'boring' and that some of the patients were so hopelessly crippled that it was a 'waste of time' trying to treat them. The sisters were unhappy that there was no textbook on the Kenny treatment available for consultation, no treatment sheet made out for patients nor any attempt made to monitor progress. It appeared that the Brisbane clinic lacked guidance and seemed to be fulfilling the prophecy made by Cilento and other critics that Kenny's presence was vital to the viability of any institution using her methods. Chuter urged her to return from England as soon as practicable. In New South Wales a medical committee recommended that the clinic at Royal North Shore be closed because of 'inconclusive evidence' about her treatment, and in Victoria the Minister of Health, in response to the public clamour for a clinic in that state, claimed that it was not necessary because 'Sister Kenny has not made any radical changes in the treatment for polio'. In the Victorian Parliament, Dr Shields (UAP) warned Victoria's parents to have nothing to do with 'quacks' in Melbourne who were offering to cure children by miraculous methods. It was not, he said:

> A case of the medical profession being jealous of a nurse and believing her incapable of doing any good but that Dame Jean Macnamara's knowledge was recognised throughout the world and was an example of a prophet being honoured in every country but her own. Everything possible should be done to prevent deformities, and that included the use of splints. Sister Kenny had fulfilled a useful service by arousing the interest of Government authorities and public bodies by her efforts to organise treatment for cripples.[572]

When the London report was released it was inconclusive, but Menzies recommended that the arrangements with Kenny be extended to July 1938 to further evaluate her method. However, the report of the Queensland Royal Commission was damning, and ignored the London findings. Although the evidence given and the report itself were not published or submitted to Parliament, the findings were made public. The Commissioners believed that her method showed a radical departure from orthodox treatment and recommended that all the clinics be closed. They found that the Kenny treatment had caused:

> Additional damage to the patient, and that the abandonment of immobilisation was a grievous error and fraught with great danger, especially for very young children. If the Government saw fit to reject the advice and decided the Kenny clinics should remain open then the Commission strongly urged that the clinics be placed under the control of a competent orthopaedic surgeon with the object of rejecting hopeless cases, thus avoiding the cruelty of disappointed hopes. Public money would be saved, and a sane and balanced view of the patient's possibilities would be obtained.[573]

Kenny had made a grave error of judgement with her early agreement to abide by the findings of the Commission. She had made some extravagant claims in 1935 of being able to bring about a significant, even full, recovery in old paralysis cases,[574] and had harboured the unrealistic expectation that, because the Queensland Government had supported her method, the BMA would do likewise. Kenny further damaged her image with the medical profession by contending that the Commission had been influenced in its findings by the political antagonism that existed between the BMA and the government. By 1938 she had well and truly modified her public utterances on possible cure rates, but her earlier rash claims continued to haunt her. She was becoming more selective, and was refusing to treat patients that past experience had shown her would not benefit from her treatment.

The new Sister Kenny Clinic and Training School[575] had opened on the corner of George and Charlotte Streets in Brisbane in June 1935, and was equipped with treatment tables, some beds, baths and office furniture. Dr Abraham Fryberg was appointed as Director, Dr Jean Rountree as Medical Superintendent, Kenny as Supervisor, along with two Sisters and two trainees from the Townsville clinic and two office staff. It was specifically designed as an outpatient clinic, with no provision for acutely ill children and would be open only during daylight hours. In March 1938, six badly paralysed children arrived for treatment in Brisbane, and all were in the early, contagious stages of the disease. Kenny requested beds for them at the Brisbane General Hospital (BGH), but was refused. She knew she would be breaking the rules of her agreement by admitting the children to the clinic, but was also aware that this was her chance to prove that her treatment was more effective if implemented in the early stage of paralysis. When she saw the condition of the children, who 'cried bitterly with pain from large bed sores' caused by immobilisation in splints, she admitted them.[576] Charles Chuter was furious and ordered her to discharge the children, but Kenny refused, informing Chuter that several specialists from the BGH had agreed to supervise the treatment of the children. Reluctantly, he conceded. In all, seventeen children in the acute stage of paralysis were treated at the Brisbane clinic, and all made an excellent recovery.

The good results and a positive assessment from the hospital doctors paved the way for the opening of Kenny Ward 7 (Wattle Brae) in June 1939 at the BGH. Hospital authorities decided that newly admitted patients would be given a choice of treatment, Kenny or orthodox, before being sent to an isolation ward for three weeks. If patients elected to receive the Kenny treatment, hot packs were immediately commenced. Ward Sister Mary Luddy remembered constantly running back and forward to wring out the woollen packs. According to her, the passive exercises were never forced, because the limbs were very tender, but pain never increased despite the exercises.[577] It was a testament to the strength of the relationship between Kenny and Chuter that their former dispute did not lead to a complete breakdown. Just before her patients were transferred from the clinic to the BGH, Kenny wrote, 'I regretted having to refuse your commands owing to your humane view of this work, and the admiration I have for your unbiased and unprejudiced attitude which, unfortunately, is so rare'.[578] Elizabeth Kenny had finally achieved her wish, to treat patients with her method in the early stage of paralysis.

The General Superintendent of BGH, Dr Aubrey Pye, was 'greatly impressed by how well her cases did than those treated in the hospital by the orthodox method'.[579] In his opinion, Kenny was a 'brilliant re-educationalist and a very competent observer'.[580] Pye was a powerful and influential friend to Kenny along with Abraham Fryberg who continued to support her after he joined the Queensland Health Department.[581] Dr Jarvis Nye had been a member of the Royal Commission that had condemned all aspects of Kenny's treatment the previous year, but now admitted that she now knew 'more about muscle origin, insertion and function than any of the men here'. Furthermore, he concurred that results with some of her Brisbane Hospital patients were 'truly amazing', and that Elizabeth Kenny 'wasn't the quack that we had believed she was'.[582] Nye tried to convince the other members of the Royal Commission to reconvene and reconsider their verdict, but they would not listen. By the end of 1939, Kenny believed there was little more that she could achieve in Australia without the support of the BMA, and turned her attention to the United States. She had been successful at gaining a foothold in Victoria at the Hampton Children's Hospital, where she was given a proportion of cases, with the others treated by two orthopaedic surgeons, Drs Forster and Price. Their report expressed the opinion that Kenny had made a definite contribution to the treatment of polio.[583] However, the report was ignored. Jarvis Nye convinced five other medical supporters[584] of Kenny to lobby the Queensland Government for financial help to fund her trip to the United States and, according to several accounts, Premier Forgan Smith was very glad to see her go.[585] It would be in America that Elizabeth Kenny finally found, for a few years at least, the support she needed.

Chapter 6

SISTER KENNY GOES TO AMERICA

In April 1940, Elizabeth Kenny and her 23-year-old ward Mary Stewart Kenny arrived in California,[586] where they then set off for New York armed with a letter of introduction to Basil O'Connor[587] of the National Foundation for Infantile Paralysis (NFIP) from Queensland Premier Forgan Smith who supported her by declaring 'my Government has been much impressed with the results of the Kenny system ... particularly the treatment of the disease in the acute stage'.[588] Kenny was determined to demonstrate that she was a professional, respected figure in her homeland and one worthy of respect in America. She was also optimistic that donors and believers in her treatment would be less beholden to the medical establishment than her supporters in Australia.

Kenny realised that the NFIP was becoming a critical force in funding the treatment for polio cases and that its director, Basil O'Connor, was a powerful player in the medical and legal establishment. A former law partner of President Franklin Delano Roosevelt, he was also a close associate of Morris Fishbein, the pugnacious editor of the *Journal of the American Medical Association* (JAMA) and was a vocal critic of socialised medicine and of any government intervention into the relationship between medical practitioner and patient. O'Connor believed that medical care for polio patients should be met by contributions to the Foundation, and that no state or government funds should be used until all other avenues of funding had been exhausted. That was in contrast to the majority of voluntary agencies in the United States that believed that their role was to supplement and not to 'displace public financing in health and welfare'.[589]

Kenny was not encouraged by the early response to her lectures on her methods to physicians in New York, Chicago and Rochester. When she arrived at the University of Minnesota in the summer of 1940 she was feeling despondent and ready to return to Australia. In contrast to previous presentations, the reaction from her Minneapolis audience seemed more positive. In particular, Miland Knapp, the Chief of the Department of Physical

Medicine, appeared willing to hear her out and invited her to see one of his own paralysed patients. In July 1940, Kenny was given Station K, a ward at Minneapolis General Hospital, after gaining the support of local lawyer Henry Haverstock and Drs Knapp and Cole[590] who obtained a grant from the NFIP to cover Kenny's living expenses.[591]

In January 1941, the NFIP arranged for several physical therapists to visit the University of Minneapolis hospital to observe Kenny's treatment. One of the physical therapists attending was Alice Lou Plastridge, the assistant director of physical therapy at the Warm Springs Foundation in Georgia. In 1931, Jean Macnamara had thought the staff at Warm Springs were 'poorly trained, skilled at handling fractures but did not know how to care for paralysed muscles'.[592] It was possibly the only time that Kenny and Macnamara agreed on treatment, although their reasons were different. Kenny had told Plastridge that the 'puddles' [hydrotherapy pools] at Warm Springs should be turned into gardens and that she wouldn't have anything to do with 'any place that used massage, pools or splints'.[593] During the two days she spent in Minneapolis, Plastridge found Kenny to be not a good lecturer or teacher, neither scientific nor logical and found her theories about the effect of the poliovirus so 'radically different from our teachings that they cannot be accepted at face value'. Plastridge thought that part of the problem was that if anyone questioned her method, Kenny took it as a criticism rather than a simple query and became antagonistic. She did, however, respect Kenny's 'sincerity and honesty of purpose', describing her as a woman with a 'mission in life'. Plastridge was very impressed with the way that Kenny taught her patients self-awareness about their own bodies before commencing exercises, and her own work at Warm Springs had shown her the benefits to patients of heat and exercise in the thermal spring pools. Plastridge concluded:

> Whether her theories are scientifically sound or not, only time and further investigation wll prove; but the fact remains that she is getting such unusually good results that it does not seem possible they could all be a matter of chance. One thing is certain. Her controversial theories have given a tremendous stimulation to further research in this field, and made many of us take serious stock of ourselves, and the type of physical therapy we are doing.[594]

Plastridge and another two technicians from Warm Springs left Minneapolis before the end of the course and, by so doing, they incurred Kenny's wrath. She was incensed when a new course of treatment at Warm Springs was advertised as the 'Kenny Treatment', prompting the Director to write to a fellow physician. 'We are doing a grand job here at Warm Springs. In fact I would be at peace with the world if that fool National Foundation hadn't spread the word that we were teaching the "Kenny method". What a mess of misunderstanding has come from that.'[595] Florence and Henry Kendall also attended the demonstration of Kenny's methods in Minneapolis. Both were respectable leading physical therapists and proponents of the orthodox care and treatment of polio. They were opposed to the use of hydrotherapy and were conservative, basing their therapies on the principles of rest, immobilisation and the protection of muscles endorsed by Jean Macnamara in Australia. The Kendalls were not at all impressed with Kenny's methods, particularly her rejection of muscle testing, the standard tool used by classically trained physical therapists to assess the amount of damage to muscles.[596]

A constant theme throughout the letters that Kenny exchanged with Charles Chuter during her time in the United States was her bewilderment at the attitude of the Australian medical profession towards her treatment. On several occasions she asked Chuter to arrange publication of the results of her success in America in the Queensland newspapers because the 'BMJ will not publish anything from me'.[597] In May 1942, she wrote to him from Minneapolis:

> Why are the people of Australia debarred from the benefit of my research? Although I am not over anxious to return to Australia and leave the country where I have proved my work, I think of the little children; and I think of those who are supposed to be doing the Kenny treatment, and I want them to do it as it should be done in the interests of humanity. There are always plenty of complaints when I do return about the staff not doing as they do when I am there. I do not blame the staff. I do blame the medical men who ridicule them for doing my work. I hope this is all over now, and the patients will get the correct treatment. I am willing to return at any time to teach in Australia. When I think of all the damaged lives from the epidemics in 1937–38 my heart is torn with sorrow.[598]

Throughout her early career, Elizabeth Kenny was bedevilled by a lack of communication skills. Teaching her method to others was integral to her success but a poor grasp of language and the inability to express complex physiological concepts to a sophisticated medical audience proved problematic. In 1942, one medical practitioner wrote to a colleague about Kenny's book, *The Treatment of Infantile Paralysis in the Acute Stage*: 'I don't wonder that you have had difficulty in obtaining any information from EK's book. I have had it since it was first published [September 1941] and I am of the opinion that it is one of the worst attempts to describe a technique that I have ever encountered.'[599]

Most practitioners, be they from medical orthodoxy or from the allied health professions accepted that the current methods for treatment of the disease were far from satisfactory. Most were deeply concerned about the suffering of polio patients and were open to the idea that the Kenny method should be given a fair trial, but many were confused by her inept attempts to explain her interpretation of the effect of the poliovirus on the human body.

In 1942, the NFIP issued a formal approval of Kenny's method for treating polio paralysis and, in December, the Elizabeth Kenny Institute was opened in Minneapolis.[600] Postgraduate courses were set up at the University of Minnesota to teach Kenny's method to physicians, nurses and physical therapists. Many who visited Minneapolis to observe her demonstrations were impressed:

> Most dramatic demonstration I have seen in a good many years … Everyone is 100% favorable. Many of our physicians who were formerly skeptical have come over 'whole hog' and a number are planning to register for your course for physicians in Minneapolis … I knew the course was good but I had no idea it was so very good … The ideal situation would be to have every child who is attacked by the disease treated by your method … The lecture was a very valuable experience for all of us.[601]

However, the NFIP refused to give financial support to the Institute and it was subsequently registered as a non-profit charitable organisation.[602] In the United States, Kenny had finally found the support she needed, and believed that her seven years of battling with orthodox medicine to have her polio treatment accepted was at an end. Victory, albeit for a few years only, was hers, and the public in particular took Kenny and her Institute to its heart. As Naomi Rogers argues in her insightful book on Kenny's American years, Kenny took advantage of her nascent popularity to reiterate her claim that polio was not solely a neurological disease, but one that also affected muscles and peripheral structures: 'But as the Institute prospered and Kenny was feted as a saviour, she began to argue that her work embodied a new knowledge of polio drawn from a close reading of the body'.[603]

1944 was a very bad year for polio in America and a very bad year for Elizabeth Kenny. The American Medical Association[604] featured prominently in a campaign to discredit Kenny by claiming that 'the public and many doctors' had been misled about the effectiveness of her treatment, in particular the use of hot packs to lessen pain and that there was nothing new about her methods. The continuous use of the packs was described as of 'questionable value and a waste of man power and hospital beds'.[605] They criticised her recovery rates, saying she did not separate out 'spontaneous recoveries' in her statistics. How could she? At that stage nobody knew how polio was transmitted, or its epidemiology or aetiology. The symptoms and subsequent consequences of exposure to the poliovirus were so wide-ranging from patient to patient that comparing the results of different treatments was almost impossible. Some patients recovered quickly or spontaneously while in others the paralysis remained obstinate and difficult to treat.

In July 1944, the Kenny Institute applied for a grant from the NFIP for funds to train teachers in the Kenny method and also to 'establish a clinical research centre' in Minneapolis.[606] Kenny did not believe the Institute would be successful, suspecting that it was part of an 'organised endeavour to get rid of me' because her visa was due to expire the following May. At the headquarters of the NFIP, Basil O'Connor knew that hundreds of letters from anti-vivisectionists and others had been written to President Roosevelt asking that more funds from the March of Dimes appeal be assigned to the Kenny Institute and not wasted 'on experiments on helpless monkeys when Sister Kenny's method works' or for 'keeping children in iron braces'.[607] O'Connor was furious when he received the grant application. The NFIP considered itself to be the premier body funding scientific research into poliomyelitis and it would brook no interference into its territory. O'Connor commissioned a report from the National Research Council (NRC) into 'the potentialities of the Kenny Institute for (a) teaching the concept and methods of Sister Kenny, and (b) research in this field'. The committee (composed entirely of medical men) found against the Institute and recommended that 'no grants be made to the Kenny Institute for research either basic or clinical'.[608] The NRC believed that the greatest problem for the Kenny Foundation was that the national officers were, for the most part, ignorant of organisation standards in the USA. They were a group of 'starry-eyed crusaders.' Ironically, the NFIP itself was later judged as not meeting the standards of 'trusteeship, organisation, administration, educational work and financing' stipulated by the National Information Bureau (NIB).[609] From 1928 to 1936, John D. Rockefeller Jr made anonymous donations totalling $110,200 to the Georgia Warm Springs Foundation (the forerunner to the NFIP) until he withdrew his support after the President's Birthday Celebration committee took over Warm Springs.[610]

The NIB reported that they had never seen a consolidated statement on either the fund-raising costs or the resources of the national and local chapters of the NFIP, said to aggregate some millions each year. Between 1939 and 1947, the NIB estimated the income of the NFIP and its chapters was approximately US$75,000,000. The Rockefeller family privately directed its lawyers to make no further contributions because of concerns about the 'secrecy by the foundation about their finances'.[611] In October 1949, the Foundation wrote to the Rockefeller family pleading for a significant contribution to the March of Dimes campaign because it was in a 'grave' financial state.[612] The previous year one of its medical directors intimated that the Foundation's administration costs were 'very high',[613] a statement that appears to be backed up by the previous year's figures published in *The New York Times*.[614]

It seemed that Kenny was destined to relive her Australian experiences as yet another report in November 1944 by a committee of medical men attacked her integrity and credibility. Chicago academic and orthopaedic surgeon, Dr Philip Lewin later commented:

> That was a crooked deal that committee, some people were on it who should not have been, and others left out who should have been on it. No I wasn't on it. I was sold out. Ghormley was the finest guy in the world. But, he should have had a minority report. There were some punks on that committee and I've got that in writing from their peers.[615]

In characteristic fashion, Kenny counter-attacked, using the media as an ally, and once again the people flocked to support and defend her.[616] The NFIP was forced to defend itself as hundreds of letters from all over the country flooded into the Kenny Institute. Most of the letter writers either attacked JAMA Editor Morris Fishbein personally, or the AMA, the medical profession or the pharmaceutical industry:

> You have found a way to relieve the suffering and tortuous crippling of our little children, while our great scientific medical specialists stood by helpless, hand on chin, brow wrinkled and no doubt rubbing their schnozolas at the same time. You have given our great medical fraternity with their self-coined technical terms, their few latin words to make them appear very scientific, and their monopoly on medicine, handed to them on a golden platter in the form of a licence, such a

staggering wallop on the aforementioned proboscis that I doubt very much if they will fully recover. Why is your Institution not getting the greater proportion of the proceeds from these 'March of Dimes' campaigns? God give us more Sister Kennys and deliver us from the Fishbeins.[617]

Another Californian wrote:

take it from me that the reputable physicians in many parts of the USA look on Fishbein for just what he is, one step above a quack ... he did not come across the office of the AMA by ability, but he wormed and chiselled his way into the editorship. He is a cheap, unscrupulous Kike who has become very objectionable to the medical fraternity.[618]

Edward Smythe, Chairman of the Protestant War Veterans association in New York was incensed at her treatment, and wrote:

America needs you more than it needs Morris Fishbein and his ilk. You stay right here ... I am asking friends of mine in Congress to invite you down there for a talk before that body of outstanding Americans. A thousand Fishbeins and names like that do not represent the sentiments of true Americans, these are but guests in this country who has [sic] outstayed their welcome, and are about to be requested by force if necessary to get the hell out of here. The AMA is dominated by these alien shysters.[619]

A pattern of prejudice against Jews had emerged during the late nineteenth century in the USA and reached an apogee during the 1940s. Anti-semitism was part of everyday life, particularly between 1941 and 1944, despite press reports about the acts of genocide being carried out against European Jews. Jewish cemeteries were often defiled, slogans and swastikas appeared in public areas and anti-semitic literature was widely available. Many Americans believed that Jews were too influential, especially in civic life.

While conceding that the AMA was a 'very strong organisation', another mother urged Kenny 'not to give up ... don't let the Pill Slingers Association beat you'.[620] Many writers used the campaign to keep Kenny in America to express their frustration with a powerful, arrogant and authoritarian medical establishment, citing a belief that doctors 'should put up a sign, 'Pay as you enter' on their doors', and that 'they are all jealous of each other'.[621] J. Hall of New York believed that 'it's a shame the way the medical profession have acted towards you ... the AMA is too contemptible for words. Some day you will be fully vindicated ... the rank and file of this country value your work.'[622] Mrs Roberts of California urged her 'not to pay any attention to the doctors, they have fought everything good that ever came along ... they fought the chiropractor and every drugless method we have.'[623] For Cosette Dexter, Kenny's gender was the key to why she was being 'persecuted':

> It's a man's world, don't give up. The women of America need you. Just realize what is against you. You are a woman, you don't have a college degree but Jesus Christ wasn't a MD, and the money interests who are reaping a harvest from the manufacturing of braces are against you. Buck up, there are thousands like me who believe in you.[624]

Some writers appeared also to harbour suspicions about the NFIP, its goals and its close association with the AMA, suspecting that its purpose was to benefit certain sections of the population at the expense of others. Other letter writers were angry when they realised that the money they donated to the March of Dimes did not go to Kenny. Mrs Bonnell of Minneapolis was not going to contribute 'any more dimes to the NFIP of which Basil O'Connor is head ... because I didn't know before that you didn't get a nickel of it'.[625] Several letter writers referred to the Ghormley report — 'a ridiculous and monstrously unfair attack' published by the AMA in June 1944. Mrs Rich had 'never been so disgusted in my life to realise that an intelligent group of men such as the AMA should underrate and make such statements about one who is giving so much to humanity', and reminded Kenny that 'jealousy apparently causes some folks to do mean, dirty and uncalled for things'.[626]

Support for Kenny crossed social boundaries, and rich and poor offered money to keep her in America. A 'soldier's wife' in San Francisco was 'more than happy to donate $5 a year to keep you here among us', while a socialite in New York promised that 'many of her friends would send donations ... if a fund for you is started here'.[627] Early the following year the press ran a scurrilous story alleging that Kenny had received a large personal payment (US$49,535) from the NFIP. What the article failed to mention was that the payment spanned three years, that wages for all the Institute staff were deducted from the total, and that Kenny herself probably received around $6400 over that period.[628]

In 1942 there were few Kenny clinics left in Australia, with a handful of Kenny-trained nurses who were not up-to-date with current treatment. In Minneapolis, Kenny heard from Charles Chuter that 'by December there will be nothing left of the Kenny clinics in this State'.[629] Cairns, Toowoomba and Townsville had been shut down, as well as the wards in Brisbane Hospital.[630] The clinic at Newcastle, the only one in Australia operating within the auspices of an infectious diseases hospital and treating patients in the acute, infectious stage, had disappeared in June 1939 when the Superintendent, Dr Kenneth Starr, re-introduced splinting, removed Kenny's name from the clinic, and announced that he had introduced 'modifications' to her treatment. Starr also admitted that Kenny's appointment as a consultant had been a mistake because of the 'most adverse reaction on the consultant medical staff of the hospital'. Chuter dismissed Starr's attitude as being on a par with the general attitude of the profession.[631]

In Brisbane, the George Street Clinic was barely functioning, with just two nurses remaining from the original staff of thirty-one. The remainder had enlisted for war service, fearful of losing their jobs at a time when memories of the Depression years were fresh. The clinic continued to operate for a few years in a 'lifeless fashion', a 'mere shadow' of its former self. In 1945 Kenny was upset to hear that her name was still used in conjunction with the Brisbane clinic because 'the work is not what it should be'. She was correct. Kenny had refined and improved her method of treatment in the years since she left Australia, and the staff at Brisbane had fallen behind. No one knew how to treat patients in the early stages of paralysis, and that failure to give appropriate treatment gave her detractors further corroboration of their case against her.

Sir Raphael Cilento was still 'deprecating the Kenny method',[632] and Health Minister Hanlon had deserted her, 'speaking of her in Caucus in degrading terms'. Chuter believed that 'hostility' towards Kenny 'still lurked in high places' despite the fact that the NFIP had informed Hanlon earlier that year that it had endorsed her treatment of the disease in the acute stage, and Basil O'Connor had written to thank Hanlon for 'referring Miss Kenny to us'. In 1942, the Australian-American Association wanted to publish an article in its Australian journal about Sister Kenny's success in America, but was warned 'to exercise caution' by a close friend and medical associate of Cilento. The Association decided not to publish the article.[633] That same year, Professor Philip Lewin published a report stating his opinion on the Kenny treatment: 'There is no doubt that her treatment abolishes pain and stiffness and minimises the occurrence of deformities. It prevents contractures, lessens the degree of paralysis, and, by treating the symptoms in the acute stage, procures a higher percentage of full recovery than any other method.' Furthermore, Lewin believed that Kenny's patients were in

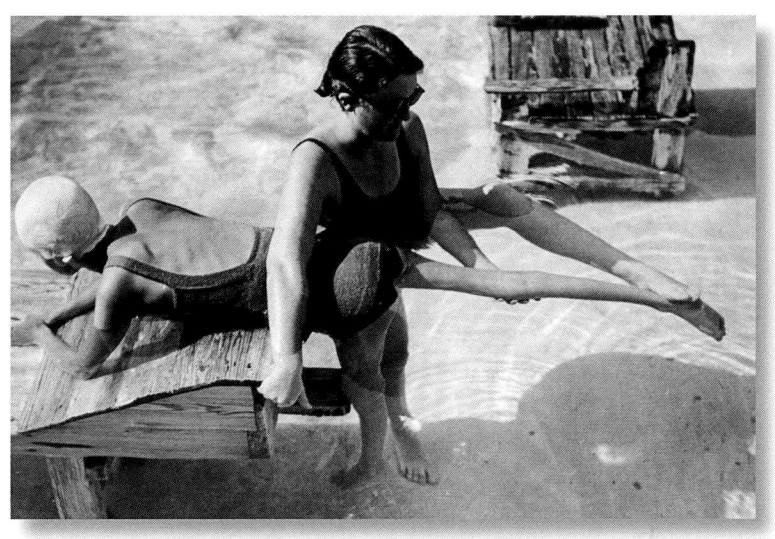

Hydrotherapy, Warm Springs, 1933.
Reproduced with permission from the National Library of Australia

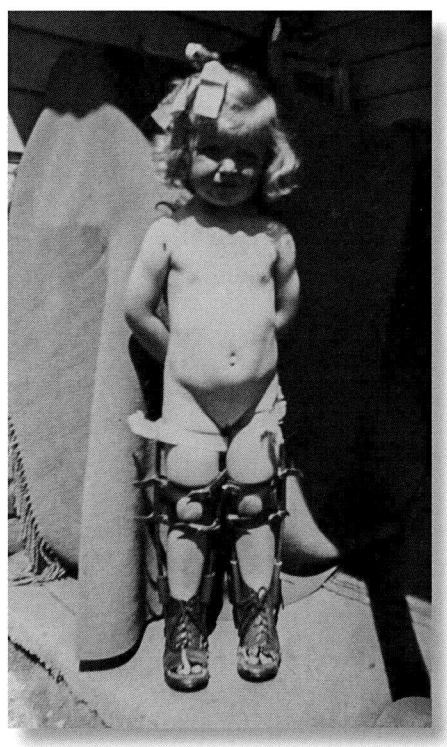

Child in splints to correct knock-knees, Melbourne, Victoria, circa 1938.
Reproduced with permission from the National Library of Australia

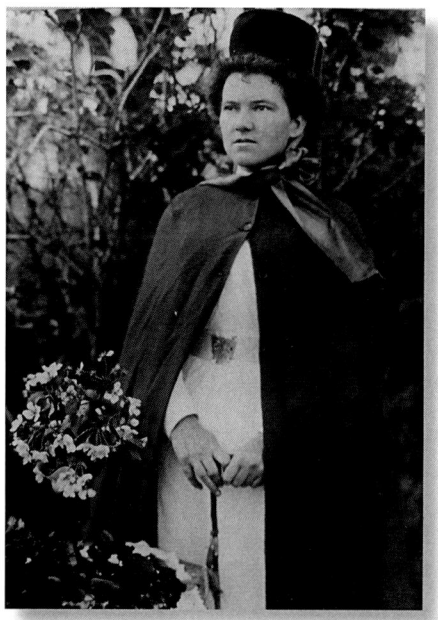

Elizabeth Kenny in nurse's uniform, Clifton, Queensland, circa 1912.

Reproduced with permission of the John Oxley Library, State Library of Queensland

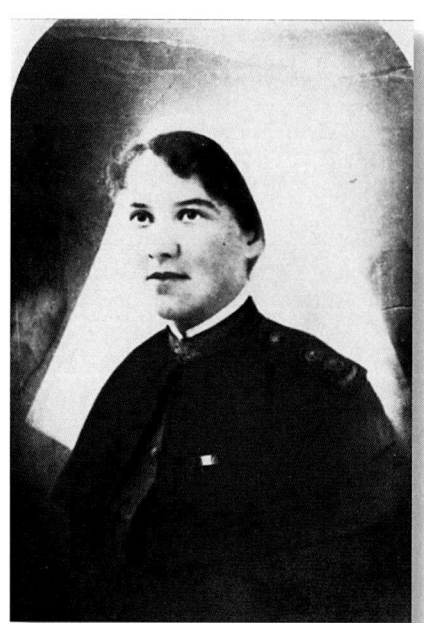 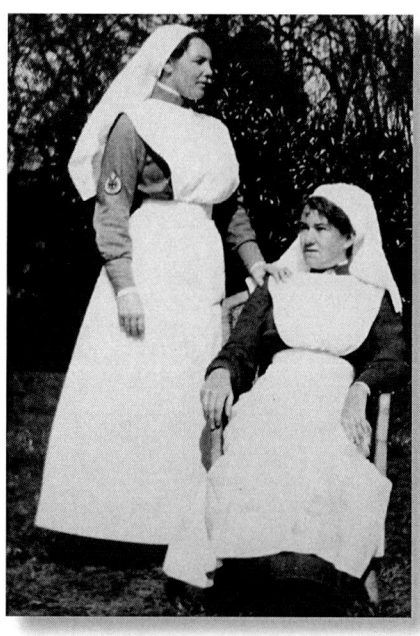

Left: Sister Elizabeth Kenny, circa 1917.
Right: Sister Ella Morphett and Staff Nurse Kenny in the grounds of Harefield Hospital, circa 1916.

Reproduced with permission of the John Oxley Library, State Library of Queensland

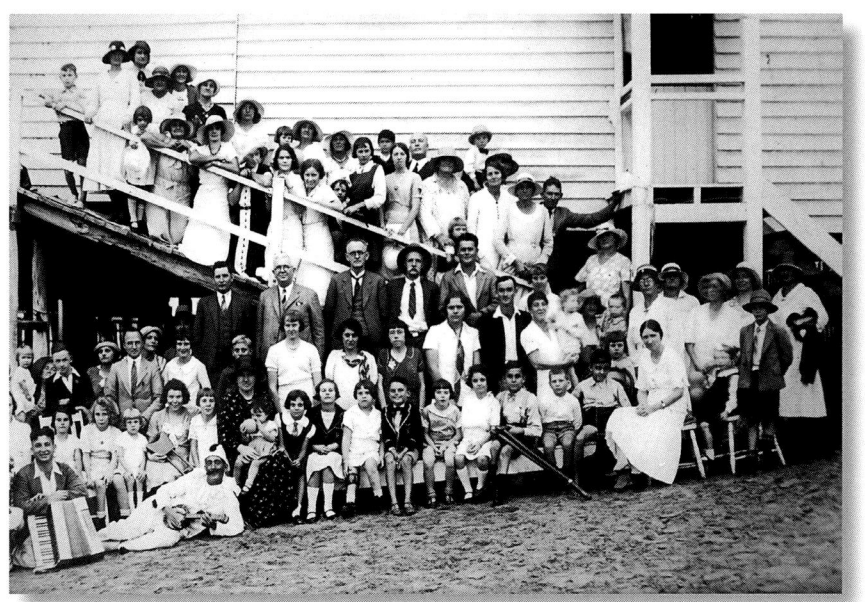

Picnic to celebrate the first anniversary of the Townsville clinic.
Reproduced with permission of the John Oxley Library, State Library of Queensland

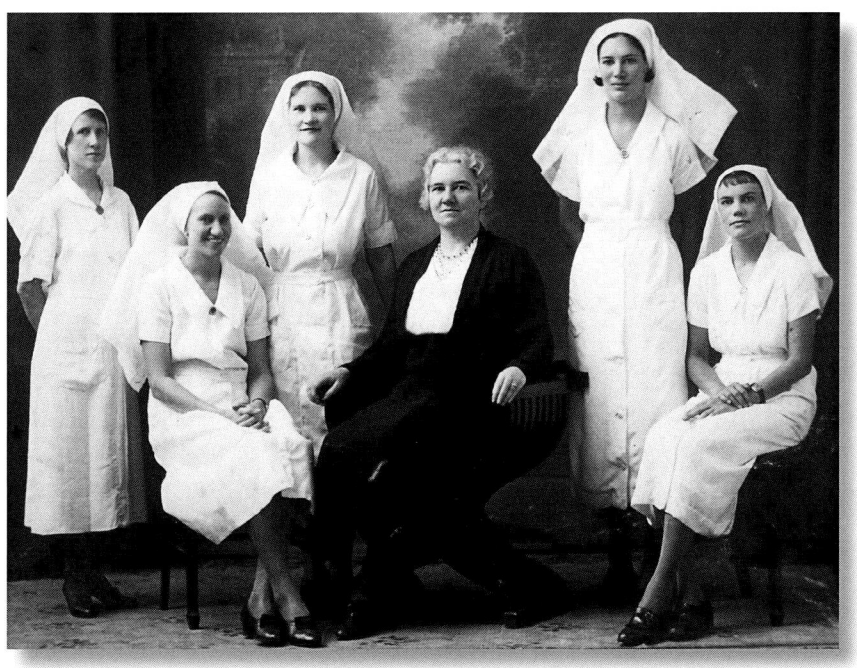

Nursing staff at the Townsville 'Experimental Muscle Rehabilitation Clinic', circa 1935.
(L-R) Sr Leila Cooper, Sr Carmella Jensen, Sr Mary Lynch, Sr Elizabeth Kenny,
Sr Alice Groth, Sr Annie Steele.
Reproduced with permission by the John Oxley Library, State Library of Queensland

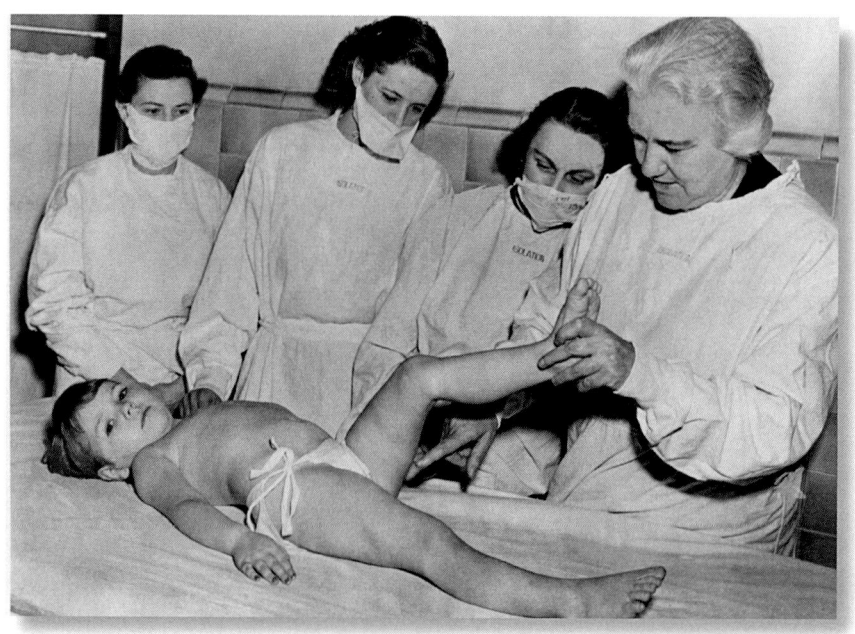

Sister Kenny demonstrates her therapy techniques at the Kenny Institute, Minneapolis.
Reproduced with permission of the Minnesota Historical Society, St Paul, MN, USA

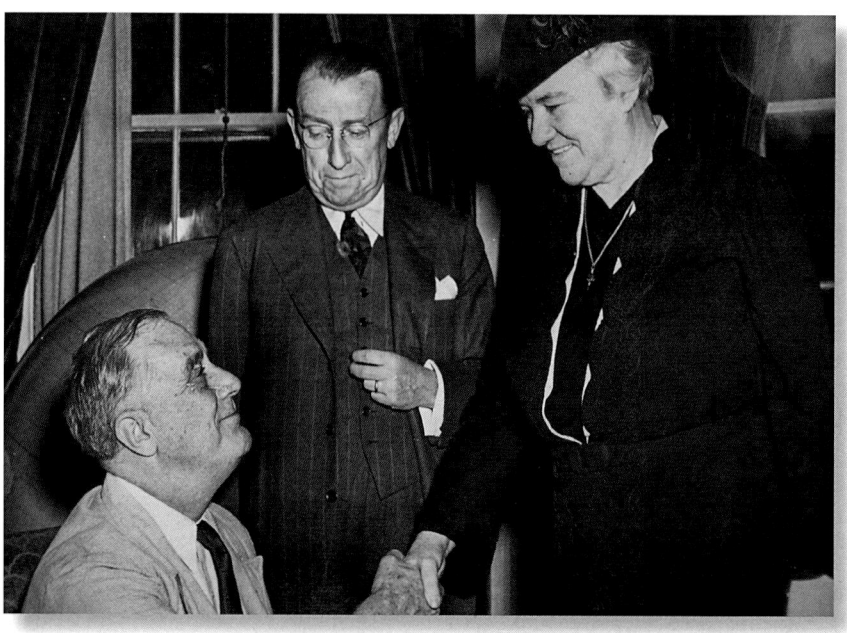

Sister Kenny meets President Roosevelt at the White House, 8 June 1943.
Basil O'Connor is in the background.
Reproduced with permission of the Library of Congress, Prints and Photographs Division, FSA/OW1 Collection

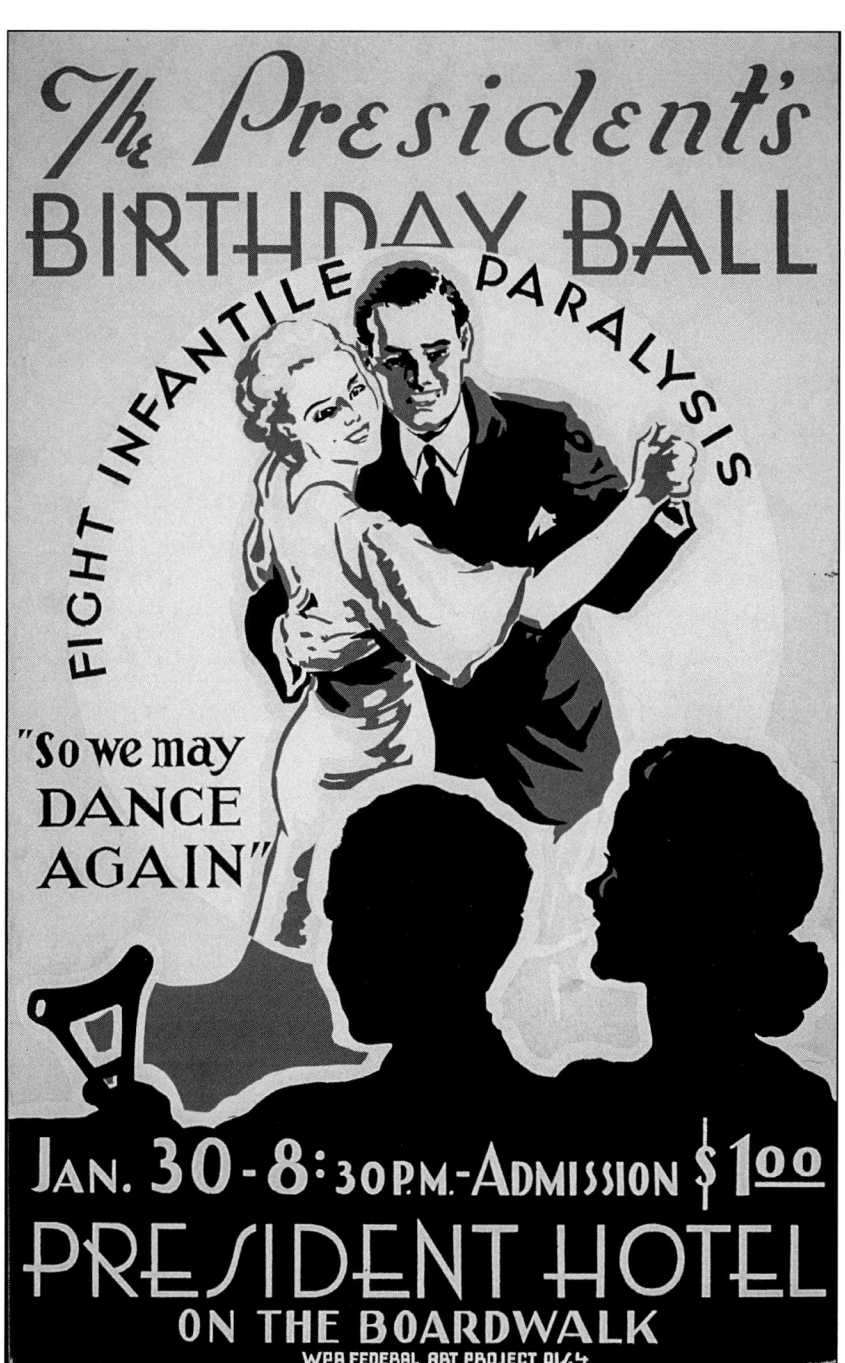

Poster for the President's Birthday Ball.
Reproduced with permission of the Library of Congress, Prints and Photographs Division, FSA/OW1 Collection

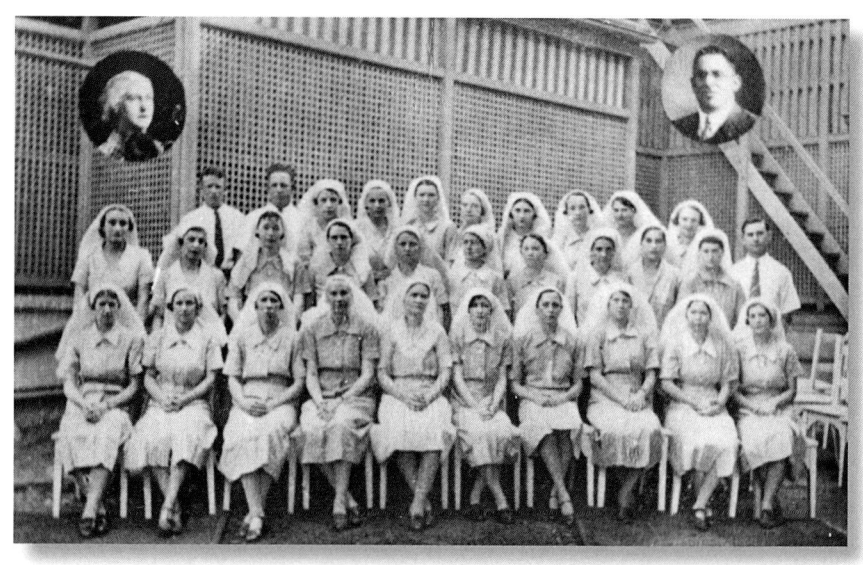
Students in training at the Elizabeth Kenny clinic in Brisbane.
Reproduced with permission of the John Oxley Library, State Library of Queensland

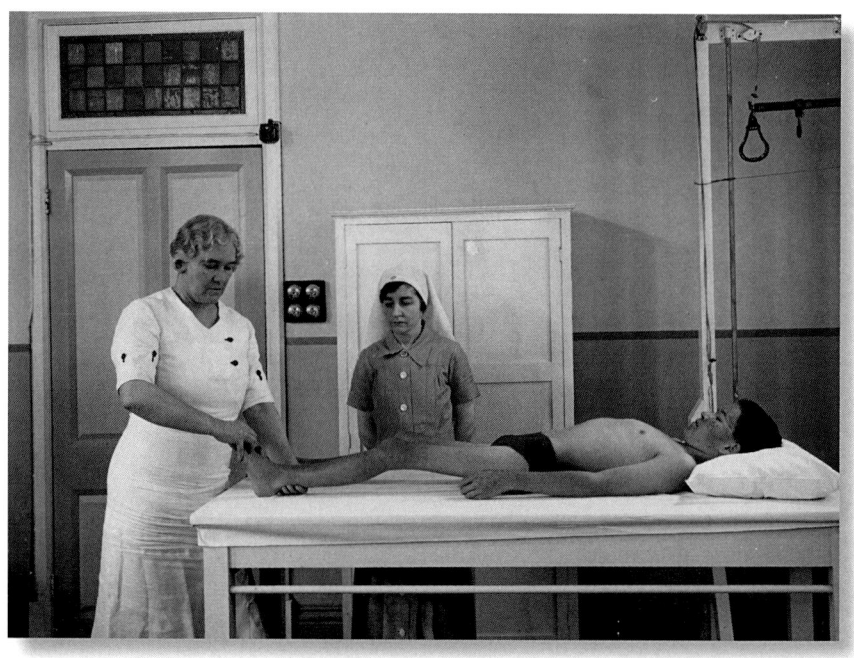
Sister Kenny demonstrating her therapy in the Brisbane clinic, 1937.
Reproduced with permission of the John Oxley Library, State Library of Queensland

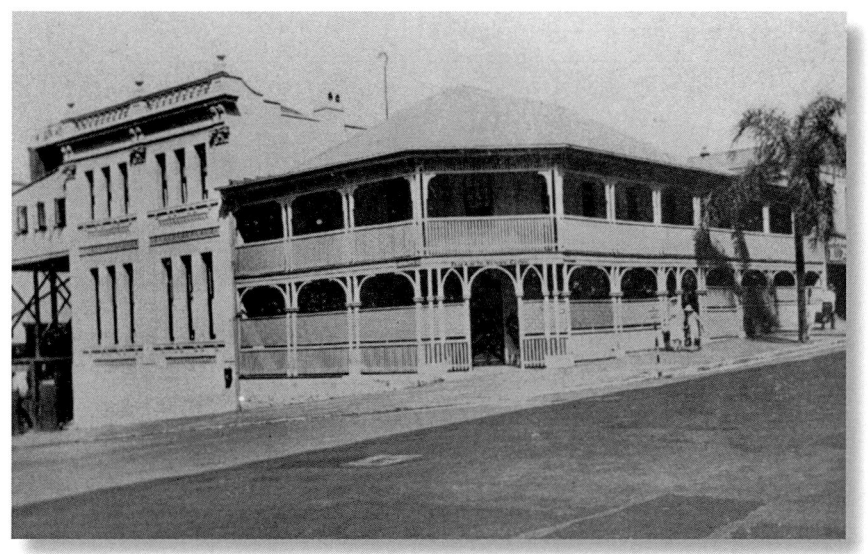

Elizabeth Kenny Clinic on the corner of George and Charlotte Streets, Brisbane 1937.
Reproduced with permission of the John Oxley Library, State Library of Queensland

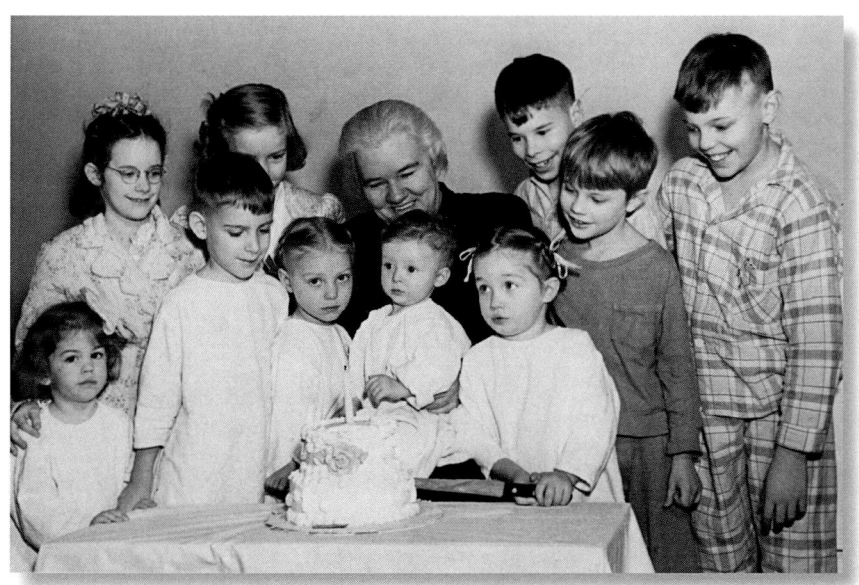

Sister Kenny Institute patients celebrate the Institute's first birthday with Sister Kenny.
Reproduced with permission of the Minnesota Historical Society, St Paul, MN, USA

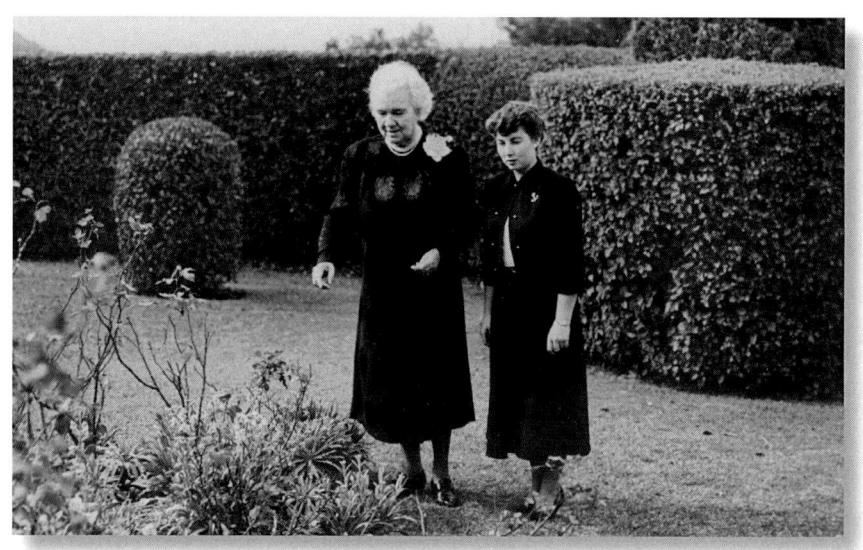

Sister Kenny with her secretary, Miss Betty Brennan, in her garden at 'Struan', Toowoomba, circa 1952.

Reproduced with permission of the State Library of Queensland (Negative 108121)

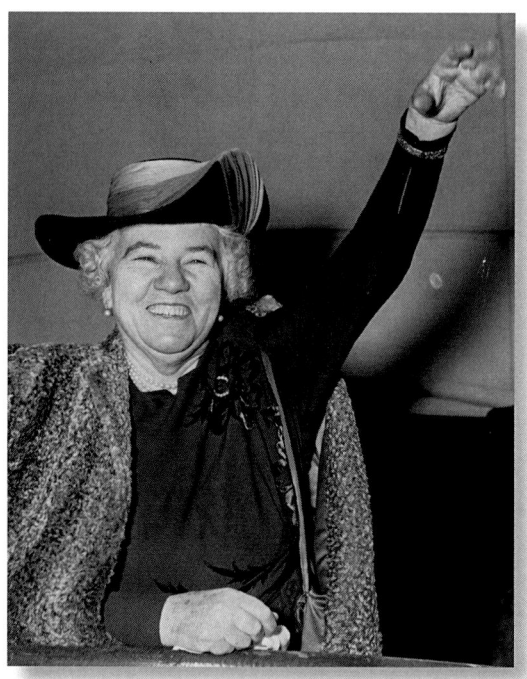

Elizabeth Kenny waving from the deck of the *Queen Mary*, New York, 1950.

Reproduced with permission from the Library of Congress, Prints and Photographs Collection, FSA/OW1, LC-US262-119197

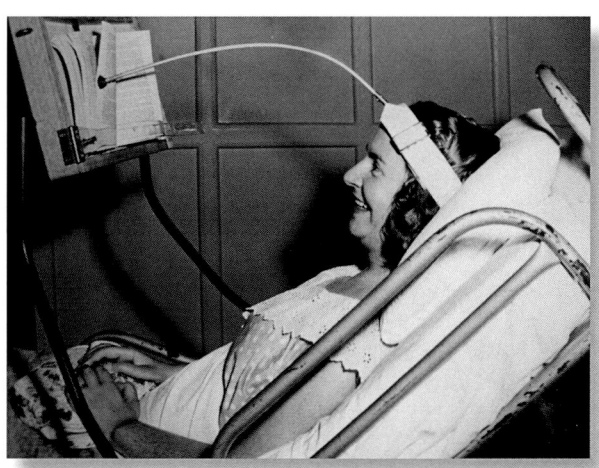
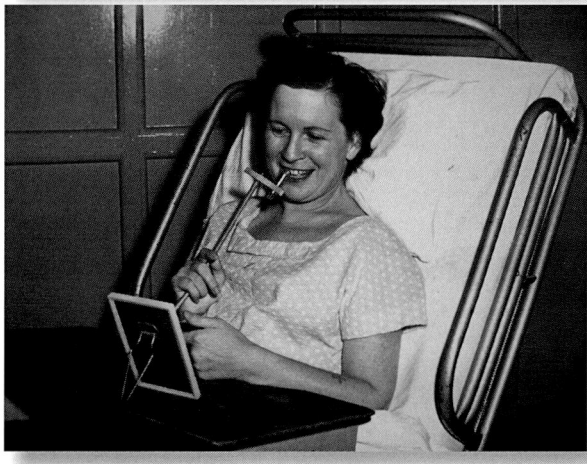
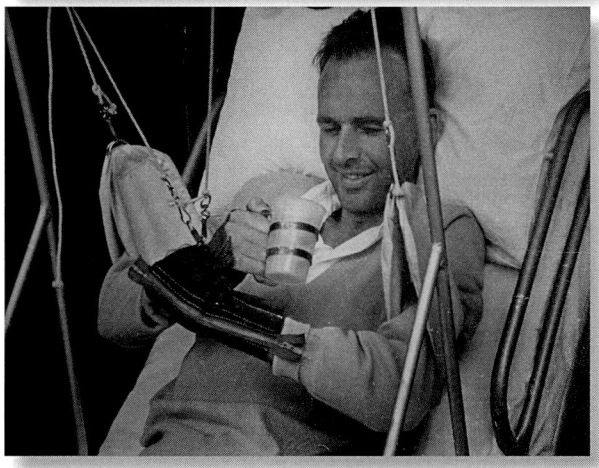

Patients achieving short-term goals at Fairfield Hospital, Melbourne, circa 1950s.
Reproduced with permission from the Fairfield Hospital Archives

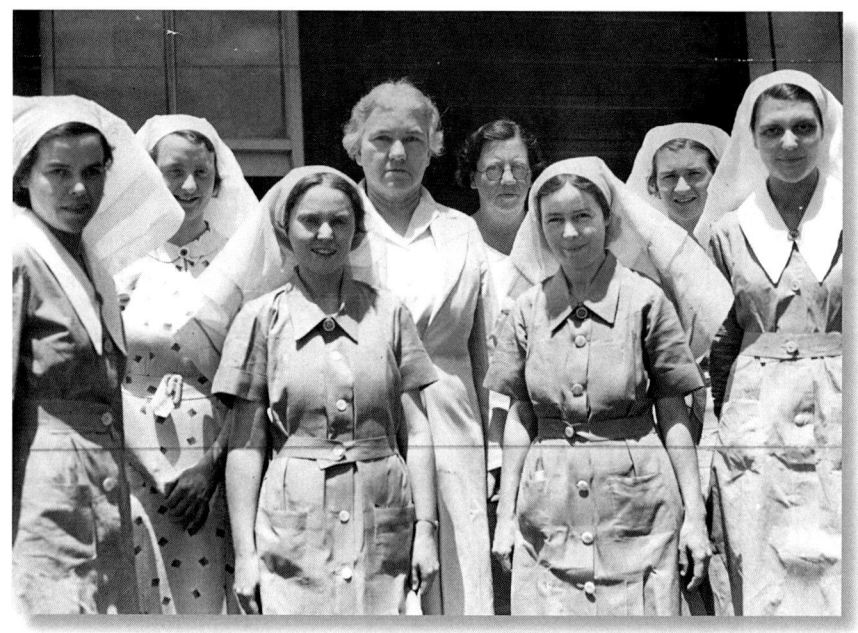

Sister Kenny and Kenny nurses at Hampton Convalescent Hospital, Victoria, 1938.
*Reproduced with permission of the State Library of Victoria
(Herald and Weekly Times Limited Portrait Collection).*

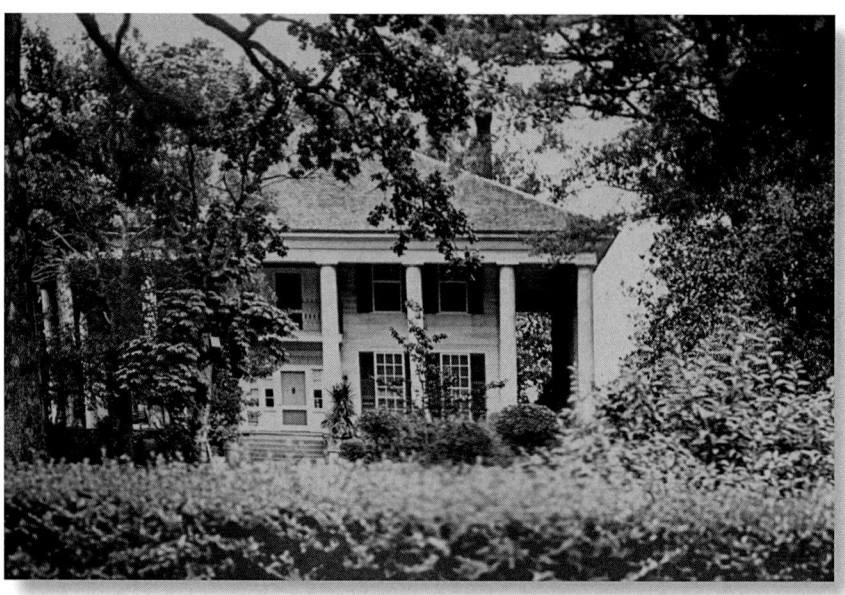

The Little White House, Warm Springs, Georgia.
Reproduced with permission from the National Library of Australia

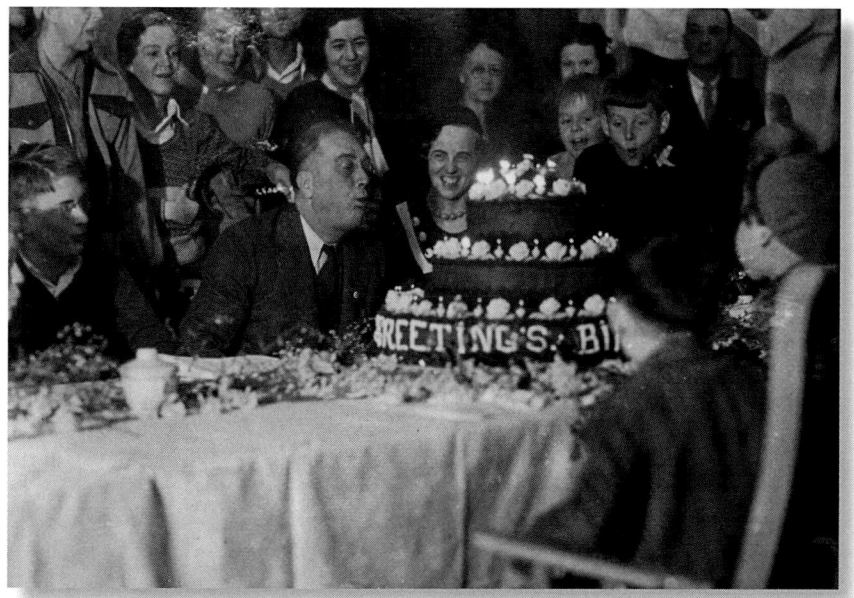

President Roosevelt celebrates his birthday at Warm Springs.
Reproduced with permission from the National Library of Australia

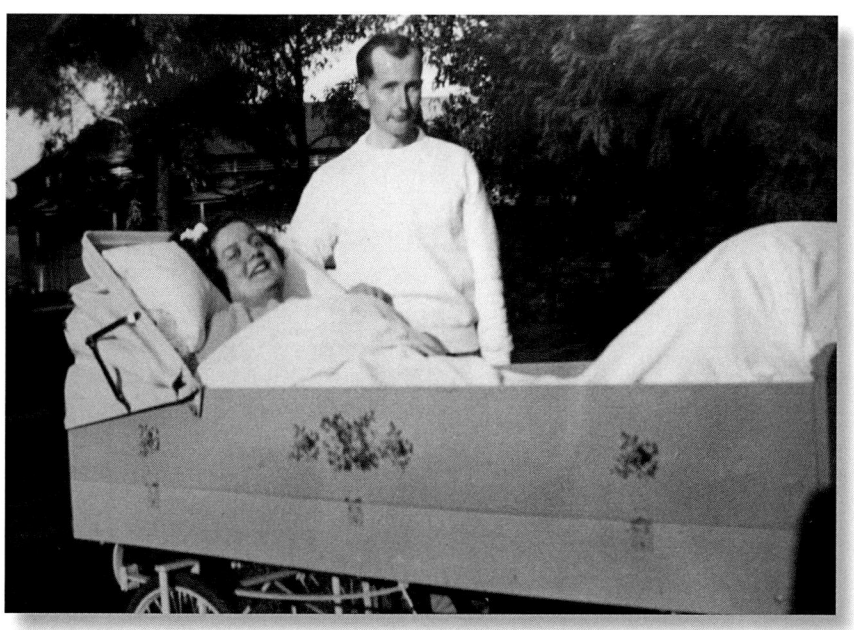

June Middleton with Vern Draffin in the grounds of
Fairfield Hospital in Melbourne, circa 1950.
Reproduced with permission from the Fairfield Hospital archives

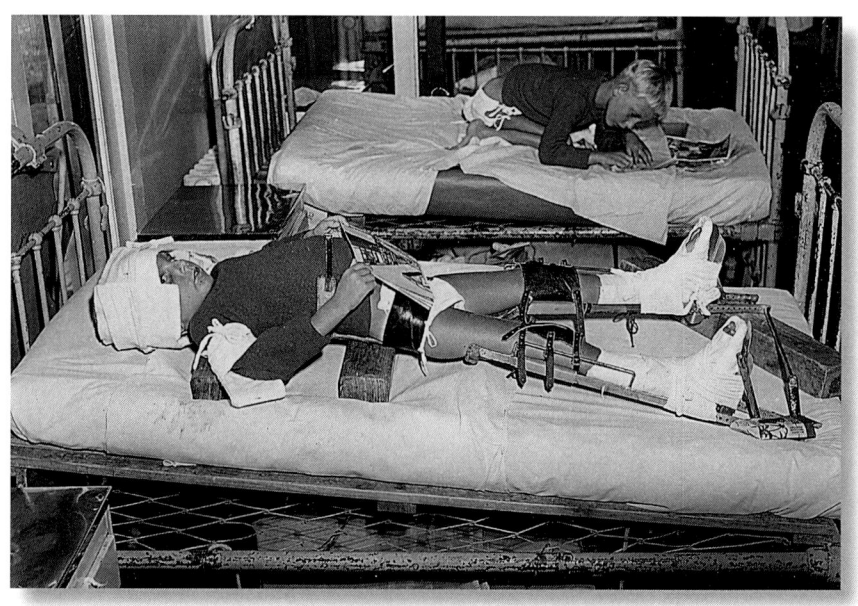

Children at Hampton convalescent hospital.
Reproduced by permission of the RCH Archive

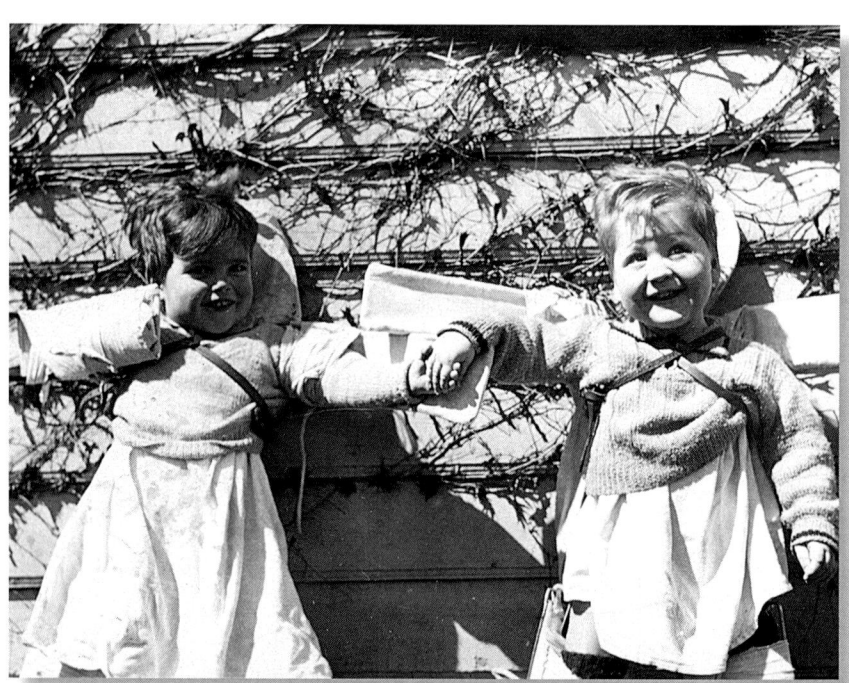

Children at Hampton Convalescent Hospital.
Reproduced by permission of the RCH Archive

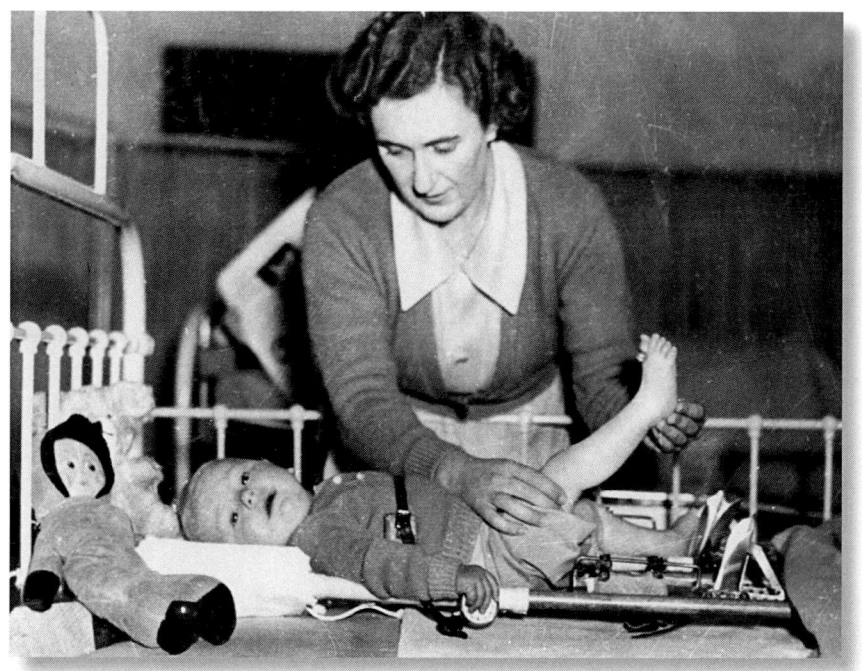

Miss Davies, physiotherapist, with a polio patient.
Reproduced by permission of the RCH Archive

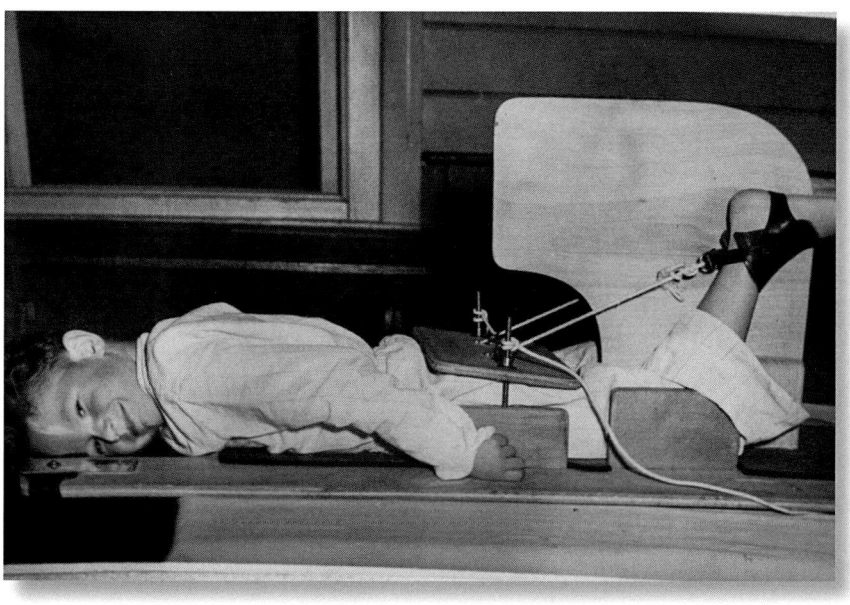

Homemade frame for stretching muscles. Melbourne, Victoria, circa 1938.
Reproduced with permission from the National Library of Australia

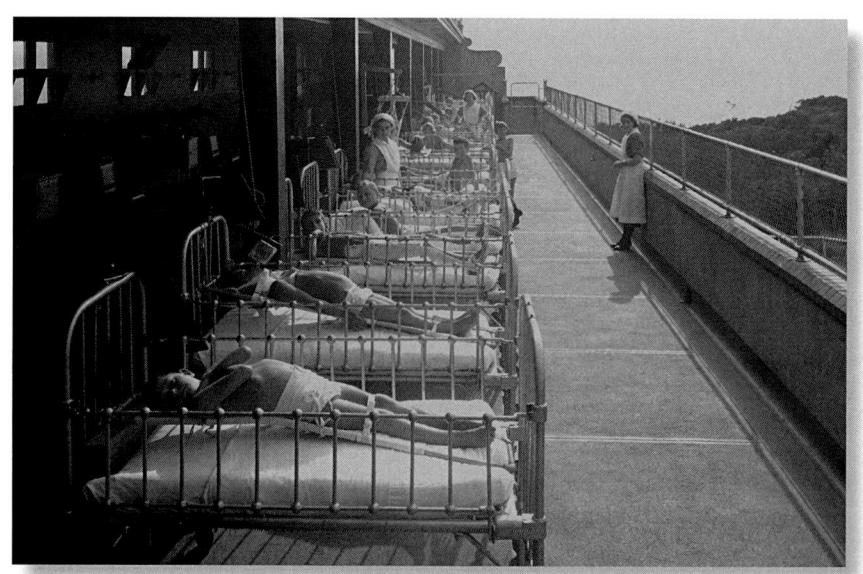

Heliotherapy on the balcony at Frankston Orthopaedic Hospital, circa 1938.
Reproduced with permission from the State Library of Victoria

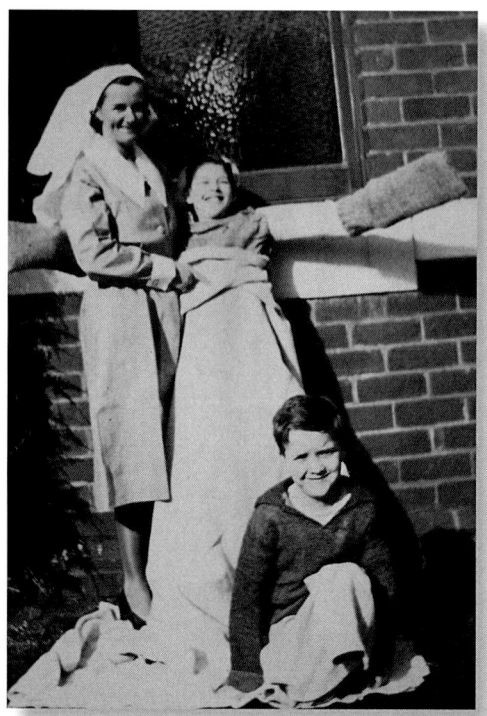

Fairfield staff with two patients in Thomas splints, 1940.
Reproduced with permission from the Fairfield Hospital archives

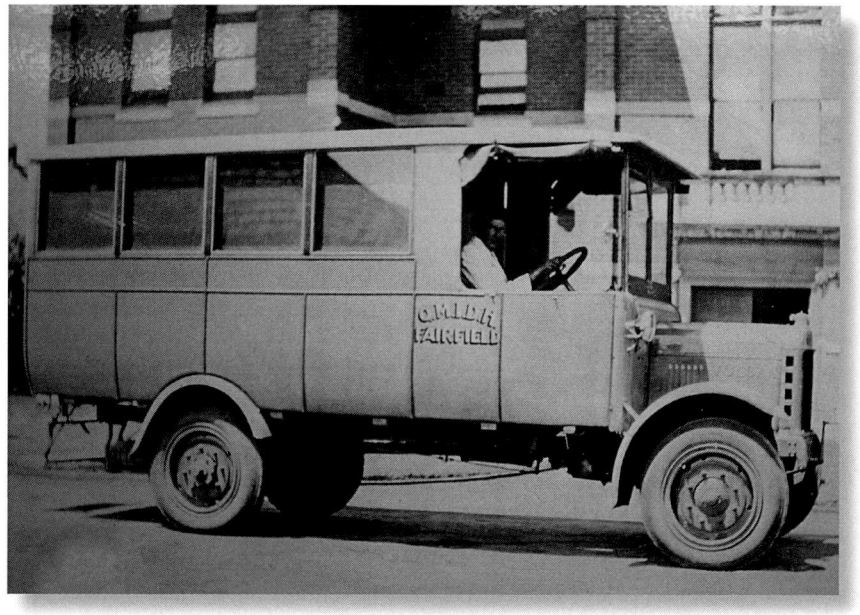

Fairfield Hospital ambulance, 1937. The floor was lined with rubber to allow up to six children to be taken to after-care treatment.

Reproduced with permission from the Fairfield Hospital archives

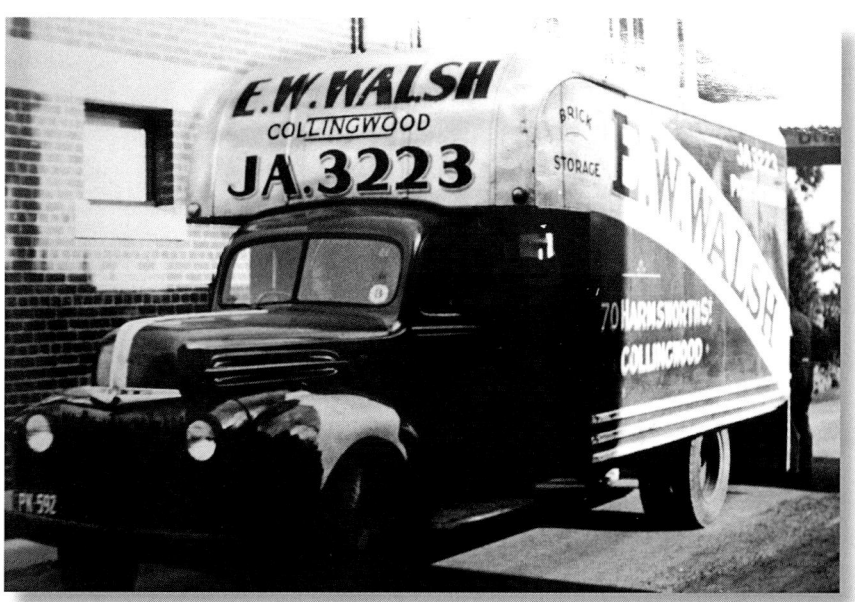

Van for transporting patients in trolley prams to the Melbourne Cricket Ground for AFL games, 1950s.

Reproduced with permission from the Fairfield Hospital archives

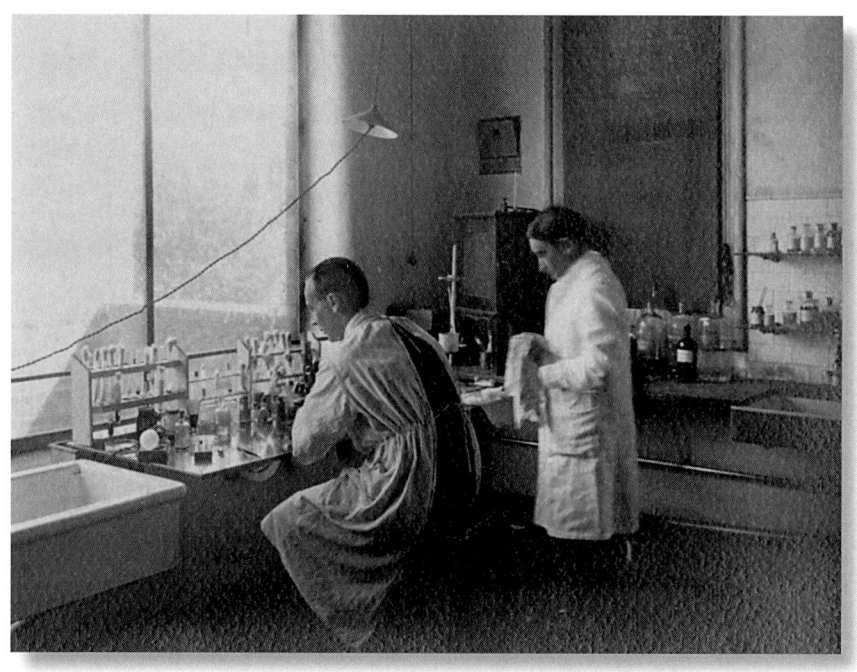

Reginald Webster in his pathology lab at the Royal Children's Hospital in Melbourne, circa 1923.

Reproduced by permission of the RCH Archive

better condition 'than any similar group I have seen anywhere in the world'. Kenny was delighted.[634]

In May 1945, the war in Europe ended and the following month Kenny travelled to London to meet up with Mary Stewart Kenny who had travelled there earlier to meet up with her fiancé, Flight Lieutenant Peter Jennings, a New Zealand pilot with the RAF. Sadly, shortly after Mary's arrival she was given the devastating news that Jennings was missing, presumed dead after his plane had been shot down. As was the case with so many men listed as 'missing', it took many months for his death to be verified. Kenny arrived in London with her latest film on her treatment, *The Kenny Concept of the Disease of Infantile Paralysis*, eager to show it to the Royal Society of Medicine in London and to involve Mary as much as possible because she 'will be pretty lost and very sad'. After showing the film she wrote to Henry James in Minneapolis that 'the committee is of the opinion that everyone should see it, that it was a great triumph'. However, she cautioned James against quoting her, stating that she would 'make a dignified and definite statement on my return, as I do not trust my enemies'. Later, Kenny visited the hospital in Carshalton where her treatment method had been implemented in the late 1930s. To her dismay she found that the children in the wards were once more being placed in splints, due no doubt to the 'untruthful and inaccurate statements published in the *American Medical Journal*'. According to Kenny her work in England had 'gone back years and so has the teaching program'.[635] In *Polio Wars*, Rogers points out that, in fact, the reception to the film by the British medical establishment was far from favourable. Both the British Association of Physical Medicine and the Royal Society of Medicine 'disclaimed all responsibility for any views expressed in the film'. However, while a few physicians had found her treatment methods 'interesting and suggestive' all firmly rebutted Kenny's theories on the pathology of polio.[636]

In a letter to Charles Chuter in May 1945, Kenny offered a copy of *The Kenny Concept* to the Queensland Government, but Chuter, worried that the film would be relegated to the 'mud of oblivion' decided to show it himself to a 'representative audience'.[637] Drs Pye and Arden accused Chuter of 'hawking the film around' but he repudiated the suggestion, stating that he had no 'desire to force the film on anyone, but was agreeable to anyone seeing it'.[638] The response to the film in Australia was mixed. Lay people were enthusiastic, some nurses and physical therapists were favourably impressed, while the reaction from medical practitioners remained sceptical. In December 1945, Kenny wrote to the Secretary of the Australian Legation in Washington about her concern for Queensland polio sufferers in the epidemic that had resurfaced in her home state. She pleaded with them to intercede for her and send a delegation to Minneapolis to study the work being carried out at the Institute. The letter was passed on to the Acting Director General of Health, A.J. Metcalfe, in Canberra but he declined, blandly stating that 'it was not possible to agree to Sister Kenny's suggestion'.[639]

The Perth Children's Hospital was one of the few institutions in 1940s Australia where the Kenny treatment was used. Orthopaedic surgeon Reg McKellar Hall told a physiotherapist working there in 1948 to 'forget everything Dr Jean Macnamara has told you'. When Macnamara visited the hospital later that year on the invitation of public health authorities, she referred to the hospital as a 'cripple factory' and declared that she would not 'send any of her girls [Victorian physiotherapists]' to work in Western Australia, whereupon the Public Health Commissioner retorted that 'it had been a waste of time and money bringing her here'.[640] Jean Macnamara was convinced that maintaining orthodox treatment was the only way to prevent deformities developing, and her considerable influence in the field of after-care treatment in Victoria meant that she also commanded the respect and attention of the rich and powerful to have her beliefs on treatment officially endorsed.[641] Uppermost in her mind were two factors. The first was the need to rescue children from entering the 'cripple factory' by treating childhood 'chassis' problems like knock-knees, flat feet and curved backs with corrective splints.

> The need for expensive centres and schools for older 'spastic' children will increase if priority of care is given to older children who have spent years in the cripple factory, while at the same time the babies, whose parents are less vocal in demanding care, are busy manufacturing needless deformities which will enable them to qualify for admission to special schools.[642]

The second was the obligation to 'minimise crippling' by enforced rest and immobilisation of those affected by the poliovirus. Both considerations would, in her view, result in a significant economic saving to Australia by reducing the number of invalid pensioners.[643] Adults should be kept in the 'optimum posture position' by plaster of Paris splints, wood or wire outlines but the natural activity of children was better 'controlled' or 'rationed' by the double Thomas splint. Macnamara believed that the American surgeon Robert Lovett had been correct when he wrote in 1917, 'The number of cases in which recovery is to be obtained is very greatly extended by keeping the patients from walking during the first year, and in many cases during the second year',[644] and that his judgment remained valid.

Not all agreed with her, even former colleagues. In 1946 Macnamara censured Burnet for his attitude of 'apathy and hopelessness' when he wrote, 'Maybe we shall have to recognize the possibility of infantile paralysis as one of the normal perils of childhood — one, by the way, which is far less important in regard to loss of life and permanent crippling than the chance of a road accident'.[645]

Some Victorian physiotherapists did go to Perth and although they were 'horrified at first at the methods used', it didn't take long to convince them that active management on 'common sense lines' was better for the patient than the 'passive system' used in Victoria.[646] As a consequence, many of the polio survivors in Perth who would have been 'rigorously splinted in Melbourne' were given minimal supportive therapy, a decision 'that was proved correct'.[647]

Elizabeth Kenny returned to Australia in 1947 and was ignored by most medical and government officials with the exception of the loyal Charles Chuter, who delivered her report to Queensland Premier Edward Hanlon.[648] In a cable to Chuter, Kenny Institute doctors backed Kenny's report:

> Please advise your government and the Australian people that we wish to state the eminently satisfactory results obtained in treating approximately 2000 acute cases of poliomyelitis during the past seven years by staff of the Elizabeth Kenny Institute. The treatment regime ameliorated suffering, minimized deformity and tended to abolish the need for corrective surgery. The contribution of Miss Kenny saved the United States from a national disaster during the recent epidemic and she has been presented with the Gold Key Award by the American Congress of Physical Medicine for her outstanding contribution to the knowledge of poliomyelitis.[649]

The only organisation to welcome her home was the Country Women's Association, a reception strangely at odds for a woman who was accorded a police motorcycle escort in major cities in America. In Toowoomba, Kenny was 'disgusted and disappointed' when she saw the foundry busy making 'steel braces and jackets for the unfortunate children in hospital' and remarked 'how different things were for the children of Minneapolis'. She wrote, 'sometimes I think that the bitter tears and broken hearts of the mothers of Australia and the broken bodies of their children should haunt these people the rest of their lives'.[650] The silence that greeted her report to Hanlon was deafening, and polio survivors in Australia continued to be denied any freedom of choice in what treatment they would receive.

By the end of 1948 and back in Minnesota, Elizabeth Kenny had admitted to many of her supporters that she had grown 'weary of the unnecessary bickerings, untruthful reports and the futile attempts to give the necessary help and knowledge concerning this disease' and that she intended to retire: she had 'done her best'.[651] Charles Chuter's death from a heart attack that year had left her without her most influential supporter with the health bureaucracy in Queensland but the support of the CWA had given her some new allies.

Kenny knew that many doctors in the United States supported her but that the enormous power and political influence of the NFIP was against her. At no point in the history of the the Kenny Foundation and the NFIP had relations been cordial; they had remained competitive, hostile and uncooperative. Kenny was worn out, her health was beginning to break down and her legendary energy and drive were deserting her; the 'old war horse' wanted to go home to Queensland to live out her remaining years. Some time during 1949 she was diagnosed with Parkinson's Disease and that strengthened her resolve to return to Australia the following year. She returned to the United States for a brief visit in August 1951 against doctor's orders and a shadow of her former self physically, but still capable of firing a broadside at anyone who dared criticise her method of treatment. Kenny then returned to Australia and poured all her remaining energy into working on a new film and writing a new autobiography, *My Battle and Victory*, a title that aptly summed up her struggle to gain professional accreditation and recognition for her method for treating polio paralysis. In January 1952, a Gallup Poll asked American women which of several famous women they would most like to be and they ranked Elizabeth Kenny first, above Eleanor Roosevelt. Her native country Australia continued to ignore her.

On 30 November 1952, Elizabeth Kenny died at home in Toowoomba, Queensland. Hundreds of people lined the roadside as her funeral cortege moved slowly along the route from Toowoomba to the small cemetery at Nobby where she was laid to rest beside her mother. One cannot help but feel that Elizabeth Kenny would have been very pleased with her final journey. She was seventy-two years old, but insisted to the end that she was six years younger and, until a few years ago when it was rectified, her tombstone did not challenge that falsehood.

The last letter she wrote was to Minneapolis: 'I think I will have to pay another visit to the United States of America to straighten things out a bit, and get the book written for the World Health Organization which is so very necessary … I have improved and am taking my medication. Please remember me to all enquiring friends, with kindest personal regards.'[652]

Perhaps it is just as well that she did not live to see two of the directors of the Kenny Foundation charged[653] with conspiracy in 1965 to defraud the Foundation and its contributors. One can only imagine her reaction to that revelation.

Polio was not the localised disease it was once thought to be and by 1950 it was accepted that it involved not only nerves, but also muscle and skin.[654] By then most leading hospitals in the United States had incorporated most of the Kenny treatment into their programs, but other treatments still remained available. Polio patients in the United States of America, Canada, the United Kingdom, New Zealand and many European countries were given the option to choose what treatment they would have. That choice was largely denied to polio survivors in Australia.

The year Kenny died, Sir Earle Page, the Federal Minister for Health, rose to his feet in the Australian Parliament to announce that he had received 'certain requests from certain authorities for an investigation of Sister Kenny's methods, to bring Australia abreast of a treatment that had proved successful overseas', but that he could see no reason for a fresh investigation because her treatment 'had done very little compared with orthodox methods'.[655] Two other eminent men, one Australian and one American, gave antithetical appraisals of Sister Elizabeth Kenny. In 1951, she had met Burnet during a brief stay in Melbourne. He later wrote,

> I had a talk with her in 1951, under rather special circumstances. She had retired and was returning to Australia to end her days — she was suffering from Parkinson's disease and the fact that I was the best known virologist of her native land moved Kenny to call on me … it was the most interesting and concentrated opportunity I have ever had to sense the quality of another human being. On this occasion she had stipulated that the Press should not be present. She told me she had treated more cases than anyone else in the world — she gave the precise number, 7828 — and no one else was in a position to speak with her authority … She is now almost forgotten by the world. But there was an air of greatness about her and I shall never forget that meeting.[656]

In 1968, Dr John Paul maintained:

> Sister Kenny's ideas and techniques marked a turning point, even an about-face in the after-care of paralytic poliomyelitis. By determination and sheer willpower she helped to raise the treatment of paralyzed patients out of the slough into which it had sunk in the 1930s.[657]

Elizabeth Kenny shook the complacency of the medical establishment which firmly believed that muscles affected by the poliovirus remained frail and vulnerable for a lengthy period, and that gentle movement of limbs in the early stages of paralysis was dangerous. That dictum became more and more entrenched in the 1930s and '40s, with the result that polio survivors were encased in plaster casts for many months. With its introduction of early, active treatment the Kenny treatment discouraged attitudes of passivity in patients, and encouraged independence and acceptance of the disability. Keeping the affected limb or chest warm with hot packs undoubtedly helped to relieve pain, and gentle passive movements helped keep joints mobile and prevented deformities. Kenny encouraged her patients to remain autonomous, to retain agency over their bodies and to work with the Kenny therapist to bring about recovery. That relationship was far removed from accepted medical practice of the era where the active care-giver gave medical treatment to the passive care-receiver.

By the early 1950s many orthodox treatment programs in the United States and elsewhere had adopted significant, if not all, features of the Kenny method, even if they did not understand or accept her definition of the aetiology of the disease. In 1947, the Medical Director of the NFIP, Dr Hart Van Riper, set out on an extensive tour of the country to visit towns and cities where polio outbreaks had occurred. Van Riper reported that he 'did not see the "orthodox" or immobilisation technique used anywhere I went', but added that in many cases 'the treatment was not called the Kenny treatment' because it had been modified in small ways by the doctor who prescribed it.[658]

Although many prominent physiotherapists in the United States were opposed to Elizabeth Kenny's treatment,[659] she did gain some support. Not all were against her. In England, Pauline Osborne treated patients at Queen Mary's Hospital in Carshalton, the major centre for cases of crippling in London. She believed that 'Kenny's method was fantastic, and that children recovered in one tenth of the time'.[660] When Jim arrived at Carshalton he remembered that staff 'ripped off my plaster cast and threw it away … they told me that I wouldn't need it any more'. Simon actually 'looked forward' to treatment because the 'physios were more affectionate … they held you more whereas at the Western [Hospital, Fulham] they were very distant and unpleasant'.[661]

Sister Elizabeth Kenny's concept of treatment was not fully integrated with the orthodox but rather the two methods began to relate to each other in a different way, to wind around each other in a synergistic relationship instead of being locked in a battle for power, and it was the polio survivor who benefited from that cooperative interaction.

That was the story throughout the world, except for one country — her homeland, Australia.

Chapter 7

DANCING IN MY DREAMS: CONFRONTING THE SPECTRE OF POLIO

Then came the glorious era of physiotherapy, where there are all those beautiful — even at that age I realised it — buxom ladies with belts of different colours like karate belts which linked in complicated ways in the middle, and sort of pushing and pulling.[662]

Because I was bandaged in the splints and could not move except for my hands, I would imagine my inner self leaving my body and dancing above myself. I can still picture it. I have on a beautiful coloured shirt fringed with lace, and my limbs are lithe and free like those of a fairy being.[663]

Once you have spent two years trying to wriggle one toe, everything is in proportion.[664]

The convalescent stage of treatment of polio paralysis usually lasted around eighteen months and depended on the initial severity of the disease. For the polio survivor, the transition from acute care or isolation to a rehabilitation ward was a significant moment. Restrictions on hospital visiting hours were, to some extent relaxed, and parents and children, wives and husbands, and friends and relatives were allowed to visit the ward and see for themselves how the patient had progressed since being admitted. Often, no improvement was visible and the realisation dawned that recovery was to be a long, slow process. Some patients were shocked to discover that, despite the many medical advances made during the Second World War, there was still no medical treatment for polio:

> When I first came to Fairfield Hospital [in 1954] I rather imagined that people would give me injections of penicillin or something ... I was shocked to discover that it was just a matter of lying in bed drinking orange juice and waiting for the polio to cease attacking vital nerve centres, paralyzing limbs, muscles and organs.[665]

Many patients grieved at the loss of their former self and became depressed, a normal reaction to the personal trauma of having polio that mirrored the 'grief cycle' later described by Elisabeth Kübler-Ross.[666] Although her seminal work focused on death, the four stages of anger, bargaining, depression or sadness, and acceptance are recognised as a common response to profound despair. Also acknowledged is the fact that the stages described by Kübler-Ross are neither predictable nor linear; polio survivors would often bounce back and forward from one stage to another. Some never expressed their anger at becoming paralysed, quickly accepted what had happened to them and moved forward, while others never reached the point of acceptance.[667]

Long stays in hospital were a common experience for polio survivors worldwide, and life in the ward was made more bearable by the fellowship and sense of belonging that developed between patients as they dealt with what had happened to them — they consoled each other during painful therapy, shared treats brought in by family and friends, joined in conspiracies to play tricks on nursing staff, laughed and rejoiced at their achievements, and supported each other when they failed.

At the beginning of the rehabilitation process, emphasis was placed on the attainment of short-term goals like holding a cup, or a pencil, attending to personal needs or sitting up in bed. Small triumphs mattered: 'Being able to move the fingers of my right hand as well as my left, then being able to lift my left arm by myself. Then — a very big event, a moment of freedom — being able to turn over in bed by myself'.[668]

In Western Australia in 1954, twenty-two-year-old Vivienne Overheu recalled her initial lack of interest when her nurse announced: 'You are going to feed yourself today'. To her surprise, she found that the effort required was worthwhile: 'I had peach juice, bits of peach, bits of scrambled egg, toast crumbs and dribbles of tea all over me. But there was a strange satisfaction in having done something for myself, and the food definitely tasted better.'[669]

Tony Gould could clearly remember the day when he, 'stood up for the first time in months, holding onto the parallel bars for dear life, I was almost overcome with vertigo. Not long afterwards, when I took my first steps on my own, with a caliper on one leg and elbow crutches for support, I was as uncertain as a novice on stilts.'[670]

The ward community provided an important link to the world outside, and patients who had understandably been preoccupied with themselves and their illness, were given the opportunity to recapture a feeling of empathy for others and to regain social skills. Rehabilitation means acceptance of social as well as personal responsibility. Self-pity was frowned upon. Hugh Gallagher told of his experience at Warm Springs in Georgia where: 'The new patient, surrounded by many in the same situation and some in a worse situation, casts off his self-pity or soon has it forcibly torn from him by his neighbors, who will tolerate practically anything but pity or despair'.[671]

There was little privacy in the ward; patients were helped onto bedpans, given sponge baths or enemas behind a screen if they were lucky, or seated on bedside commodes in a hospital gown that flapped open at the back. Many older men found the complete dependence on nursing staff 'demeaning', especially when staff 'dressed them in a nappy' and 'treated them like children', using phrases like 'naughty boy' when an unfortunate accident occurred and bedclothes were soiled.[672] Patients in Fairfield Hospital in the late 1940s remembered the 'nightly sponge baths on freezing cold nights' and the joy they felt when they could progress to having a warm bath. When Clem was taken down to the hydraulic bath in Fairfield he was 'amazed how happy and jovial' the other patients were. Completely paralysed, his naked body was 'placed on a stainless steel table and lowered into the water to be washed by the nurses, no privacy any more'.[673] Some young girls going through puberty found it 'so embarrassing to have nurses attending to personal needs',[674] and older women also lamented the lack of personal privacy: 'we weren't allowed to have screens around the bed when using a bedpan, Sister said it was too much work for the nurses'.[675] The more mobile patients were encouraged to become less dependent on hospital staff, and were happy to help overworked nurses with routine tasks, and gained satisfaction from feeling they were becoming a little more independent. In Prince Henry Hospital in Sydney, Lynne Ellis remembered the 'absolute bliss' of her first hot bath in months, and of 'giving each other home perms from time to time, crossing over to another's bed on a bed table, or illicit wheelchair'.[676] 'Not all experiences of hospital were negative … there was a camaraderie on the ward and many of us developed life-long friendships … the older girls who could walk around helped change the babies and feed the little ones. It was like one big, happy family.'[677]

Although visiting hours were slightly more liberal in the convalescent wards, they were strict by today's standards and especially punitive for rural families in Australia who were obliged to travel hundreds of miles on weekends to spend an hour with a partner or child. Most parents agreed that being able to see their child at frequent intervals helped to allay their natural fears about their welfare, but the inflexibility of hospital bureaucracy generally made that impossible. Many families tried to visit regularly, but some eventually gave up because it was just too difficult, especially with other young children at home. Relatives and friends were often too afraid of catching the disease to volunteer to look after siblings while parents visited their sick child. In addition, weekends were generally the only time when farming families could snatch a few hours' respite from their gruelling daily schedule by recruiting school age children to help with farmyard chores. One interviewee recalled: 'My parents were farmers outside Launceston and they were not wealthy people. To begin with they used to come to see me every weekend, then once a fortnight. Very few people came to see me in hospital.'[678]

Some mothers travelled on a motorbike to the hospital, while another 'rode a bicycle the fifty-two miles from Railton to Launceston, every Sunday for three years'.[679] In Minnesota, Arvid Schwartz's parents made the 'seven-hour trip' to the Sister Kenny Institute 'every Sunday with the exception of one time when they got caught in a snowstorm'.[680] In many instances, small children did not recognise parents or siblings when they came to visit after an absence of several weeks.[681] A mother in Perth was allowed to see her fourteen-month-old son for two hours a week: 'He didn't know who we were when we went in to see him. By the time we were about to leave he was beginning to recognise us and then we would have to go, and he'd scream, and all the children would scream.'[682]

Children under seventeen were not allowed in the wards. Pamela Solomon remembered when her brother came 'with Mum and he had to stay outside the gate, all we could do was look at each other'. Not surprisingly, Geoff Golding thought Fairfield Hospital was 'like a prison'.[683] It was not until 1953 that visitors were allowed into the wards, because of the fear of spreading the various infections the isolation hospital housed within its walls. Before then, patients who were both ambulatory and well enough to leave the ward (criteria that excluded most polio survivors) were 'escorted by staff' to a 'covered Visiting Station':

A facility which boasted a wire-netting fence to ensure a separation between patient and visitor and thus contained the infection. The visitor, out in the open and some yards from the patient, was also behind wire netting — with a sort of no-man's land in between. The whole rather unsavoury and demeaning set up was, not surprisingly, known as 'the pens'.[684]

Some hospitals discouraged parents from visiting because it was 'disruptive'. Elaine Theodore's parents were not allowed to see her for six weeks in the Children's Hospital in Melbourne because nursing staff told them 'she would fret', so they climbed up a nearby wall and waved to her.[685] At Queenstown in Tasmania, 'parents stood at a fence and, across an expanse of grass, tried to glimpse children held up at hospital windows'.[686] However, if the Matron or Supervisor was sympathetic, change could occur:

> When I was a student nurse, a child came into hospital and did not see the parents again for two weeks. I thought that was perfectly horrible and as soon as I became a supervisor I began to make a change. In the Respirator Centre [Mount Sinai, New York] we allowed visitors in the morning, afternoon, or the evening, whichever was convenient for the relative.[687]

The pregnant Dulcie Black initially thought that the pain in her back and legs were labour pains but her doctor diagnosed polio and sent her to Fairfield Hospital where she gave birth to a son who rapidly developed symptoms of the disease:

> I didn't see my newborn baby for twelve months. Then he was moved to the convalescent home at Mt Eliza, and we used to travel from Warburton every six weeks because that was all we could afford. We didn't have a car and we had to get a taxi. I used to nurse him in his Thomas splint for about an hour and a half. He came home when he was three years old and it was only then that I realised that I had a son … I don't know how long it took him to realise that we were his mother and father.[688]

When they were first moved to the rehabilitation ward, many patients were still experiencing painful muscle spasms. Polio patients, unlike those who suffered a spinal cord injury, retained full sensory awareness — they might not yet have been able to control their muscles but they could *feel* the pain in their limbs. Despite the considerable pain experienced by many survivors, in other aspects the retention of sensation was a bonus, for it meant that patients also retained control over many important bodily functions. For many young men, the realisation that they could still 'perform' was a huge relief. Fourteen-year-old Michael Davis remembered mixed feelings of 'acute embarrassment and joy' when he 'suddenly developed an erection' during a sponge bath, but consoled himself with the thought, 'well, there's at least one muscle that still works'. Mercifully for Michael, the middle-aged nurse who was bathing him 'carried on as if nothing had happened'.[689] The retention of the ability to feel muscle movement in their limbs also meant that polio survivors could sense and learn to activate adjacent stronger muscles to take over the role of those weakened and damaged by the poliovirus.

Mending the body was not simply a matter of straightening limbs and rebuilding muscle tone. For most, it meant readjusting themselves to life in a body that was no longer familiar: one that had endured not only severe pain from the physical effects of the virus, but also significant emotional and psychological trauma, and physical change. Survivors had to cope with a loss similar to losing a loved one, and many were not given sufficient time to work through the grieving process. The physical effects of the virus were but one aspect of a larger dimension of disability, and ethnicity, class and gender all played a part in the individual response. But everyone connected with the polio survivor was affected by the experience:

> Polio belongs not just to those of us who were paralyzed by it but to our mothers and fathers, our sisters and brothers, our partners and our children; to those who cared for us, to those who brutalized us — not mutually exclusive categories; to those who saw us as palimpsests on which to write their discomfort, their fear, their pity, their admiration, their empathy.[690]

It sometimes took years for survivors to give up their dreams of complete recovery and a return to a pre-polio life, and to come to terms with their disability. For men, the weakening of their body by the poliovirus threatened innate values of masculinity: strength, virility, leadership and independence; while public opinion often viewed disabled women as being non-sexual beings, no longer suited for the conventional mid-twentieth century role of wife and mother.

In Australia, the iron lung was commonly referred to as the box and, for the lucky ones, their intense feelings of relief and joy at being free of the respirator were soon tempered, as the realisation that many weeks, months and possibly years of hard work and more physical pain lay before them before they could regain a sense of identity, and purpose about what the future held for them. Some survivors remained dependent on respiratory support; those who learned to 'frog breathe' by using their neck muscles to force air into their lungs became a little more independent than those who had to rely on the rocking bed, or on the cuirass respirator.[691] Some remained apprehensive about leaving the security of the iron lung. When Jim Marugg was allowed home for Christmas he 'felt like a glass man that might break, or come apart at a touch'.[692] Others were worried that they would 'get seasick' on the rocking bed, and Louis Sternburg was relieved to discover that it was straightforward, and offered him 'another way to breathe'. Furthermore, it meant that he was 'finally weaned from the womb of the iron monster'.[693]

Survivors had to come to terms with their feelings and conceptions of self-image, especially if they had previously shared widespread stereotypical and cultural views about the disabled body and its place in society. As Daniel Wilson has explained in his study: 'Most, if not all polio patients had very conflicted emotions about iron lungs, braces and wheelchairs. To assent to using them was a certain sign that one had left the world of the able-bodied and crossed over to the world of the crippled, the handicapped and the disabled.'[694]

Jim Vickers-Willis had 'often wondered' what it would be like to have paralysed limbs. In Melbourne in 1954, he found out: 'You look at your arm and you say to yourself: "I'm going to move that arm." You try your darndest to move it but it just will not budge.'[695] Some patients had ongoing breathing problems that prohibited the use of an anaesthetic, thus affecting other aspects of treatment. In Fairfield Hospital, eight-year-old Noel Spurr retained vivid memories of the hospital dentist: 'He worked on our teeth without pain killers or anaesthetic. Having my teeth out like this with my mouth propped open with steel frames and blood spilling out everywhere stays with me forever.'[696]

The myth of total recovery, perpetrated to a large extent by the American 'polio' president, Franklin Delano Roosevelt,[697] and based on an expectation that patience, hard work and adherence to exercise regimes would bring about improvement and a return to a normal body, was exposed as a cruel illusion. As the sociologist Irving Zola pointed out, Roosevelt was a wealthy, powerful figure with access to the type of support services of which the average polio survivor could but dream. In 1924, FDR had become attracted to the idea of hydrotherapy for paralysed limbs after hearing about several successful recoveries from friends and, after visiting Warm Springs in Georgia to bathe in the warm mineral waters at the rundown resort, he was convinced the treatment would help.[698] In 1926 he bought Warm Springs, much to the relief of the owner, who received twice what he had paid for it a few years previously, and made plans to turn it into a facility for polio treatment — albeit one for white sufferers, as it transpired, since no African American was admitted to Warm Springs during the segregation years in the South. FDR's illness sparked an enormous revival in public and scientific interest in polio research and treatment, and promoted the visibility and growth of the profession of physical therapy in the United States. Nevertheless, the abiding message that the Roosevelt myth imposed on other less fortunate survivors, be they black or white was, 'if Franklin Delano Roosevelt could overcome his handicap so could, and should, all the disabled. And if we fail, it is our problem, our personality defect, our weakness.'[699] As a consequence, many American survivors experienced feelings of guilt that they had been unable to live up to the example of their President and overcome polio as he had done. However, Roosevelt's message of conquering polio was ambivalent. By refusing to acknowledge publicly his disability,[700] FDR inadvertently supported society's view that the disabled should continue to live their lives on the fringes as passive recipients of charity, forever reliant on the goodwill of family and friends to survive — to all intents and purposes historically invisible.

The growth of physiotherapy[701] in Australia had initially been influenced by the experience of nursing Allied casualties during the First World War, and later by the return of disabled soldiers. The profession dominated the provision of care and treatment for those who survived exposure to the poliovirus, and rose to prominence during a period of great social change in this country: two world wars and the Great Depression formed the context within which polio epidemics waxed and waned in Australia.[702] By the mid-twentieth century, American physiotherapists had sent out a clear signal to the medical profession that, although they wished to maintain close ties with the medical profession, they expected to control their own training and curriculum, and to be accepted as professionals in their own right within the medical field, and not as subordinates.[703] Following the end of the Second World War, physiotherapists in Britain began to challenge the orthopaedic surgeon for control over the rehabilitation of patients.[704] In Australia, this came somewhat later. The physiotherapy profession did not become recognised as a fully separate and independent association within the practice of medicine until the 1970s. Before that, 'hospital physiotherapists … kept a low profile in wards to avoid upsetting the doctors or nurses'.[705]

Convalescent patients were given exercises to stretch their contracted muscles, and descriptions of that process varied from 'not too bad' to 'intensely painful'. If they were given hot-pack treatment before therapy commenced, it usually lessened the pain. A great deal depended on the skill of the therapist and the zeal with which they approached the challenge of getting a muscle to stretch just beyond the point where pain occurred. In Hampton Hospital in Victoria, four-year-old Joan Smith remembered 'Miss B, a thin, hard woman who would stretch me and weigh me down with sandbags', an experience she described as 'excruciatingly' painful.[706] In St George Hospital in Sydney, Gary Golding encountered something similar, but he was older than Joan and reluctantly accepted the pain as an inescapable part of the process of getting better:

> Every day a physiotherapist, Miss T, would come and undo each of my limbs from the iron frame and try to get them mobile. It used to pain like the dickens and I used to scream the place down and call her for everything, yet it was Miss T who got me walking. She sent me Christmas presents for the next ten years. When I finally left hospital, I had a caliper on each leg, a steel body brace and walked with the aid of crutches. A true man of steel.[707]

Many referred to the Physiotherapy Department as the 'torture chamber' or the 'screaming ward' and admitted to being 'scared of the physios'. One therapist threatened eight-year-old Ruthanne Werner, telling her she would 'put her in the pool and hold her head under water' if she didn't stop crying during stretching treatment.[708] Others were luckier: Beatrice remembered her therapist as 'wonderful. She would stretch my muscles like nobody's business. I'd get tears in my eyes, but I still looked forward to my time with her because she was just such a nice person … she'd had polio herself.'[709] Most polio survivors agreed that therapy hurt, and many children cried. In the Bronx in 1955, Edward O'Connor was treated in the 'torture chamber … They had this inclined plate and they would slowly move it up a couple of degrees and then you would sit there for half-an-hour and that would hurt. They slowly progressed it until you were sitting up.'[710]

Ian Dury was a musician in the 1980s and the lead singer of his band *The Blockheads*. He contracted polio as a young child and, along with many survivors of polio, he raged against the idea that he was a 'victim' of the disease. He loathed the patronising idea that pain was somehow ennobling, and that he or any other disabled person should be viewed as a 'good cause'. His 1981 song 'Spasticus Autisticus' was an angry musical rebuttal to those who sought to frame disability in those terms, and his descriptions of the physical reality of being disabled led to a nervous BBC banning the song:

> *I dribble when I nibble*
> *And I quibble when I squibble*
> *... I wibble when I piddle*
> *Cos my middle is a riddle.*

Ian's song was a feature of the 2012 Paralympics opening ceremony, an electrifying performance by the disabled performers who belted out the lyrics in a style akin to Dury's performance in 1981. Ian recalled his own physiotherapy in 'the screaming ward, and you could hear people screaming on the way there, and screaming on the way back ... This geezer used to get hold of my left ankle and my left thigh and, kkkkkkkrrrr, put my heel up to my arse ... and then it was you [screaming] when you was there'.[711]

Many associated the period of their hospital convalescence with treatment with hot packs. The reaction to these seems to have been mixed. Some thought they brought relief from pain, while others loathed having them applied. Charles Mee thought the treatment was a 'bizarre, disgusting procedure',[712] and Jim Porteous could 'still remember the smell of wet wool for years afterwards, and the itching'.

Our human sense of smell is directly connected to the brain and the association between memory and smell can trigger long-forgotten memories. Smelling wet wool transports Michael Davis back to the summer of 1944 and having polio:

> There were the other typical sickroom smells, but that of hot wool has been everlasting. While we were quarantined in isolation, the hot pack treatments continued day and night, with changes every hour. We learned to catch snatches of sleep between changes. After a while we were hardly even awakened by the process of unfastening diaper pins, rolling us around, removing cooled packs and replacing them with those fresh from the boiler.[713]

The packs were a comfort for a short period while they were warm, but once they cooled down Jim felt the experience was 'like having a wet nappy on'.[714] J. Downham of Delaware thought that the packs, 'from his shoulders to his knees, helped wonderfully' with the pain in his limbs.[715] In the early 1940s, the nursing staff in New York State:

had no equipment to use for this new method, so they rigged up two towels with sticks in the ends and they squeezed the packs between them. This proved to be unsatisfactory as it left too much water in the wool. So then they got a table with washtubs and an old-fashioned wringer in the middle and put the packs in boiling water in one tub and then squeezed them out in the other. After a brief cooling they were applied to my entire body and then wrapped in pieces of rubber to keep the heat in. The packs were on 24 hours a day for two weeks.[716]

Busy nursing staff sometimes applied the wool packs while they were still too hot, burning hapless patients. Patients and staff alike dreaded the treatment — patients because they were terrified of being burned, and staff because it was hard, unrewarding work, and the majority had no desire to inflict additional pain on survivors: 'It was very trying using those hot, steamy packs on a hot day, we had no airconditioning in the hospital and we had to run the packs through wringers and then wrap them up in a waterproof covering so that the bed wouldn't get too wet'.[717]

Most patients who were treated at the Kenny Institute in Minneapolis or at other centres in the United States were positive about their experience, and many letters can be read in archives[718] from grateful patients or parents. Mrs Danielson wrote: 'When my daughter Betty was stricken with polio in 1939, she was treated unsuccessfully at the University of Virginia and Warm Springs, before being transferred to the Institute in 1944, and she improved'.[719]

Another mother wrote saying that she was 'so glad the Kenny method was used on our boy ... it took away some of our terrible fear'.[720] Rose Fitterer worked as a nurse at Washington Park Hospital in Chicago during the 1949 polio epidemic, and treated 'many patients with the method, who blessed Kenny for her contribution to science'. Fitterer believed that 'many, many of our children and adults are walking today because of Kenny, an Australian nurse who gave of herself so unselfishly'.[721] Michael Davis believed that his 'life changed' when Kenny-trained therapist John Untereker appeared 'with a huge pair of shears' to help his mother treat him at home, cutting up the 'ingredients for a Kenny "sandwich" custom-fitted for me':

> John showed my mother how to build the layers of cotton sheet for my sensitive fair skin. Doubled blankets, rubber sheet, and outer cotton blanket for each of my body limb parts, and how to fasten them around me every hour with huge, diaper-sized safety pins.[722]

When Michael was admitted to Kosair Children's Hospital in Louisville, Kentucky, he continued with the treatment for four weeks before being discharged. Some time later, he returned for muscle re-education treatment under the care of Untereker. In contrast with the above, two second-hand accounts painted a different picture of undergoing the Kenny treatment. In her book, Anne Finger described a telephone interview she had with a man who claimed he was treated as a young boy at the Kenny Institute in Minneapolis, where 'male physical therapists — gorillas — forced his body to bend forward while he screamed with pain'.[723] Charles Mee, in his book, included a similar account from a patient in Nebraska, who claimed he saw: 'one of Sister Kenny's disciples stretch out the hamstrings of a fellow polio patient by pushing down on his foot as hard as she could until he screamed. She didn't stop until the foot was stretched straight out … tearing some tissues.'[724]

Both those experiences were at odds with everything that Kenny believed in, and taught to her students. In a letter to Sister Dryden in New Zealand in 1948 she wrote: 'Acute cases require very gentle handling, any stretching that is to be done must be done very mildly. The patient, on no account must be put in any pain, gentle stimulation is desirable'.[725]

Of course, Kenny had no direct control over individual therapists who claimed to be applying her method, and the same applied to therapists who used more orthodox treatment. There is little doubt that ill-treatment by certain therapists did exist, and although most patients reported that therapy was painful, there is a vast difference between the deliberate imposition of pain upon someone and the often unavoidable side effect produced by stretching a muscle that has contracted. Time and time again, Elizabeth Kenny emphasised that stretching was not to be carried beyond the point where pain was felt.

A few parents rebelled against hospital regimes and treatment and, despite the fact that many respected the expertise of medical staff, some were willing to try another approach. The father of a patient in Sale Hospital in Victoria said:

> We got fed up with the lack of treatment. At first her arms were tied to the back of the bed. Then Mr Lee the specialist came and put her in a Thomas splint. She wasn't treated for weeks so we met Matron Buller and Mr Lee and I told them I could give her better treatment. They told us 'If you take her out of our control the child will never walk again'.

> We took her home and massaged her legs every three hours and within three months she was walking.[726]

Others who had earlier agreed to have their child treated by the Kenny method were sometimes shocked to find that hospitals might now refuse treatment. One family was told by the family doctor, 'what would she [Kenny] know about it, she was only a bloody woman'.[727] Shirley Barnett's parents refused to give permission for her to be placed in a Thomas splint. When they asked hospital staff if an alternative to splinting existed, they were told: 'Sister Kenny has a small hospital in Hampton' but that her treatment 'was not acceptable'. Nevertheless, and despite being told by the orthopaedic specialist that their daughter 'would never walk again if they removed her from Fairfield Hospital', they decided to place her under the care of Kenny.[728] Some parents were so overawed by the prestige of medical practitioners that they dared not question treatment, fearing that their child would be in some way disadvantaged if they were viewed as 'uncooperative' by hospital staff.[729] Most of those fears were not justified, but there were some exceptions. Simon Parritt claimed that he was 'punished for wetting the bed' by strapping him down so that he could not move:

> The nursing care was just appalling. I was largely incontinent unless I had someone there to give me a bedpan or a bottle the moment I needed it, because I couldn't move at all. Looking back now, I can hardly believe that young kids, some of whom couldn't have been more than a year old, were smacked for wetting themselves.

When Simon's parents complained to the staff nurse at Queen Mary's Hospital in Carshalton about the standard of nursing care, 'he suffered for it in all sorts of niggling ways: the hot packs were put on a little bit too hot; he was handled more roughly than usual; and if he asked for a bottle, he was told to wait for his turn.'[730]

Dissatisfaction with the physiotherapy treatment provided in hospital was not confined to Australia. In England, Jim Porteous' parents were not happy with his progress and requested his transferral to Queen Mary's Hospital where the Kenny treatment was used. Their consultant warned them that Kenny's treatment was 'fanciful', and declared that the 'best bet for their son was to remain in a plaster cast'. But his parents contacted an orthopaedic surgeon at Carshalton, who advised them to tell their consultant 'to take a running jump and bring your son down here'.[731] In 1955, Dr Richard Metcalfe, a consultant orthopaedic surgeon at Queen Mary's remarked:

> We have been laughed at here for sticking to her [Kenny's] principles, but we get amazing results even after others say nothing can be done. Maud Forrester Brown [an orthopaedic surgeon at Bath] has stated that people who don't use splints in the early stages of polio are nothing more than quacks or charlatans despite the fact that it was universally accepted at the 1951 Copenhagen Conference [on Poliomyelitis] that immobilised patients developed tightness or contractures.[732]

George Durr was eighteen months old in 1931 when he contracted polio in New York State. After four years in hospital in Westchester, his father told doctors he was taking him home, 'because they weren't doing anything for me':

> I remember leaving the hospital and I could not walk. I was completely paralysed from the neck down. They had to strap me into the car. This was my first experience in being outside — seeing trees and corn. The ride home was very exciting. It was just amazing to see houses and roads and cars. It was just unbelievable to a five-year-old kid who had been literally strapped and locked into a bed his entire life.[733]

By the early 1950s most overseas experts had conceded that, to be truly effective, stretching had to be started in the early stages of rehabilitation, and strict immobilisation of the body had been abandoned. Across the Tasman, some hospitals in New Zealand had been using the Kenny treatment since 1943 when the Health Department had decided that there was 'something in it'.[734] In 1945, the Duncan Hospital at Wanganui was under the supervision of a physical therapist who had been trained at the Kenny Institute in Minneapolis, and Kenny herself visited in December 1947. The attitude of the Health Department in New Zealand stands in stark contrast to its Australian counterparts. It negotiated with the Kenny Institute in Minneapolis for the exchange and training of several physical therapists during the 1940s, and arranged for a surgeon, Dr Walter Robertson, to visit there in 1947 'to study Kenny treatment and other orthopaedic matters to see what could be usefully applied in New Zealand'. On his return, Robertson said that he knew 'of no better treatment' than the Kenny method, and that 'it was a good and rational method in both acute and convalescent stages, with much to be gained and little to lose, and he recommended that training be given to nurses and masseuses, to be held in readiness for epidemics'.[735]

However, the Department of Health in New Zealand did not choose to implement all of Robertson's recommendations — probably because staff numbers were inadequate. One of the major criticisms that health authorities had of the Kenny method was that it was highly labour intensive, and there were simply too few physiotherapists to call upon. However, by the 1950s, the Kenny treatment was widely available throughout New Zealand and, in another breakthrough in rehabilitation treatment, the care of polio patients had been transferred from the orthopaedic surgeon to the physiotherapist.[736]

A paradigm shift in the treatment of the paralysed body had occurred, not only in New Zealand, but globally. In the 1940s, what the profession of orthopaedics had most feared from the Kenny treatment was losing control over the rehabilitation process. By the 1950s, that jurisdiction had largely been lost, as authority for the care of the paralysed body shifted from the medical profession to para-health professionals.

While polio survivors in New Zealand and elsewhere had a choice of treatment in the late 1940s, that was not the case throughout most of eastern Australia.[737] It appears that the more things changed globally on the treatment of polio paralysis, the more they stayed substantially the same in Australia. Barbara Watson was fourteen in 1951 when she was taken by ambulance to Fairfield Hospital. Once admitted, she was put into plaster casts from her feet to her knees, with her upper body strapped into a metal and leather double Thomas splint twenty-four hours a day. The lower part of her right arm was left free 'to eat or read'.[738] In 1954, eight-year-old Gailene Stock 'was strapped from head to toe into a full-length body frame for twenty-six months'. The young girl, whose sisters 'grew accustomed' to seeing their sibling 'in a cage', was unable to 'sit up to eat, drink, or use the toilet'.[739]

In the early 1950s, Fairfield Hospital was desperately in need of more physiotherapists. Some patients recalled that they 'had no treatment for weeks' or, at the most, once every three or four weeks during their daily bath in warm saline. Les Corneille had, 'no treatment for three or four weeks and I stiffened up quite badly during that period. By the time the physiotherapist got to me just doing passive exercise was quite painful.'[740]

Una White suffered from 'bad bed sores from the coconut fibre mattress ... I didn't get moved or turned over because the nursing staff were so flat out'.[741] The situation had improved by the end of the decade. Patients in Fairfield went to the physiotherapy ward 'each day' where they were 'strapped into our double Thomas splints' and had 'strength tests every week on every muscle' that were then scored on individual 'muscle charts ... there was also the salt water bath where four or more of us kids were strapped in together by our shoulders'.[742] Children learned not to expect sympathy:

It was so hard on me emotionally. We weren't allowed to complain or be upset, it just wasn't allowed. If I ever showed I was lonely or frightened, the nurses either ignored me or I got into trouble. It was so hard, so I just learned to never show how I was feeling ... As I got better, they started physio on my limbs and I started to learn how to get about a bit in the leg irons. That seemed so heartless too. No-one ever helped, or picked me up when I fell over. It was all up to me, if I wanted to get better, then I had to do it. I guess that's where I got to be so determined.[743]

After-care therapy for polio survivors in the 1930s and 1940s was based on an economic model aimed at producing employable members of the workforce, and on social integration through a vocation-oriented rehabilitation system. The conviction existed that the disabled had to be 'normalised' by becoming productive members of society, in contrast to an institution-based life of dependence on charity. Some of the training began in the wards. Any occasion that interrupted the long tedious hours was welcomed: even the dreaded physiotherapy was a respite from the boredom of staring at walls and ceilings.

In England, the earliest organised social interest in care for the disabled had commenced in the eighteenth century and coincided with the emergence of orthopaedic medicine. The aim of reformers was to offer shelter to the disabled by confining them to institutions, thus achieving the equally important goal of removing them from the streets, and far from the gaze of the more fortunate members of the population. In line with broader concerns about social reform and a growing awareness and understanding of how 'normal' children developed, the British Government had assumed responsibility for the training and education of crippled children in 1899. The topic of segregation of the disabled in special schools versus integration with the able-bodied in ordinary schools was widely discussed in Britain and, in 1918, education for the disabled became compulsory.[744] Education programs were dominated by the overriding economic conviction that educating the disabled was a 'cost-effective prophylaxis against a lifetime of dependence on public welfare'.[745] That attitude was still evident in Australia in the 1930s. By 1930, twenty schools in London catered for crippled children, with free transport provided by the London City Council. Before the First World War, treatment and care for the crippled child in the United States of America and Britain was far in advance of that available in Australia. In America, hospitals, convalescent homes and asylums were available for residential care, and outpatient clinics or orthopaedic dispensaries provided after-care for children discharged from hospital.[746] The earliest attempt to provide education for crippled children in the United States was prompted by charity workers,[747] but as the twentieth century dawned there was a gradual transition from private to public responsibility as the conviction grew that the state should provide educational opportunities for the crippled child. Massachusetts was the first state to introduce public education in 1906, and by 1915 special classes for crippled children were provided in New York.[748] In 1931, a committee set up by President Roosevelt estimated that there were 300,000 crippled children in the United States, with at least one-third needing education.[749] Following a joint research project in 1951 with the New Zealand Crippled Children's Society, that country's Education Department concluded:

> A visit to orthopaedic wards would convince most people that it is possible for children to live a reasonably happy life in such surroundings. In the best equipped wards children had lessons from a hospital teacher, and were given books, handiwork, outings, and entertainment. Older children had correspondence lessons, listened to talks over the radio, and had pen friends.[750]

Although a census of crippled children had been carried out in New York in 1915, no attempt had ever been made to find out just how many crippled children there were in Australia. The sight of badly crippled children on the streets in cities and country towns in the twenties evoked pity in the population, but little constructive effort. Long periods in hospital gave children and adolescents little hope for the future, apart from the possibility of an invalid pension once they reached the age of sixteen.

For the Australian parent of a crippled child before 1920, there were no after-care homes or special schools for children apart from Yooralla Hospital School in Victoria which had been established in 1917 by Sister Faith, who was motivated to do something about the plight of the disabled after she had found a 'crippled child spending her days penned under a chicken coop while her parents were at work'.[751] In Australia, a philanthropic ethos did not exist to the same extent as in the United States and Britain, but it must be recognised that in the early part of the twentieth century there was no large wealthy class, nor was there a centralised system of direct, uniform taxation to fund national welfare programs until after the Second World War. New Zealand was in a similar situation, and parents of crippled children had to rely on charity from churches and other organisations.[752] The care of the crippled child was regarded as 'the responsibility of parents and guardians' and, as was the case in Australia, the crippled child was often hidden from sight. A sense of family shame abounded: 'In the twenties, there existed a deep sense of stigma about having an "odd" child, and ignorance about where to turn for help for the handicapped made an already complex problem into a seemingly insoluble one'.[753]

The question of how to set up a system to care for crippled children was exacerbated by the fact that nobody knew how large the problem was. When a child was discharged from hospital, further help was given only if parents sought it, and many did not know where to turn to find that help. No education department, medical practitioner, or hospital had any idea of the number of crippled children in Australia. During the period from 1850 to 1900, the Melbourne Ladies Benevolent Society had carried out some important surveys of 'physically impaired children and adults' as part of the duties of its 'lady visitors' to working-class homes in central Melbourne and four adjoining suburbs, and those figures had revealed that approximately thirteen per cent of the disabled were children, with the highest number having a 'crippling condition'.[754] So authorities would have suspected that those findings would be replicated elsewhere in Melbourne.

The first concentrated campaign to identify the number of crippled children began in Sydney at the end of 1928, following a proposal by the President of Rotary International in California that Rotary Clubs throughout the world should survey the needs of crippled children within their community.[755] Sydney Rotarians took up the challenge with enthusiasm. They issued a brochure announcing that the main activity for Rotary for the following year would be initially to identify just how many crippled children there were in the city of Sydney, and then to work towards the goal of providing them with educational and vocational training.[756] Well before the survey was completed, word filtered through the community of its aims, and more and more parents brought their children forward for assessment.

During the survey,[757] Rotarians came up against a problem they had not envisaged, and that was the humiliation of many parents at having a crippled, or 'odd' child, as many were described. They found that many children were concealed from inquirers, especially if the child also had an intellectual disability. Callers found hundreds of crippled children living out a lonely and hopeless life in the back rooms of houses, children for whom no rehabilitation treatment was then available. Their lives were not documented in the public record, they lived in the shadows, dependent on the goodwill of parents and kin to avoid being sent to an institution. When the Rotarians called, the door was often slammed in the caller's face, but many persisted and insisted on seeing the crippled child that anecdotal evidence indicated was hidden within.[758] As a general rule, it appeared that most parents relented, and allowed entry to the house: 'Whenever a visit was made to Joyce's home she was just sitting doing nothing. She was 12 years old and could neither read nor write. Her family had not made any plans for her and her future seemed to be one of mere existence. Both her legs were crippled and she could only shuffle.'[759]

Apart from the problem of a parental sense of shame, there were other examples where a child was exhibited on major thoroughfares in the city to elicit sympathy from passers-by.[760] However, it must be acknowledged that most working-class city families in early twentieth-century Australia had to sell their labour in order to survive, and the disabled beggar on the street corner was a common subject for journalists and writers.[761]

There were other cases in Sydney where, with the best of intentions, a child was excessively sheltered by parents who exercised complete control and refused any social contact. Some parents believed that the best and only security for their child was the invalid pension, available at £1 per week from the age of sixteen, while others did not want to forfeit it by allowing an eligible child to take up an offer of work. One of the major goals for all Societies for Crippled Children in Australia was to stress to parents the importance of education, instead of looking to the certainty of a pension.[762] Some health workers unjustly suggested that parents struggling to make ends meet had accepted the crippling of their child as 'inevitable'.[763] It was understandable that some parents complained that they 'could not afford to buy the boots, irons and braces that were recommended',[764] for times were tough and money scarce; a pair of orthopaedic shoes fitted with calipers cost four pounds in 1932.[765] In 1918, Sister Faith[766] visited the home of a crippled child and found the father, a returned soldier, 'absolutely incapacitated. The mother is dying upon her feet, one boy has both legs in irons, other children of four and two claim constant attention, and the hunger wolf is in the house … the mother's face reveals a world of such exquisite suffering and tragedy.'[767]

Little had changed by 1930 when Welfare Officer Margaret Watts reported: 'There was poverty in many homes, and many children needed nourishing food and warm clothing. After-care following hospitalisation was impossible for there was nowhere for the children to go.'[768]

The majority of the children had received little, if any, education. A local headmaster told her of a 'severely crippled child' who lived in an isolated farmhouse in a nearby valley, and when Watts and her companion had negotiated 'the perilous, winding track in her small car' she discovered:

> A woman and a crippled boy, a polio case, who came hobbling towards them. The visitors were made welcome and invited into the earth-floor dining room where the husband was. The mother had 'dropped her bundle' because she felt that life was quite hopeless, but the visit by the two women gave her new heart and she agreed to bring her son to the Society's next orthopaedic clinic in Wollongong. Two months later the son entered Margaret Reid Hospital for surgery and made a reasonable recovery.[769]

The tremendous effort by Rotary stirred an enthusiastic response from government and from the British Medical Association in Australia, but that was overshadowed by the reaction from the general public, who contributed over £15,000 in a few months to the appeal for the formation of the New South Wales Society for Crippled Children. This was a remarkable effort when viewed in the context of tightening fiscal policy following the October 1929 market crash in the United States and the global Depression that followed. The Society set up Women's Auxiliaries in all metropolitan areas of Sydney to visit the children and evaluate their needs.[770]

Victorian health authorities were increasingly concerned that a large-scale social problem was evolving because of the lack of after-care facilities. No formalised system existed to care for children once they had been discharged from Hampton, the convalescent hospital near the beach at Brighton, or from the newly constructed orthopaedic hospital at Frankston.[771] Outpatient clinics operated in some hospitals, like the Royal Alexandra Hospital for Children in Sydney and the Children's Hospital in Melbourne, but there was no organised service for transporting children to and from their homes to the hospital. Existing outpatient clinics overflowed with parents and children seeking massage treatment and realignment of splints. In 1890, Grace Jennings had described the scene at the end of the century as 'a string of characteristic-looking folks, hospital bent' making their way up the street to the Children's Hospital:

> Often the means of locomotion consist of nothing better than a deal box on wooden wheels or the cast-off tire of an old-fashioned perambulator. Children on crutches, in go-carts drawn by their brothers or sisters, or limping painfully along unaided; draggle-tailed mothers, in many coloured garments, dawdling by with infant chronics, and exchanging

confidences in high key as they make their way, in a leisurely fashion, to the great hospital at the corner ... Into one large room they all pour pell-mell while the forms fill up and the air becomes thick and charged with many odours, the while begins a perfect Bedlam of cries and ejaculations and explosive scoldings or entreaties. Poor little children![772]

Thirty years later, not much had changed. However, in the late 1920s, the efforts of hospital administrators to alleviate the problem of overcrowding in hospital outpatient clinics led to the development of several allied health professions, including physiotherapy, occupational therapy and social work. The Children's Hospital in Melbourne responded to the polio epidemics by implementing some major new developments aimed at looking after patients. The physiotherapy department was upgraded and moved to the new outpatients building, and Jean Macnamara was appointed to the position of Honorary Medical Officer (HMO) in Physiotherapy in 1928.[773] Some parents refused to bring their children to the clinic because they disputed the diagnosis of polio, while others just ignored letters from hospital staff asking them to attend.[774] It was not an easy task to bring a crippled child to the clinic. Mothers had to cope with travelling on the slow, inaccessible public transport system with children constrained in cumbersome braces and heavy boots. Some children were still confined in the Thomas splint. Elaine Theodore's mother recalled how she had to carry her twelve-year-old daughter, 'in her plaster from the train platform at Flinders Road Station up the ramp and right down to where we could get a taxi to the hospital. Nobody ever offered to help me.'[775]

Mothers often spent many hours waiting in the various departments of hospitals, where an almost 'endless line of children, suffering from many and various forms of gross crippling, including muscle weakness and paralysis following poliomyelitis',[776] waited for consultation, x-rays, blood tests, physical therapy, and the fitting and removal of splints and calipers. It is not surprising, therefore, that many mothers failed to bring their children back for treatment after the first three or four weeks; it was just too difficult. In her notebook, Jean Macnamara described some of the problems she experienced with getting children to attend the outpatient clinic:

> John A of South Melbourne had 'attended for a while but not since his splint was fitted' while another 'was not attending the clinic because the diagnosis of polio was disputed by the parents'. Joseph B of Brunswick was walking about 'with severe paralysis' because he was 'allowed to

walk too early'. Ruth B's mother was 'very deaf' and refused to bring her child in to the hospital despite her 'badly wasted calf muscle'.[777]

Macnamara appreciated the fact that having exhausted mothers and children waiting hours for treatment was detrimental and, in 1931, she lobbied successfully for the introduction of an itinerant physiotherapy service based at the Children's Hospital.[778] The new service would have a twofold approach. Children could be treated in their homes and their mothers taught by therapists to carry out simple daily treatment. Massage therapists also visited country areas once a week and held clinics in 'a local hospital, medical clinic, or even in the lobby of a hotel'.[779] Slowly, in Victoria at least, the situation for after-care treatment of polio began to improve.[780]

In 1930, the Committee of the Melbourne Children's Hospital decided to build Australia's first orthopaedic hospital for children at Frankston to cater for long-stay hospital patients up to the age of sixteen who were still in splints or plaster casts.[781] In Western Australia in 1936, there were three hospitals offering treatment, but no convalescent homes. South Australia treated patients at the Adelaide Children's and the Royal Adelaide Hospital, and Tasmanians received treatment at Vaucluse Hospital in Hobart and the Launceston General Hospital. Wingfield House in Hobart was erected by the Tasmanian Society for the Care of Crippled Children in the late 1930s to supplement the services offered by St Giles Home for Crippled Children.[782] In Queensland, George Marchant of Montrose donated his home and five acres of land in 1932 to the Queensland Society for Crippled Children.[783] A public appeal raised £5000 in two months and the Government made a grant of £500 to assist in the first year of operations. Rotary carried out a survey in Brisbane and 200 children were discovered to be in need of help.[784]

Some important work on determining the number of crippled children in country areas was carried out in New South Wales in 1926 by the Far West Children's Health Scheme, a non-sectarian organisation founded in 1924 by the Reverend S.G. Drummond for the purpose of giving indigent country children orthopaedic treatment, and a holiday at the beachside suburb of Manly. In travels covering thousands of miles, from the border with South Australia to as far north as Tamworth, Reverend Drummond and his wife discovered hundreds of crippled children. Most had never been seen by a doctor or received any kind of treatment for their condition, whether the cause was congenital, or resulted from an accident, or from disease. Various reasons, based on fear and ignorance, were given by parents for not consulting a doctor about their children. Friends had told them that the child 'would grow out of it', or that they had known 'children who had died under treatment', or that the medical cost would be exorbitant.[785] Some parents said they had been trying to save money for the trip to Sydney to see a specialist. In Broken Hill, eighty-six children were identified and sent to Sydney for specialist treatment and, following their own return to Sydney, the Drummonds organised a team of orthopaedic surgeons to travel out west. In forty-five days the group travelled over 7000 miles and identified over 600 children in need of treatment in New South Wales alone. Some of the children needed immediate treatment and, in the vast majority of cases, the condition was chronic. Many parents mistakenly believed that nothing could be done. Clearly, many more children would be scattered throughout Australia.[786] By 1932, the needs of the country child in New South Wales had come within the jurisdiction of the Society for Crippled Children.

As was the case in urban Australia, a disabled child was often a source of further hardship for rural families. A child unable to work on farmyard chores was a drain on meagre household budgets. If the need for after-care for crippled children was serious in urban areas, it was critical in country Australia where vast distances between settlements and towns made it harder to locate children and bring them in for assessment and treatment.

In Victoria, the *Education Act of 1872* had made schooling compulsory for all children, but it did not make any provision for those who were unable to attend school because of 'sickness, fear of infection, temporary or permanent infirmity or any unavoidable cause'.[787] Because many children were kept immobilised in bed in hospital or at home for many months, many fell behind in their education. Where Australia was concerned, the education of children in hospital appeared spasmodic, despite the best efforts of various state Societies for Crippled Children.[788] Some children had no schooling, books or games unless provided by parents, while others remembered a teacher coming in for reading lessons.[789] During the 1920s, efforts were made to introduce some form of vocational training for the disabled, but that training was usually in the form of needlework for women and young females, and basketwork for men and young males. Many of those occupational therapies would have reinforced a feeling of inadequacy and hopelessness in many of the disabled, for their training was so limited that the future would hold few prospects for them outside the charitable sheltered workshop.[790]

In New South Wales, the first school for disabled children was opened in 1930 at the Royal Alexandra Hospital for Children, and the Society for Crippled Children arranged a transport system to take children from home to the school, and to public hospitals for orthopaedic treatment.[791] Before then, children from the Royal Alexandra Hospital were taken to 'Canonbury' in Darling Point for rehabilitation. 'Canonbury' was run by the Australian Jockey Club; it provided free accommodation for the children, and a large, warm saltwater pool was constructed for hydrotherapy. For six-year-old Pat, the best thing about life at 'Canonbury' was:

> the one-teacher school run by the Department of Education in a cottage in the grounds. At first, I was wheeled into the classroom in my bed. The standard of teaching must have been reasonable because, although I had only been at school for three weeks before catching polio, when I returned home after two and a half years I came third in class and thereafter topped my year.[792]

By 1933 children occupying the eighty-eight beds at Frankston Hospital were receiving schooling and occupational therapy. Tasmania, Victoria and Queensland all formed Societies for Crippled Children between 1932 and 1935 and carried out surveys of crippled children in their state. All found children in great need of help either for treatment, care or access to education. In Tasmania, thirty per cent of crippled children were not attending school in 1932.[793]

In 1938, the Society for the Care of Crippled Children in Tasmania forged a close relationship with the Education Department to improve education standards of children in hospitals and convalescent homes throughout the state. As well as receiving tutelage in the basic skills, children were encouraged to save the money they received from the sale of their handiwork[794] — 'woollen mats, kettle holders, tapestry pictures, small toys, wood-fibre flowers, baskets and trays'. The Hobart Hospital almoner also noted that children undergoing long periods of treatment for polio paralysis 'presented a serious behavioural problem' for nursing staff if they were not kept occupied and amused. She also commented on the 'appalling lack of education among older cripples', some of whom had spent years in hospital with no tuition provided. A few older patients in Tasmania were given the opportunity to develop skills that were more in keeping with earning a future living: 'six patients were receiving instruction in commercial work, accountancy, typewriting and shorthand', and the Society managed to place two as apprentices in Hobart.[795] But it was often an uphill battle to change entrenched cultural views of the disabled, as the Hobart Hospital almoner reported in 1939. She thought that many people still believed that 'if one possessed a crippled body one must be in touch with the devil', and denounced those potential employers who 'refused to give young cripples a trial'. It was her opinion that Hobart businessmen should 'give thanks' that their children and grandchildren had been spared 'the scourge' of infantile paralysis, and should each undertake to employ one disabled person during the coming years.[796] Still, the majority of the disabled appeared destined to spend their time doing handicrafts. Gary Buchanan was taught how to

> weave cane baskets and trays, then later how to make leather wallets then how to knit a scarf. I remember when I started basket weaving and was getting positive comments from the visitors who came to my ward that I had a flash of marketing initiative and set myself up in business as a supplier of all my hand made goods. The baskets I charged five shillings for, the trays seven and sixpence and the wallets were nine and nine pence. When I was finally discharged I had amassed a fortune of just over twenty pounds, almost enough to buy a block of land with![797]

By the mid-1940s, the Education Department had provided greater access to the basic skills of reading, writing and arithmetic for children in Tasmania's hospitals.[798] In Victoria, the Education Department provided a teaching service for children in hospital, correspondence lessons for children at home and teaching staff at Yooralla, and the Victorian Society for Crippled Children and Adults arranged for the education and training of disabled children and adults on its register. In Western Australia, education and training for polio survivors in hospital was provided at the Princess Margaret and the Royal Perth hospitals.[799] Attitudinal change towards the disabled came about as more and more people became aware that the crippled child or adult was more than just a problem and responsibility for hospitals; that families and the community needed to become involved as well. Future prospects for the disabled would improve only if hospitals, families and the community worked together to formulate and operate a comprehensive scheme to help them achieve their full potential.

Despite that viewpoint, some family members and friends were convinced the polio survivor would never live a 'full' life, and exhorted them to lower their expectations about the future. Viewed as being incapable of real community participation or of usefully directing their own lives, polio survivors were often regarded as the antithesis of all that was healthy and normal in society. When a friend of Roosevelt's mother visited the family home after FDR fell ill, she observed: 'Now he is a cripple … will he ever be anything else? His mother is wonderfully plucky and courageous, but it's a bitter blow.'[800]

Rick remembered that his parents 'were embarrassed about me ... they didn't want to talk about my polio. It was ignored. They said quite a few times that they wished I died ... they put me in a closet when they had company.' Rick wonders whether it would have been a 'better thing ... if I had [died]'.[801] At home in Western Australia, a young polio survivor 'had to do [my] exercises in the hallway of the house while everyone else was having dinner, due to the shame they felt'.[802] The effect on relationships and on the ebb and flow of family life was often far-reaching. Sometimes the trauma experienced by young children at the forced separation from family lasted well into adulthood, and the relationship between parent and child never fully recovered. Often it was the parent who now felt rejected:

> I'd hear the car coming up the drive and I'd go to the door, like I'd greet anybody — more so a family member — and I'd go to kiss him. He'd turn his face right away ... stabbing me in the back ... those were things I found very hard to handle. I couldn't understand why he would do that to me [his mother].[803]

When her son was discharged from hospital in Western Australia, doctors told another mother that it 'was up to her if he ever walked again'. Every day she had to give her son 'five hours of exercises, and I had to go back to Princess Margaret [Hospital] three times a week to see the physios there ... we didn't see friends, we didn't go out ... our complete life changed.'[804]

According to Barbara Watson, her mother 'never coped with the fact I had polio — she was embarrassed'. The fourteen-year-old Victorian remembered going home for the weekend in a long pram with the double Thomas splint:

> My father took me out in the pram, my mother wouldn't come. She tried to get me into a nursing home as she didn't want to look after me at home, but I was too young. She always referred to me as 'my other daughter' but only when she had to refer to me at all. I lost my name when I got polio. She would always walk several paces ahead of me if we were out and tell me to hurry up. When I turned sixteen, my mother wanted me to look for a job, saying that I could not expect them to keep me.[805]

Disabled young women were often stigmatised as being unsuitable for a future role as wife and mother. When Valda Heath was growing up her mother told her: 'Always stand with your back to the wall, it's crooked and no one will ever want to marry you'. And, when she turned twenty-one, her parents gave her 'a sapphire ring and told me "no man will ever want you … you've got a crooked body."'[806] Some tried to hide their condition by carrying on as though they had never had polio.

> The tears I shed trying to get the washing done, trying to cook the meals, trying to do those things for the children and act as a 'normal person' … because it didn't show. They didn't see the brace on your back and I always wore slacks so that I hid the caliper and then people expect you to do everything that a normal person does.[807]

June Middleton had been preparing for her wedding to another young Victorian when she suddenly found herself with polio and confined to an iron lung. After five years in Fairfield Hospital, she told her fiancé to, 'go out and find someone else who had some future … it was a good thing that it happened six months before the wedding and not six months after. His parents stuck by me … lovely people but dead now.'[808]

June Middleton remained in her iron lung at the Yooralla Ventilator Support Service in Melbourne until she died on 30 October 2009. She holds the Guinness World Record for the person who survived for the longest time in a respirator. June believed that 'she has lived a happy and positive life', and that 'it doesn't pay to be miserable'. She had no movement in her limbs apart from her little finger, but could 'type a reasonable letter in two hours … it gives you some independence'. An only child, she remembered her father coming to visit her in Fairfield Hospital, 'three times a week by public transport until he was well into his 90s'.[809]

In the United States, a young wife wrote about how her marriage had been adversely affected by her disability:

> I had been married a little over seven months when I was stricken in 1939 … not a very promising future for my husband, and in the past few months he has sort of given up on me. I can walk by myself on the level but it takes very little to throw me off balance and down I go. I have to wear a steel back brace which has two steel bars the length of my back and one across the hips and a long leg brace on my right leg.[810]

Society has placed great value on certain physical attributes such as sexual attractiveness and physical symmetry. Jean Johnson had been 'a pretty child', who had grown up accustomed to the 'admiration of her boy cousins'. Catching polio 'knocked out her high opinion of herself', and when she had left hospital and enrolled at Miami University, she discovered:

In this kind of culture, men like perfect women. They like their arms and legs to match. And that was quite a shock to me because I still thought of myself as quite a catch. Right away, you knew where you stood with men and it was just devastating. And nobody ever talked to me about it, nobody ever said, 'This is what you should expect now'.[811]

From the time they were admitted to isolation, most polio survivors dreamed about the day when they would hear the words, 'You can go home', and, although the majority would leave in braces, on crutches, or in wheelchairs, most were excited and happy at the thought of leaving the hospital. The decision to send survivors home was generally made when medical staff decided that no further recovery in muscle power could be expected. Brian Caulfield was discharged from Fairfield 'in a Thomas splint and was wheeled around by his family on a modified pram'. Louis Pruscino was seven when he came home from Sale Hospital in Victoria, 'with two calipers and two walking sticks as well as a brace for the spine … therapy was severe'. At night he was tucked into a splint, spread-eagled and unable to move, with his hands and feet tied. In Melbourne in 1951, Marguerite Swann was also discharged in a full Thomas splint, 'totally confined so that all I could move were my hands'. Her father 'placed her in the family car on a plank of wood that went from the back seat to the front'.[812] Another boy had to continue sleeping in his Thomas splint, but sometimes he could convince his brother 'to untie the straps for me' and he could escape.[813] When twenty-two-year-old Una White went home from Fairfield Hospital in 1950, she wore 'a brace with steel bars with calipers on my legs and on crutches. I couldn't do anything. If I let go of the crutches I'd fall. It was better when I got the wheelchair, and I'd carry the kids and the shopping on the chair back to the house.'[814]

Adults were often understandably apprehensive about returning to a world they had known as a physically different person. Society in the mid-twentieth century expected the disabled to adjust to their altered physical state, and made few concessions.

> I was constantly tired [after going home] and I was never allowed to say that I was tired. We lived at the top of a hill and we would walk down to the shops with my mother. I remember being so tired that I just didn't know how I was going to get back [home]. I used to say to my mother, 'I'm tired, I'm tired' and she used to say, 'You can't say that'. That fatigue is for me, the thread that runs through all my life and it has been a really debilitating force for me. The lack of treatment, the lack of being

able to rest, and to recover, and to recuperate and to be treated with a sort of respect, in a way that a serious illness demanded.[815]

Buildings and public transport were largely inaccessible. Some children were very anxious about leaving the confines of the hospital walls. Many had never known another life, and looked upon ward staff as their family. Five-year-old George Durr 'met his brothers and sisters for the first time' when he went home, and Cindy Bernstein admitted that she 'should have been happy but I was terrified about going home because the hospital and the other children there were my family. I had forgotten who my real family were.'[816] Some children thought they never had a normal childhood because they spent so much time in hospital: 'Then I went home. Boy, was that weird. I had hardly seen my family for years and suddenly I was supposed to be part of them again. I really didn't know how to handle it, and I don't think they did either.'[817]

Other children felt that they settled back fairly easily into family life, learning to play again with siblings and neighbourhood children, although not able 'to do everything they did'. One boy 'managed to ride my bike again, but I kept falling off, and climbing in the backyard was really hard'.[818] Reflecting on his post-polio life, a Western Australian interviewed by John Smith observed: 'I never had the chance to play team games, and I think I missed out on a lot in learning the ethos of a team. That's my biggest loss. I never learned to share victory and defeat in team sports that other boys of my age would have had. I think that was the biggest loss.'[819]

The financial burden on families did not end with the return of the survivor. Homes had to be altered, physical barriers erected or removed, and arrangements made for after-care therapy. Hazel Atkinson went home in 1952 to Narrandera, NSW, and her three children under five years, 'strapped to an aeroplane splint for fifteen months ... it was somewhat like a horse's harness'. The family had no 'home care or financial help' and the young mother had 'two paralysed hands, as well as her left arm'. They employed a girl to help around the house but dismissed her after coming home to find their baby 'covered in bruises from ill-treatment'.[820] If at all possible, the extended family helped out with care of the disabled child. Marguerite Swann's grandmother would take her for walks around Melbourne,

> on a long flat pram bandaged in the Thomas [splint]. She wheeled me along streets where houses were being built, and we used to pause by an old hedge which was full of singing birds. Nan had the thoughtfulness to buy me a pair of sunglasses because she said I was looking at the

sky all the time. I remember them well, they had white plastic frames. Another time she took me across the road to a huge paddock. It was full of bright yellow daisies and she made daisy chains for my head and neck. The perfume was potent and life giving. I remember these as happy times.[821]

In Melbourne, the Children's Hospital accepted the responsibility of providing outpatient after-care for all children under the age of fourteen if they could pass a stringent means test. The medical profession was opposed to admitting anyone to a public hospital who could afford to pay private fees. Private physiotherapists treated those who could afford to pay for the treatment (10/6 per visit) three times a week for several months or years. For those who could not afford to pay a physiotherapist or who failed the means test, the Department of Health paid a panel of therapists to provide orthodox treatment for cases approved by the Consultative Council on Poliomyelitis. The Council was set up in Melbourne in 1945 to provide physiotherapists, accommodation, transport of patients and the necessary treatment for the after-care of polio patients in Victoria, and it subsequently provided after-care at five institutions.[822] Dr Jean Macnamara was convenor of the Splint Sub-Committee of the Council and the only treatment method sanctioned was the immobilisation treatment that she endorsed. In 1947 the Council announced that the 'prompt provision of splints' was an essential part of its treatment program, and believed it was an 'urgent' matter that the inventory of splints be increased because of the likelihood of another epidemic of polio in Victoria.[823]

A Craft Centre under the supervision of the Children's Hospital was organised at Frankston and 'every effort was made to find employment' for the older polio survivor. At Christmas, a group known as the 'Polio Aunts' organised gifts for paralysed children living at home. Not only dolls and books, but also practical donations like 'mattresses for long prams, pillows, blankets, hot water bags and swivel mirrors so that little patients lying on their backs could see what was going on around them'.[824] One suspects that the children would rather have been given a toy. In South Australia, one full-time physiotherapist was appointed by the Crippled Children's Association 'to organise and service all country clinics' and itinerant services for Adelaide were begun in 1951 by each of the hospitals.[825] The workload of those dedicated practitioners must have been arduous. In Victoria, Wards 9 and 10 at Fairfield Hospital were set aside for the after-care of longer-term patients but not for 'hopeless cripples', and the Red Cross declared it was willing to help with older polio cases who did not require heavy nursing. It had been intended that Victorian country children would be given care at hospitals with a physiotherapist on the staff,[826] but that rarely eventuated because the overworked therapist was so busy with treating other general patients that there was 'very little time' to attend to the needs of the polio cases. More physiotherapists were needed in country areas, but it had proved 'very difficult' to induce them to leave the city to work in country hospitals.[827] In 1949 there remained large areas in Victoria where no adequate after-care was available for the paralysed child, adolescent or adult.[828]

The power of orthodox medicine lies in its potential ability to return a person to full health, but that model often fails when confronted with chronic illness. Some parents recognised that fact and decided not to use the after-care provided by authorities but instead to seek out alternative healers to help their child. Some of the treatments used were bizarre. In Hobart, some children were taken to the Tattersalls Hotel where the 'Wrestlers, Fouché and Felice' 'threw you around like rag dolls'.[829] In Victoria, Val Heath's parents took her home after forty months in Fairfield Hospital and arranged for a so-called 'Kenny-trained nurse' to treat her,

> twice a week on the kitchen table where my naked body was slapped with the outside leaves of lettuce (for the iron content) and then she would rub my back, legs and arms with dugong oil, which was very hard to get in wartime Melbourne. I smelled like a fish. Then she would put me in a bath and hose me with cold water ... I hated that woman.[830]

Louis Pruscino went to an osteopath who worked on his spine, and told him to wear his leg caliper on alternate days because daily use would 'further weaken' his leg.[831] In Australia, the BMA took a very dim view of medical practitioners who took up the practice of homeopathy. It excluded them from membership until 1916, and forbade its members from consulting with alternative therapists.[832] When Louis' specialist discovered that he was seeing an osteopath, he threatened to have nothing to do with him if he continued with the alternative therapy.

Fortunately, the outcome of polio paralysis was resolved in many patients within six to eight months, but others underwent surgical intervention to repair damaged tendons, or a spinal fusion to correct a curved spine. Valda Heath's memories of that experience were chilling:

> Every year from the age of eleven till eighteen, I used to go to St Andrews Hospital [East Melbourne] and there I would be hung by the

chin from the roof with my hands on a nurse's shoulder till my feet were just off the ground ... that would get my back reasonably straight, and then they would slap Plaster of Paris around ... I was naked and I hated it ... then they would cut the plaster off and make a celluloid model with laces down the front ... every time I breathed the laces squeaked so I was conscious of it ... I had a very poor image of myself.[833]

When Valda was eighteen,[834] Dr Eric Price told her 'now that you have finished growing, we'll fix your back'. Valda woke from the anaesthetic to find she was 'in plaster down to my knees'. Soon after:

They cut a hole in the plaster at the back and put in a turn buckle ... it became a torture rack ... don't think I have ever gone through such pain ... every morning the doctor would turn the screw, and as he turned it I twisted and stretched ... the pain was shocking ... after four months I had stretched six inches and my spine was pretty good ... so then they operated and cut some bone from my left shin and put it down one side of my spine. I thought that was it, but then three weeks later they did the other side. I was happy in hospital though.[835]

Gareth White's leg was treated at the Children's Hospital in Melbourne in the mid 1950s. His mother told how surgeons, 'wanted to slow down the growth of his good leg, so they smashed the bones in it, so the other leg could catch up. He had a builtup boot all the years he was at school.'[836]

Stories of pain, both before and after surgery, were common, especially where contracted muscles had to be stretched before corrective surgery or where curvature of the spine was straightened before spinal fusion. The experience of survivors worldwide was consistent. In the United States:

Many surgeons used casting to straighten the spine prior to surgery. Some patients were 'hung' or 'lynched' ... a strap around your neck and head pulled you up as you stood so that your feet were barely touching the ground or some platform and then the cast was applied. This process could take some time before all the plaster had dried sufficiently to maintain the stretched spine.[837]

In 1957, Gary Buchanan was admitted to St George Hospital in Sydney to have his spine fused. Once he was settled into bed, Gary was then 'harnessed in a steel frame with weights on each end ... to stretch me. That session on the rack lasted three months before the doctor realised that I hadn't stopped growing, so sent me home.'

For the next two years, Gary had to wear a full plaster cast from his neck to his hips which he found was 'agony in summer', especially when the cast became 'soaked with perspiration and I couldn't scratch the unbearable itchiness'. His cast was changed every six months by suspending him 'from the ceiling by a support under my neck … once it was removed you couldn't get too close to it as it was really on the nose'.[838] Polio survivors overseas also remembered the body cast as an 'awful experience' and the 'terrible itching' and 'sores that developed' where the edge of the cast rubbed on bare skin. Many added that they did not feel any better after the surgery; sometimes they 'felt worse'.[839]

After negotiating the emotional upheaval associated with returning home, the next big hurdle for polio survivors was assimilation into wider society. For children, that meant either returning to the school they had previously attended, or enrolment in a special school for the physically disabled. Survivors had to become accustomed to the stares and comments of the general public: 'when you have a physical disability you become used to people looking at you with a mixture of sympathy and disgust'[840]. Other schoolchildren could be particularly cruel and insensitive. One girl recalled:

> School was torture, I was left by myself in the class-room at recess. Sometimes the teacher would ask some of the children to play with me at recess — but they would run off as soon as she was gone. Later, when I was in the schoolyard the other children would make fun of me if I tried to join in. They would imitate my 'funny walk' and would smack me and laugh if I tried to run after them. I could never use the toilets because some of the older children would gang around the entrance and say, 'You're too ugly to come in here'.[841]

A boy remembered: 'I used to get teased a lot at school because I had a caliper on my right leg … got called names like 'Football boots' or 'Limpy' or 'Hopalong Cassidy'.[842]

In contrast to the cruelty of some of their peers, older school children were sometimes protective. 'One day I got into a fist fight with a boy and someone rushed up and said, "Cut it out John, don't hit him, he's a polio sufferer"'.[843] Even getting to school was an ordeal — Pauline Corrigan recalled how her 'brother and sister had to push me in the long pram up the hill every morning'. Her desire to go to school in Traralgon, Victoria, with her brothers and sisters was so strong that several times she 'crawled across the highway in her calipers, but the police always got me at the Caltex service station' and took her home. She couldn't understand why the school would not allow her to attend: 'it was my legs that didn't work, not my brain'.[844] Some girls desperately wanted to look 'the same as everybody else' and hated 'being different, forced to wear warm socks and leggings to keep the polio bits warm'.[845]

Adults went back to their previous workplace if they were lucky, or tried to find new employment. Mothers went home to their families and many tried to act as if nothing had happened. Marguerite Swann recalled the joy she felt when, years after contracting polio, she 'gave birth in turn to five healthy little babies who grew freely and energetically towards adulthood. I found something miraculous and healing in bringing forth those perfect little bodies from my own imperfect one.'[846]

Many children and adults who had experienced grief and trauma when separated from family found themselves in a similar set of circumstances when they were released from hospital. Friendships forged over months and years were abruptly terminated, and many polio patients missed the warmth and companionship of the polio convalescent ward where everyone had faced the same difficulties and challenges. When they went home, some felt alienated from family and friends, when all they really wanted was to fit in, and to be accepted as they were — the same person inside as they had always been. It was just the outside bits that had been irrevocably altered by their confrontation with the poliovirus.

Chapter 8

A TALE OF BRAINS, GUTS, AND A VIRUS

> There are times when workers of great scientific repute continue to misconstrue the meaning of their data or will not admit inadequacies in the techniques employed by them ... when this happens progress in science may be materially impeded.[847]

The search for the truth about the aetiology and transmission of the poliovirus, and the quest for a possible vaccine, was not an easy or a smooth road to success. There were many paradoxes. Epidemics of polio increased as sanitation and public health methods of prevention of disease increased; the disease was known as infantile paralysis, yet by the early twentieth century morbidity and mortality rates in adolescents and adults were increasing; and, by no means least, the conviction that polio was a disease that affected only the nervous system diverted researchers from the truth that the poliovirus gained entry to the body primarily through the gastrointestinal system. The history of the research into the poliovirus is one characterised by a chronicle of errors, at both the clinical and scientific level — a tortuous journey punctuated by dead ends, scientific obfuscation, time-wasting and expensive deviations, and an inexplicable disregard of some very strong evidence that the mouth was the portal of entry for the virus into the body.[848]

From the discoveries of cell physiology, anatomy and pathology in the mid-nineteenth century grew the new science of bacteriology, and it transformed the relationship between the physician and the laboratory. Pasteur, Koch, Lister and others were able to demonstrate that the cause of disease lay within the aegis of the micro-organism. Although some physicians and surgeons were slow to comprehend the potential of the new discoveries, most realised the prospects for improving therapeutic outcomes for their patients, and embraced the new knowledge on teachings as diverse as Listerian antisepsis and pathogenic specificity, to the new techniques of isolation and purification of blood products for transfusion and serum therapy, antibiotic use and chemotherapy.[849] In addition, many people believed that the germ theory and the discovery of the bacteria that caused common diseases such as typhoid, tuberculosis and diphtheria offered a credible alternative to the contemporaneous assumption that dirt and poverty were the principal causes of society's ill health. Furthermore, many hoped that the revolution in bacteriology would provide both the means to prevent disease through isolation and prevention, and improve prognosis of disease outcomes through better, more targeted medical treatment.[850]

The articulation and coalescence of various germ theories in the late nineteenth and early twentieth century proved a powerful force in influencing the practices of clinical medicine and surgery, and the principles of public health and their application. In itself, the use of the word 'germ' was a loose construction, a nebulous term that embraced many forms of particle believed to be contagious:

> The terminology used to identify the microbial agents of disease varied dramatically in the 1870s: 'vibrio', 'algae', 'fungi', 'cryptograms' … as well as the more familiar modern word, 'bacteria'.[851]

The discovery of bacteria and fungi provided the basis for new programs of public health that focused on sanitation, quarantine, hygiene, and infectious disease control and notification, as well as stricter guidelines for the supply of food to the public. However, it soon became evident to researchers that common infections like smallpox, chickenpox, measles and influenza were caused not by bacteria, but by other organisms that were too small to be seen by scientists with contemporary microscopes. Viruses were everywhere; the big problem was that scientists could neither see them nor grow them in their laboratories. That conundrum made it impossible for laboratory workers of the period to fulfil Koch's postulates, the classic scientific criteria for establishing a particular micro-organism as the cause of a given disease.[852]

The early literature on polio often referred to it as Heine-Medin disease, so named for the two physicians[853] who made perceptive clinical observations about the disease in the mid- to late nineteenth century. Heine noted that the symptoms suggested involvement of the spinal cord and first coined the phrase 'infantile paralysis' to describe the disease that affected mainly young children, for polio at that time was rarely seen in adults. Medin was particularly astute when he noted during the 1887 Stockholm epidemic that paralytic cases were few, and that 'persons with only mild illnesses', or carriers, were spreading the disease to others.[854] Medin was also the first person to use the term 'epidemic' in relation to polio. Later, his assistant Ivar Wickman furthered the study, using epidemiological techniques to trace the spread of an epidemic in Sweden in 1904 and to illustrate that not all cases of polio progressed to the paralytic stage. Wickman also confirmed the hypothesis that polio was contagious, and spread from personal contact between human beings who were often asymptomatic, and along lines of communication like railway routes and highways.

In order to demonstrate that a virus was the causative agent for polio, scientists had to find a way of corroborating the link between the suspect agent and the disease. It proved to be a long and difficult process. However, a breakthrough occurred in 1908 when Karl Landsteiner and Erwin Popper succeeded in transferring the virus into two monkeys, one belonging to the species *Macacus rhesus*. They inoculated each animal via the abdomen with an emulsion of spinal cord from a young boy who had died in the fifth day of an attack of polio and, within six days, one of the monkeys died. The other developed paralysis in both legs, and post-mortem findings in both monkeys revealed that the virus had attacked and destroyed the anterior horn (nerve) cells in the spinal cord responsible for supplying the stimuli for muscle movement.[855] The findings of the two scientists meant that an experimental animal to use in studying the disease was available, as all previous attempts to transmit polio to the usual laboratory animals — guinea pigs, mice and rats — had failed. Humans and monkeys are the only species possessing the poliovirus-receptor (PVR) in the cells lining the gut.

The poliovirus is a single-stranded RNA virus and a member of the family of enteroviruses. It enters the human body through the mouth, and initially infects lymphoid tissues in the tonsils and the intestine before being carried across the gut lining by way of the PVR to the lymphoid tissue of the alimentary tract. Here, it is either killed by antibodies produced by the immune cells, or, if there is no immune response, the poliovirus replicates rapidly and passes from the lymph into the blood circulatory system where it produces a transient viraemia.[856] Viraemia is an essential step on the pathway from the entry portal of the poliovirus to the central nervous system. If the virus remains contained within the lymphoid tissue in the gut, the immunity produced is long-lasting. Finally, the poliovirus is excreted in faeces. The virus is highly resistant to environmental change, such as extremes of temperature, and survives for long periods in faecal matter and sewage. Transmission of the virus in humans is by the ingestion of minute amounts of faecal contamination, usually on the fingers.[857]

A Tale of Brains, Guts, and a Virus

The poliovirus provokes a response in humans in one of four ways: asymptomatic, abortive, non-paralytic and paralytic. When infected with the virus, ninety per cent of cases either do not develop any symptoms, or have a mild to moderate gastrointestinal illness that lasts for fewer than five days. Of the remaining ten per cent of cases, approximately eight in ten experience moderate to severe backache and headache with meningeal irritation that does not lead to permanent paralysis.[858] For the unlucky ones, the exposure to the poliovirus results in paralysis and a loss of function in one or more of the major muscle groups. Paralysis occurs when the nerve supply to a muscle disappears due to disease or trauma and, because the muscle is no longer used, it begins to atrophy. If the nerve cells supplying a particular muscle are destroyed they cannot regenerate, but other nearby cells can be trained to take over the role of stimulating muscle movement.[859] The leg muscles were the ones most commonly affected,[860] but if the respiratory muscles were also involved,[861] breathing became extremely difficult, with death occurring in about five to ten per cent of such cases.[862] The Drinker respirator[863] or, as it was more commonly known, the 'iron lung', was the preferred treatment for those patients unable to breathe on their own. For those who survived an episode of polio, recovery was complete, partial or absent.

Before the 1930s, physicians relied on their clinical judgement to distinguish polio from similar diseases affecting the central nervous system, but the diagnosis was difficult because of the co-existence of epidemic meningitis, the symptoms of which were often indistinguishable from polio. Doctors also placed increasing reliance on the examination of cerebrospinal fluid (CSF) withdrawn from patients by a spinal tap or lumbar puncture and examined microscopically for the presence of cellular material; any increase in cells indicated that an infection was present. However, whether the infection was caused by polio or another pathogen was not clear. Little was known about how the poliovirus survived within the human body or how it reproduced and, in order to increase their knowledge about polio, researchers correlated the clinical observations of clinicians with post-mortem tissue examination and laboratory analysis of antibody levels. But, despite many past attempts to correlate pre-paralysis symptoms and examination of CSF with a prognosis on the degree of paralysis expected, it has proved impossible to judge or alter the eventual outcome of the disease. Furthermore, to date no antivirals or chemotherapy agents have proved successful in halting the progress of the poliovirus through the body or in treating a patient who has polio. Like the situation that existed in the twentieth century, the medical care for paralysed patients today is mainly palliative.[864]

As research into the poliovirus proceeded, the laboratory and the scientist thus became important symbols in the eyes of the public in the 'war' against polio, and many hoped that experimentation would provide answers about the cause and the transmission of the disease. One of the foremost laboratories in that struggle was the Rockefeller Institute for Medical Research, established in New York in 1901 by philanthropist John D. Rockefeller. In 1903, Simon Flexner, Professor of Pathology at Johns Hopkins Medical School, was appointed as Director of Medical Research at the Rockefeller Institute, a post he held until 1935. An extremely intelligent, charismatic but dogmatic individual, Flexner had begun his research into polio in 1907, much of it devoted first to identifying the causative agent, and then to infecting monkeys with the virus. Flexner realised the importance of comparing and contrasting laboratory findings on polio with clinical observations of the disease process in humans, and he arranged for the newly established Rockefeller University Hospital to admit acute cases of polio.[865] Because of that collaboration, research carried out in the laboratory was no longer viewed as work done in isolation; on the contrary, it emphasised the growing importance of laboratory investigation as an adjunct to clinical observation and diagnosis of disease and, because of that, research into polio acquired a human dimension, as researchers endeavoured to prove that the disease process that occurred in experimental monkeys was analogous to that in humans.

One hurdle for scientists to overcome in their research was obvious from the beginning. Because the virus could not be 'grown' on laboratory media in the classical sense as defined by Koch, the onus was on scientists to produce the disease in one group of monkeys and then infect another group.[866] Louis Pasteur had earlier demonstrated that it was possible to study a suspected agent of disease by 'passing' it through live animals, and observing the animal's reaction to infection. But using experimental animals was expensive and time-consuming, and those 'passes' also increased the virulence of the micro-organism. In 1917, Flexner demonstrated that when the poliovirus was inoculated into the nasal cavity of the *rhesus* monkey it then entered the nervous system and caused paralysis.[867] However, it was not until a second group of monkeys developed polio after being injected with post-mortem spinal material from the first group, that researchers became convinced that the respiratory system was the portal of entry for the virus in humans. Because Flexner was, to all intents, 'growing' the virus on monkey brain tissue, the Rockefeller mixed virus (MV) strain not only became more virulent, it also became neurotropic; that is, it developed a preference for growing and reproducing in nervous tissue. That induced neurotropism of the Rockefeller poliovirus further confused the situation, and added weight to Flexner's theory of respiratory transmission and the nasal cavity as the portal of entry.[868]

Further research progress was made in 1913 when Flexner and his associate Hideyo Noguchi demonstrated that the poliovirus would pass through a filter with pores that were small enough to hold back ordinary bacteria.[869] Thus the term 'filter passer' was adopted to describe biological matter that fulfilled that criterion. The two Rockefeller scientists knew they also had to establish beyond doubt that the filtrate contained infective material and not merely toxins, soluble proteins that are toxic to humans and laboratory animals and are produced by many pathogenic bacteria.[870] They believed that the filtrate contained material capable of inducing polio, for their research with monkeys had proved this to be so; post-mortem findings in the paralysed animals had shown the typical pathological changes of the disease in the brain and spinal column. Because they could not see the virus microscopically, they realised they were dealing with a class of micro-organisms so tiny that they were not within the limits of visibility of contemporary microscopes.[871] Only the very largest viruses can be seen under the ordinary light microscope, and the poliovirus is one of the smallest.[872] Thus it was not until the invention of the electron microscope in the 1930s that researchers finally got to examine the morphology of the 'filter passer' they suspected as being the causative agent of polio.

In 1926 Flexner and Noguchi believed they had succeeded in growing the poliovirus under laboratory conditions when they observed under the microscope material they had grown on laboratory media without oxygen (anaerobically).[873] Their subsequent claim that the minute, globoid bodies they had isolated were the causative organism of polio caused a storm within the research world and, indeed, for a few years the poliovirus was known as Flexner's organism. Other researchers disagreed with the conclusions drawn by the Rockefeller scientists, and argued that the material that had been isolated was an aberrant form of the *Streptococcus* bacterium. Many of them insisted that it was impossible to grow a virus on non-living material. Tom Rivers was one who did not believe that a virus could be grown or multiply outside a living cell, primarily because he was convinced that it relied on the host cell for its reproduction and viability[874] but, during the 1920s and '30s, Simon Flexner, along with other notable scientists,[875] held sway with their belief that it was possible to cultivate viruses on artificial laboratory media. Eventually, researchers like Rivers in the United States and Frank Macfarlane Burnet in Australia would be proved correct, for the minute globoid organism isolated by Flexner and Noguchi turned out to have nothing to do with polio. It soon became increasingly evident that the disease was caused by an agent smaller than bacteria.[876]

The poliovirus is excreted by infected individuals in faeces, a fact that was suspected by Swedish workers as early as 1912, by Dr C. Levaditi of the Pasteur Institute in Paris in 1914, and in 1918 by an Australian, Dr Reginald Webster.[877] Levaditi was convinced that the digestive system was the portal of entry for the virus into the body, and believed that *Macacus cynomolgus* rather than *Macacus rhesus* should be used as the experimental monkey because *rhesus* could not be infected by feeding the virus. Although Flexner and Lewis had earlier found the poliovirus in the intestinal tract of monkeys as well as in respiratory tissues, they chose to focus on the latter as the likely focus of infection, thus lending weight to the theory that the nasopharyngeal area was the portal of entry.[878] Perhaps the two researchers were influenced by the longstanding belief that infection was commonly passed from one person to another in the air by 'droplet infection', a scientific term to describe an everyday event when small drops of bacteria- and virus-laden saliva are sprayed into the air by common human activities like talking, coughing or sneezing. Transmission of the virus by droplet infection rather than by faecal contamination due to poor personal hygiene was also more socially acceptable to the sensibilities of that era; especially when the prominent and influential lawyer, politician and future President of the United States of America, Franklin Delano Roosevelt, became ill with polio in 1921.[879]

At that time, the weight of worldwide scientific opinion supported the findings of Dr Simon Flexner and his co-workers at the Rockefeller Institute in New York. However, not everybody accepted the notion that the virus entered the human body through nerves in the nasal cavity and, in 1936, Simon Flexner agreed to consider an alternative point of entry for the virus. He repeated Levaditi's experiment, and fed his *Macacus rhesus* with poliovirus. As expected, he could not duplicate Levaditi's findings for it is impossible to infect *rhesus* orally.[880] Flexner then reiterated his belief that the nasal membrane was the obvious choice for the portal of entry of the virus.[881]

Across the world in suburban Melbourne, Dr Reginald Webster was working with two *cynomolgus* monkeys in a small pathology laboratory in the Children's Hospital in Melbourne.[882] Webster was also convinced that the monkeys could be infected with polio by feeding them the virus, but knew that because his sample size was small[883] his results would be statistically invalid. Nevertheless, he decided to go ahead with his experiment. Infantile paralysis was prevalent in Victoria and the cause of great community concern, especially when the death rate soared to eight per cent of cases.[884] Webster inoculated one monkey intraperitoneally with an emulsion of spinal cord from a six-year-old boy from Sydney, and when the monkey developed the classic signs of polio paralysis, he was delighted. To Webster it was evidence of a breakthrough in determining how the virus was transmitted. But when he attempted to infect his healthy monkey with material gathered from his diseased monkey, the experiment failed. Discouraged, Webster then decided to abandon his ideas about the oral method of transmission, and to adopt Flexner's protocol of using the *rhesus* monkey and injecting the virus into the brain cavity.[885] That decision was unfortunate. Dr Webster, in his small laboratory in Melbourne, was on the right track. *Cynomolgus* later proved to be the correct choice of experimental monkey for polio research, not *rhesus*, which could be infected only through the nasal route with the neurotropic Rockefeller MV strain. Moreover, Webster was also correct with his hypothesis that polio was a systemic infection, and that the virus could reach the central nervous system by penetrating the body's defence mechanism and entering the bloodstream. Tom Rivers would later claim that if Simon Flexner had used *cynomolgus* instead of *rhesus* in his experiments, the world would have had the polio vaccine much earlier than it did.[886]

From the time he graduated, Frank Macfarlane Burnet knew that he wanted to work in medical science. His appointment as a pathology registrar at the Walter and Eliza Hall Institute[887] in Melbourne and subsequent association with the Institute's Director, Charles Kellaway, was the beginning of a long and illustrious research career in virology. When Burnet returned to Australia after two years in London in January 1928, it was a decision that was in keeping with his view that, despite its distance from Europe and America, Australia was the best place for his approach to research. For Burnet, his new position as assistant director at the Walter and Eliza Hall Institute afforded him the best of both worlds: an awareness of 'what was happening in the great centres of research' overseas, but also autonomy. In Australia he did not feel 'overwhelmed by being surrounded with men knowing or seeming to know more than oneself'.[888] Challenging an accepted idea is always difficult, especially one advanced by an authority like Simon Flexner, and it is probable that many young researchers felt intimidated by the power and prestige of the Rockefeller scientists. In Australia, Burnet was free to pursue his ideas and, in 1928, Jean Macnamara, a fellow graduate in medicine from Melbourne University, joined him at the Institute. Macnamara was by then a consultant and medical officer to the Poliomyelitis

Committee of Victoria, and someone integral to any account of the history of polio treatment in Australia. Jean Macnamara was particularly interested in the therapeutic use and long-term viability of human serum taken from polio convalescents.[889] Serum was claimed to possess qualities that gave the recipient protection against paralysis, and was promoted by many scientists as an effective weapon against the effects of the poliovirus. Serum treatment offered hope in a time of uncertainty.

Scientific discoveries build on work done previously by other researchers in the field, and the sharing of material, hypotheses, methodology and results is commonplace, for nothing is accepted without corroboration. Simon Flexner, as head of the Rockefeller Institute, maintained a strict policy of sharing the results of research with other workers in the field and, because the filtrate containing the Rockefeller strain of poliovirus remained viable for at least twelve months if kept refrigerated under fifty per cent glycerine, it could be sent to other laboratories for confirmation or rebuttal of their own findings. When Jean Macnamara wrote to Flexner in 1929 outlining the difficulties she and Burnet had experienced in gathering a sufficient amount of virus material for experimentation,[890] Flexner agreed to send to the Walter and Eliza Hall Institute some of the Rockefeller strain with instructions on inoculating monkeys intracerebrally.[891] From experiments they carried out in July of that year, Burnet and Macnamara realised that the viral material from the Rockefeller Institute was more virulent than the local strain, and that infection with the Victorian virus did not offer protection from the American virus. For Burnet and Macnamara, that singular fact indicated that more than one type of polio existed; that the Melbourne and Rockefeller viruses were immunologically different.[892] Previously, both Flexner and Noguchi had appeared convinced there was only one type of poliovirus. Both scientists were impressed by Burnet and Macnamara's experiments and conclusion, and asked for a sample of the Victorian virus to be sent to New York when circumstances permitted.[893] Initially, the work by Burnet and Macnamara in 1929 at the Walter and Eliza Hall Institute in Melbourne was ignored, but ultimately proved to be influential, as it marked the beginning of the differentiation of the poliovirus into Types I, II and III. Type I would prove to be the causative agent for eighty per cent of all epidemics of polio, followed by Type III and then the relatively rare and more benign Type II.

A later paper by Burnet on the 1937–38 epidemic[894] in Melbourne posed an interesting question on the circumstances surrounding the importation and use of the Rockefeller poliovirus at the Melbourne institute. He commented that the characteristics of the epidemic were 'unusual' and did not follow the pattern of previous outbreaks. The epidemic had begun in winter, and the disease was much more contagious than previous episodes had been. Particularly striking was the high level of contagion within the family, and the level of paralysis in those affected, factors that indicated that a different type of poliovirus was now circulating in Melbourne. Was it possible that the Rockefeller virus had escaped from the laboratory and infected the Melbourne population? In the 1930s, laboratory work was performed under conditions that would be regarded as primitive by today's standards of biosecurity. Experimental work was performed at the bench, using test tubes with cotton wool seals, and the flame from a bunsen burner to sterilise inoculation loops. Even simple pieces of equipment such as plastic gloves and fume cupboards were rare — certainly nothing that approaches the sophistication of today's specialist isolation cabinets. In the 1930s, laboratory workers were handling a material that 'contained a thousand million or more virus units per cubic centimetre'[895] without any extra protection. Scientists did not know how long a virus could survive without a host to support its growth. If a virus can escape from a highly sophisticated laboratory in the twenty-first century,[896] surely it would be even more feasible almost eighty years ago. In 1931, notifications of polio in Victoria tripled from those of the previous year.[897] When the Melbourne virus arrived at the Rockefeller Institute and was grown by Flexner, it was found to cause 'mild facial paralysis' in the monkeys who subsequently recovered, whereas the Rockefeller virus killed them, proving that at least two strains of the poliovirus existed.

The Rockefeller Foundation's association with the Walter and Eliza Hall Institute was extended when, in 1934, it agreed to contribute funds towards Burnet's work on using hen eggs as a medium for growing viruses.[898] The Rockefeller grant was a 'great comfort' to Charles Kellaway because it ensured that 'Burnet's work would not be hampered by the lack of funds that affects the rest of us in the Institute'.[899] But the poliovirus steadfastly refused to grow in chick embryos, although later experiments to grow the influenza virus proved successful. In America in 1936, Albert Sabin and Peter Olitsky grew the poliovirus in embryonic nervous tissue and further reinforced Flexner's hypothesis that the pathway of infection was from the nose to the brain. However, because the researchers used the MV Rockefeller, or neurotropic form of the poliovirus, those findings were later dismissed.[900] In 1937, two Australians, Dr Charles Swan and Dr E. Graeme Robertson, examined the olfactory bulbs in the nasal cavity of eleven children who had died in the Melbourne epidemic and found them to be free of any pathological change. They correctly concluded that the nasal route was not the portal of entry.[901] The following year, researchers in the USA isolated the virus from the faeces of a baby they suspected of being a carrier, or 'abortive' case of polio.[902]

The 1937–38 polio epidemic in Melbourne provided the stimulus to Burnet to focus his attention on polio again, and 1939 proved to be a turning point in his research. Despite the limitations imposed by not having sufficient monkeys,[903] experiments by Burnet and his colleagues at the Institute proved that the *cynomolgous* monkey was more susceptible to polio infection by the oral route than was *rhesus*, ending the long-held belief that the respiratory tract gave access to the poliovirus.[904] In addition, Burnet showed that the virus circulated in the bloodstream, and thus proved that it was not carried on nerve pathways. In an experiment that would later prove crucial for the development of a vaccine, Burnet and his colleague Dora Lush succeeded in growing the virus in human foetal tissue.[905]

Any form of tissue culture demands that the cells used should be free of contaminating bacteria and, as human embryonic tissue is sterile, it was the obvious choice. Obtaining a supply of the tissue was difficult, but that would soon change. Dr George Simpson was then a member of the Eugenics Society of Victoria and sympathetic to its views on the sterilisation of the unfit. He had graduated from Melbourne University in the same year as Burnet, had been best man at Jean Macnamara's wedding to Ivan Connor in 1934, and was well known to the two scientists. Simpson was also in charge of the contraception clinic at the Women's Hospital and had made it known at meetings that the Eugenics Society 'should just quietly go ahead and send him cases' [for abortion].[906] Because of the personal relationship that existed between the three friends, it seems likely that the aborted embryos were then sent to Burnet's laboratory. The supply of human embryos was intermittent and unreliable, and monkeys were difficult to obtain and very expensive. Perhaps that is why Burnet eventually abandoned that line of research.[907]

Sadly, Burnet and Webster's story remains one all too familiar in the history of Australian science: a lack of government support and philanthropic funding resulting in promising scientific research either withering or going overseas. Burnet lost interest in working with polio, and turned his attention to developing the technique of culturing the influenza virus in living tissue,[908] a process that had been facilitated by the addition of antibiotics to non-sterile body tissue like kidney and liver. This freed up a greater range of tissue for laboratory use and meant that scientists no longer had to rely on the supply of controversial embryonic tissue.

In the United States, virology studies on polio had been interrupted by the outbreak of the Second World War and it was not until the defeat of Japan and the victory of the Allied Forces that funds began to flow back into scientific research. In 1949, a team comprising John Enders, Thomas Weller and Frederick Robbins at Harvard University decided to replicate the 1936 experiment of Sabin and Olitsky and grow a fresh strain of Lansing (Type II) poliovirus in embryonic tissue, instead of using the neurotropic MV Rockefeller strain used by Sabin. Copious amounts of the virus had been isolated from the faeces of polio patients and the team did not believe that such a large volume of virus could be manufactured by the nervous system. They decided to have another attempt at growing the virus in non-nervous tissue. Enders and his colleagues were overjoyed at their results: the Lansing strain grew and quickly multiplied, and convinced them that *in vitro*[909] tissue-culture cultivation of the virus was possible in volumes large enough to produce a vaccine. Previously, thousands of monkeys would have been needed to grow an adequate quantity of poliovirus *in vivo* but, by harvesting the kidney tissue from a relatively small number of animals, a practical solution was achieved — hundreds of cell cultures could be produced from one kidney. As Tom Rivers succinctly expressed it, the paper by Enders and his colleagues 'was like shooting off a cannon … and sure as hell captured everybody's attention'.[910]

That discovery transformed virus production, and the three men were awarded the Nobel Prize in Medicine in 1954.[911] It is of interest to Australia that when Frederick Robbins was awarded his three-year fellowship by the National Foundation for Infantile Paralysis (NFIP) in 1947 to study virology it was with the proviso that his last two years of research should be with Macfarlane Burnet at the Walter and Eliza Hall Institute in Melbourne. The NFIP was an organisation that evolved from the Roosevelt Birthday Balls in the 1930s to sponsor treatment and research for the fight against polio, and was funded entirely from public support and donations collected in the annual March of Dimes.[912] However, because the investigations at Harvard at the end of Robbins' first year were so promising, the NFIP agreed he should stay in the United States. As a result of that decision, we can only surmise the possible outcome for Australian science if the original conditions of that fellowship had remained in force, and Robbins had gone to Melbourne to work with Burnet, described as 'one of the world's prominent figures in virology and immunology'.[913] It is entirely possible that the Nobel Prize and associated prestige given the United States for developing the technique for producing a vaccine against polio might have instead been accorded to Australia. Burnet had, after all, developed the technique for tissue culture of viruses with his colleague Dora Lush in Melbourne ten years previously.[914] When officials from the Rockefeller Foundation visited the Walter and Eliza Hall Institute in 1948 they were impressed with the 'magnificent building', and believed that 'it possessed no great originality of insight to predict' that its director, Frank Macfarlane Burnet, 'will sometime come up with a knighthood and a Nobel prize unless something goes seriously awry. Still in his early forties, he is not only an inspired experimenter, but a wise administrator and a very nice person as well.'[915]

The succession of bitter controversies that accompanied the story of the development of the polio vaccine began with a well-known disaster, that of the failed Park-Brodie and Kolmer vaccines in 1935. Maurice Brodie, a young Canadian researcher and W.H. Park,[916] an ageing, but renowned bacteriologist, developed a vaccine using formaldehyde to inactivate the virus, and Californian officials gave permission for 7000 children to be immunised. Although it was never conclusively proven, many scientists believed that several children developed polio as a result of being given the Park-Brodie vaccine. Tom Rivers remarked that 'the vaccine was made in the most incredibly sloppy manner'[917] and doubted whether any of the children had developed any antibodies to polio as a result of being vaccinated. At the University of Pennsylvania, John Kolmer also used what he thought to be an inactivated form of the Rockefeller MV poliovirus to produce his vaccine, and the results were even more disastrous. The inactivation process failed, and several vials of vaccine were subsequently found to contain live, infective virus. Just over 10,000 children were vaccinated in the summer of 1935, an enthusiastic press spread the story around the world and an excited public revelled in the news that a vaccine against polio had been produced. However, trouble was brewing. In October, James P. Leake of the US Public Health Service presented evidence at a meeting stating that the Kolmer vaccine had caused the death of five children. Using the 'strongest language' Rivers had 'ever heard expressed at a scientific meeting', James Leake — described as being 'hot under the collar' by Rivers — accused Kolmer of being 'a murderer'. Rivers remembered that after Leake sat down 'all hell broke loose', with everybody trying to speak at once. A white-faced and shaken Kolmer declared, 'Gentlemen, this is one time I wish the floor would open up and swallow me'.[918]

Not surprisingly, 'both vaccines were dead', and so were the careers of Kolmer, Park and Brodie; after the close of the meeting, all three retreated into obscurity. For two years virologists remained sceptical about the possibility of making a vaccine at all, let alone one that was safe to use.[919] The spectre of the humiliation of Kolmer, Park and Brodie, not to mention the lost and ruined lives of the children they had injected with their faulty vaccines, would stalk many researchers who dared to venture down that particular research path.

Following the end of the 1937–38 epidemic in Melbourne, Burnet and his colleagues in Australia and overseas agreed on one point: that the only way to control epidemics of polio was to have the whole population immunised.[920] Quarantine and improved standards of hygiene merely slowed the spread of the disease, they did not prevent an outbreak. Scientific research had to concentrate on finding a safe and effective means of protecting the population through immunisation and, with that goal in mind, a modest research program was set up at the Walter and Eliza Hall Institute that culminated in the debunking of the nasal cavity theory as the point of entry of the poliovirus, and introduced a pioneering technique for tissue culture. Meanwhile, in the United States the work of John Enders and his colleagues in developing *in vitro* tissue culture for growing the poliovirus, had paved the way for the logical extension to their findings — the development of the Salk vaccine.

In the early 1950s, the desire of many scientists to develop a vaccine that would protect children from polio came closer to being fulfilled. They knew, because the virus had been detected in blood, that a vaccine would work. Finding the right one was the problem. American science, through the work of Jonas Salk and colleagues at the University of Pittsburgh,[921] was devoting its energies towards the production of a killed virus, not an attenuated vaccine, which both Burnet and Albert Sabin favoured. The controversy surrounding the issue was considerable: both the attenuated and the killed vaccine had their own advantages, and each had powerful advocates. A killed virus vaccine was technically easier and quicker to produce than an attenuated or weakened one, but the essential difference lay in the way they acted in the body. Live vaccines produced a sub-clinical case of the real disease, with better and longer-lasting immunity; the risk was that the weakened virus would revert to the virulent form, causing vaccine-associated paralytic poliomyelitis (VAPP).[922] A killed virus produced an immunity, but it was only temporary, and booster shots were necessary to maintain an effective level of protection. Finally, a live vaccine posed fewer logistical problems in poorer countries, especially those with continued circulation of the wild poliovirus, and was one of the reasons why the World Health Organization subsequently adopted the Sabin vaccine.[923]

Many in Australia rightly believed that it was vital that the country should not fall behind in vaccine research, and Burnet used his connections with Salk and the scientific community in the United States to gain a position for Dr Percival (Val) Bazeley of the Commonwealth Serum Laboratories (CSL) with Salk at Pittsburgh.[924] Bazeley took up the position as chief assistant on technical matters to Salk in 1952 and remained there until his return to Australia in 1955 to set up polio vaccine production at CSL. At the conclusion of an extensive period of typing[925] that covered two years from 1949 to 1951, scientists knew that, although there were many strains of the poliovirus, they all fell into three immunological types,[926] a hypothesis that had been proposed by Burnet and Macnamara in Melbourne as early as 1929. Researchers in the quest for a safe vaccine knew it was vital that all three serotypes of the poliovirus be included for it to be effective — they knew that immunity gained against one type did not protect from infection with the other two.

In July 1952, the 38-year-old Jonas Salk began trials of his tri-valent vaccine using handicapped children in two institutions in Pennsylvania, a practice that would be considered abhorrent today, but was not unusual for America at that time despite the revelations of Nazi atrocities at Nuremberg. Although Salk later admitted that he had been worried about injecting the Pittsburgh children with his vaccine, and 'didn't sleep very well for two or three weeks', the results were encouraging.[927] However, Salk's use of the virulent Type I strain, 'Mahoney', would later prove to be disastrous both in terms of the lives lost and the blow to scientific prestige and reputation. Over the next few months, the children produced antibodies to the vaccine, there were no side effects, and none developed polio.[928] When the statistics were published the following year about the severity of the latest polio epidemic, and word began to spread that a doctor in Pittsburgh was working on a vaccine to prevent polio, everyone sat up and took notice. No one felt safe from the polio epidemics that arrived with summer in America. Salk wrote up his findings and submitted them to the *Journal of the American Medical Association* in January 1954. The published paper received bountiful praise and was greeted with boisterous enthusiasm by the medical community. The stage was now set for a full-scale implementation of a national field trial to test Salk's vaccine, despite reservations being expressed by several scientists on the committee established to supervise the immunisation campaign, who

A Tale of Brains, Guts, and a Virus

wanted to implement a double-blind placebo trial.[929] Jonas Salk went on the offensive against those who dared criticise his vaccine and who wanted a properly conducted clinical trial. He was horrified at the thought of 'intentionally injecting children with a salt solution or some other placebo', for he believed that all children should receive the benefit of his vaccine. It was, moreover, a 'fetish of orthodoxy' to argue for the use of placebos, enough to make 'Hippocrates turn over in his grave'.[930] Basil O'Connor, Chairman of the National Foundation for Infantile Paralysis, was determined to go ahead with the trial, for he believed he had to keep faith with the thousands who had donated their dimes and dollars to the March of Dimes campaign for research into polio. He succeeded. Moreover, Salk's argument against an injected control prevailed, and agreement was reached on an observed control plan.[931] Eleven states disagreed with Salk, and used a placebo control. In the observed control in the other thirty-six states, children aged seven to eight were given the vaccine and all children aged between eight and ten years were observed for the summer 'polio' season. Thousands of parents, willing to try anything that promised protection against polio, flocked to volunteer their children as a 'Polio Pioneer' for the trial that would begin in April 1954 just before the polio season arrived. Salk expected to publish the results the following year.[932]

On 12 April 1955, amid a 'fanfare and drama far more typical of a Hollywood premiere',[933] the formal verdict on the vaccine trial was announced. Dr Thomas Francis of the University of Michigan presented results that were clearly positive against all three types of polio.[934] The atmosphere in the auditorium was electric, and reporters rushed to telephones to contact newspapers, radio and television channels with the news. Their reports hit the airwaves and the streets, and the public rejoiced. The trial of the Salk vaccine was a success. Ushering in the largest public health campaign in America's history, a six-year-old boy from Virginia was injected with vaccine. Coincidentally or not, that day was also the tenth anniversary of the death of the 'polio' President, Franklin Delano Roosevelt.

On 26 April 1955, reports began to filter through to public health officials in California that something had gone terribly wrong with the vaccination program. Five children had become paralysed after receiving the Salk vaccine and, disquietingly, the paralysis had begun in the vaccinated arm. Over the following few days, notifications increased until the whole program was halted on 7 May 1955. By then 204 children who had received the vaccine had been diagnosed with polio, 150 were paralysed and eleven had died. Small communities were devastated. Polio was striking their children once more and, even more terrifying, was caused by Salk's vaccine. All the stricken children had received vaccine manufactured by the Cutter Laboratories in Berkeley, where nine lots were subsequently found to have been contaminated with live poliovirus.[935] It was not only the immunised children who became ill with polio: family members and contacts in the community were also infected. Typing tests soon revealed which strain was responsible: it was the virulent Mahoney strain.

Public faith in the safety of immunisation campaigns was shattered, a casualty of what many viewed as a too hasty implementation after the success of the field trials. What had been viewed as a miracle of science, a triumph over infectious disease, was now revealed as flawed. The repercussions were enormous, but none more so than for the families of the children who received the Cutter vaccine. Their lives were irrevocably changed by their decision to have their child vaccinated with the Salk polio vaccine in April 1955.

Many scientists and officials blamed Basil O'Connor and his grand vision for the NFIP to conquer the 'crippler of our children' for the haste with which the immunisation program was launched. Everyone involved sought to lay the blame elsewhere. Salk insisted that the manufacturers had 'not followed his procedure properly'; the manufacturers insisted that they had followed the protocols approved by the National Institute of Health; Albert Sabin roundly criticised the whole program, but he was hardly an impartial observer; the US Public Health Service 'denied any responsibility' that went beyond the 'act of licensing', and later criticised the fact that a program normally expected to take years to implement was 'telescoped into months'.[936] In a barely disguised attack on the NFIP, Dr John Enders responded, 'we must never again allow decisions about essentially scientific matters to be made for us by people without training or insight'.[937]

> It was all too quick, said medical colleagues nationwide. Salk had gone public without first publishing everything in the journals. He rushed out a killed-virus serum without waiting for a safe live-virus one, which would have been better. Doctors walked out of professional meetings; some quit the Foundation that funded the testing. Salk was after personal glory, they said. Salk was after money … Salk was after the big prizes.[938]

In 1954, Burnet had stated that it was unwise to assume that the 'Salk vaccine was certain to be effective and free from all danger' and felt that, because the virus was killed by a 'gentle method' then it was 'possible that a living virus could persist in some batches of vaccine'.[939] That is exactly what occurred at the Cutter Laboratories in California. Opinions were expressed that the NFIP should have handed over responsibility for the program to the US Government following the field trials. After all, editorials thundered, it was the health of the nation's children that was at stake, and many opined that government, not a charitable organisation dependent on public funding should have been in charge of supply of the vaccine.[940] Bureaucratic obfuscation triumphed, for the question of who was ultimately to blame for the lapse in quality control at the Cutter Laboratories has never been resolved.

In 1954, government, medical and public health officials in Australia were well aware that large-scale field trials of the Salk vaccine were being conducted in the USA, and that supplies of the vaccine would not be available for export for at least eighteen months. As was to be expected, America was giving priority to its own citizens before considering the needs of others outside her boundaries. Australian media reports on the overseas research into a polio vaccine had appeared frequently since the early 1950s, and public expectations for a successful immunisation program were high.[941] Nevertheless, many in Australia remembered the previous disasters with vaccines that had occurred in the United States, and parents were understandably anxious about the efficacy of Salk's 'creamy white' vaccine, and its endorsement as 'the most powerful weapon' in the 'worldwide battle against polio'.[942] Public anxiety and opposition to the vaccine was fanned by ill-informed rumours, prejudice and innuendo. Various interest groups and individuals made a case for special consideration against being immunised,[943] while others pointed to the disaster in America as evidence for the likelihood of a similar flaw occurring in the production process in Australia. Prime Minister Robert Menzies and his Cabinet consulted Burnet on the options available. Burnet stated his belief that, if future trials in the United States were successful, and no harmful side effects of the vaccine detected, then Australia should produce its own vaccine. However, Burnet included the proviso that he was doubtful that protection from the Salk vaccine would last more than a few months, for he questioned the likelihood that the antibodies produced by the vaccine would create a permanent immunity to polio. Burnet and many others believed that the only way to ensure long-term immunity to polio would be by using a live virus vaccine similar to that being developed by Albert Sabin.[944] Nevertheless, and despite Burnet's reservations, Cabinet believed that it was in Australia's best interests to go ahead with the Salk vaccine, and not wait for what could be many more years for Sabin's vaccine to be produced. As a result, Dr Bazeley and his colleagues at the Commonwealth Serum Laboratories (CSL) in Melbourne were instructed to begin production of the Salk vaccine.[945]

In Australia, by the end of 1955 work had been completed at the CSL on the production laboratory and the animal house to accommodate the monkeys. Although the federal government knew that sufficient supplies of the Australian-produced vaccine would not be available until the first quarter of 1956, that information had not reached local government level and, as early as May 1955, many Sydney councils began to lobby the Commonwealth Department of Health to supply them with the vaccine.[946] Production began in mid-November that year, aimed at making quantities sufficient to begin a nationwide immunisation program in June 1956. Some parents were not content to wait for the start of the campaign and imported the vaccine from the USA with the consent of the Commonwealth.[947] Just how long private citizens were allowed to bring in the vaccine is not clear from the records, but within two years all importation by individuals was banned.[948]

Large-scale immunisation with the Salk polio vaccine started in Australia in June 1956. Its implementation was not without setbacks and difficulties. The agreement between the Commonwealth and the states had stipulated that enough vaccine for 400,000 doses per month would be available on a pro-rata population basis.[949] It was to be supplied by the Commonwealth at no cost to the states, but each state was responsible for the cost and implementation of its campaign, and the National Health and Medical Research Council (NHMRC) defined priorities for immunisation within the population.[950] Stringent safety measures were implemented at the CSL, testing procedures were carried out at many stages during production, and each completed batch of the vaccine was independently tested by both the Fairfield Hospital and the University of Melbourne.[951]

Despite most parents being terrified at the prospect of their child catching polio, opposition to the Salk vaccine did exist within the community. Some Christian Scientists wanted their children excluded because they 'relied wholly on spiritual healing',[952] and one mother wrote to the Federal Minister of Health, Dr Earle Page, demanding to know why 'if the vaccine is so safe ... were not the Royal children being vaccinated?'[953] The campaign appeared to divide the community. On the whole, the anti-vaccinationists were defending what they believed to be the freedom of the individual to decide on medical intervention, and were also influenced by the fear that immunisation would introduce disease to an otherwise healthy body.[954]

The campaign against the Salk vaccine was at times intensely anti-Semitic. Jonas Salk was described by one writer as the 'Yiddish inventor' who was 'directing the inoculation of millions of American children with this sinister concoction of live polio germ', while another, no doubt influenced by the political climate existing in 1950s Australia, was convinced that it was 'a communist plot to get the country'.[955] It appears that the campaign by those opposed to immunisation did have some effect on the Victorian public. In three local government areas of the state, fifty per cent of parents asked to fill in consent cards for the Salk vaccine declined to do so, and indicated they would not consent to any future vaccination.[956] Perhaps the reluctance of some Victorians to have either themselves or their children immunised against polio was influenced by official figures that showed that notifications had fallen between 1951 to 1954, a period when the worst outbreaks were in Western Australia, followed by Queensland, New South Wales and South Australia. However, it does appear to have been a surprising decision by the Victorian community, especially when considering the widespread emotional response to the distress caused by the epidemics of 1937–38 and 1949. Maybe many Victorians believed that the bad days of polio epidemics were behind them for, by 1964, 72 per cent of Victorian children under fourteen had been immunised with Salk vaccine compared with 83 per cent in NSW, 75 per cent in Queensland, 78 per cent in SA, and 79 per cent in WA. However, across Bass Strait the population was not so confident that polio had disappeared, and Tasmanians recorded the highest consent rate in Australia to vaccination with the Salk vaccine (92 per cent).[957]

In 1957, the Medical Council of the BMA (Australia) wanted the vaccine made available to general practitioners for them to dispense. It was concerned that the growing reluctance of young adults to line up with schoolchildren to be vaccinated was placing them at risk of contracting polio. The Council believed adults would be more likely to agree to be vaccinated if they could have it 'done by their family doctor'.[958] However, the Federal Minister of Health, D.A. Cameron, would not consent to the BMA's request, and cited 'administrative and technical' reasons for his refusal. Cameron argued that the Salk vaccine was issued by the Commonwealth 'free of charge' to the states, and he could see no reason to change that arrangement, especially as the National Health and Medical Research Council (NHMRC) had recommended that the Salk vaccine 'should not be made available' to GPs until the state campaigns had finished.[959] Cameron was aided in his resolution by the Victorian Minister of Health, H.M. Wade, who wrote to him in February 1962:

> The fact that poliomyelitis is a very serious disease and the extreme importance of maintaining the potency of the vaccine, have been the main factors which have influenced the policy of the vaccine being distributed through State and local Health Authorities and not directly from the CSL to family doctors. The policy of having available to the public a potent vaccine when required, necessitates storage at a precise temperature, something which cannot be guaranteed by every refrigerator.[960]

The war of words between Minister Cameron and the BMA continued unabated until the end of that year, when very limited permission for GPs to dispense the vaccine was granted.[961]

A possible reason for government reluctance to allow the Salk vaccine to be given by medical practitioners in Australia may well lie in an earlier immunisation campaign conducted against diphtheria in 1928. Following the introduction in the 1920s of a combined diphtheria toxin-antitoxin (TAT) solution for immunising children against the disease, the incidence had been falling. Local health authorities in Bundaberg, Queensland, decided to conduct a campaign to immunise children with the help of the local Medical Officer of Health, Dr Thomson.[962] In January 1928, twenty-one children received injections of the TAT from a bottle that had been used seven days previously to inject children, and stored at room temperature in a cupboard in Thomson's consulting room.[963] Within thirty-six hours, twelve of the children had died, and the grieving inhabitants of the town struggled to come to terms with a tragedy that was directly associated with a state-initiated public health policy. Investigations later revealed that it was not the diphtheria TAT that was to blame for the deaths of the children, but toxin produced from a common skin bacterium (*Staphylococcus*) that had contaminated the TAT solution. The tragedy occurred because of a complete lack of quality control and ignorance about the use and storage of biological material. Frank Macfarlane Burnet was part of the Royal Commission set up to investigate what had happened at Bundaberg, and he later wrote: 'Even in 1928, we were shocked at the idea of leaving a solution in which bacteria could grow for a week at sub-tropical temperatures, and then using it again'.[964]

The central issue in the government refusal to allow medical practitioners to give the Salk vaccine in the 1950s was likely the belief that rigorous quality control standards had to be maintained in a state-initiated immunisation campaign. Thirty years after Bundaberg, public health officials would have remained mindful of the tragedy, and the need to maintain control over the entire vaccination process. They had to get it right with the Salk campaign, and it was vital to the entire operation that trust be maintained between the Government and the community. The Cutter incident in the United States remained fresh in the public's mind, and authorities could not afford another tragic mistake. As one historian has argued, the Bundaberg tragedy was a 'crucial event in the history of immunisation in Australia'.[965] Community fears about vaccination brought to a halt the practice of prophylactic mass immunisation against common childhood diseases.

Almost immediately after the Salk immunisation campaign commenced in Australia, shortages of the vaccine were reported, and by the end of July 1956 there was increasing concern about dwindling supplies.[966] Public health officials organising the immunisation campaigns were mindful of public demand, and their efforts to inoculate as many children as possible led to the vaccine being used as soon as it became available. In the minds of many it became a race against time to vaccinate children before the summer season, and competition was fierce among local councils for the limited amount of vaccine produced by the CSL.[967] Problems of supply of the vaccine continued to trouble health officials until the early 1960s, when the decision that a fourth injection of Salk vaccine would be necessary to maintain immunity levels further exacerbated the situation. Sydney's *The Sun* newspaper reported on a team of British doctors who stated that a fourth booster shot was necessary.[968] Burnet had been correct when he questioned the efficacy of a killed virus in providing long-term protection against polio. By mid-1961, the Government had made the decision to look elsewhere and, in August, vaccine produced at the Connaught Laboratories in Canada was distributed to all states.[969]

Australians had to wait longer than North Americans to get their Salk vaccine but, by 1956, the revised specifications for the manufacturing process ensured it was safe. By the time the immunisation campaign began in Australia, a further twenty-five million American children had been immunised without any ill effect. Fortunately, due no doubt to the exacting quality controls employed by the CSL, and the testing of all batches of the vaccine at the Fairfield Hospital and Melbourne University,[970] there were no 'Cutter' incidents in Australia.

Polio notifications throughout Australia fell steadily after the introduction of the Salk vaccine, and public health authorities were optimistic that epidemic polio could be beaten. However, the virus was not to be defeated so easily.[971] A severe epidemic occurred in all states in the early 1960s, prompting health officials to search vaccination records for a possible explanation. Had immunity levels dropped in those vaccinated, or was there some other reason for the outbreak? They discovered that a high proportion of cases admitted to Prince Henry Hospital in Sydney had either not been vaccinated, or had not received the full dose. Officials blamed 'public complacency', expressing disbelief that 'an outbreak of such proportions should occur in a community in which the highly effective Salk vaccine has been available, free of charge to the public, for five years or more'.[972] When Queensland reported the figures on its epidemic it became clear that there was far more to the outbreak than had previously been suspected. Nearly one-third of the Queensland polio cases had received the full course of Salk vaccine.[973] It was becoming more evident to the Government and the scientific community that the fears of Burnet and others about the long-term effectiveness of the Salk vaccine to maintain immunity against polio were proving correct.

It was during the period when problems were occurring with the supply of the Salk vaccine in Australia, that moves first took place to replace it with the oral, attenuated vaccine developed by Albert Sabin. His work had captured scientific attention in 1956 when a paper was published by the Yale University polio unit describing limited trials of his vaccine in a children's home in a small village in Arizona.[974] But Sabin was aware that he would have to conduct large-scale trials to prove that his vaccine worked — the question was, where? By 1957 much of the American population had been vaccinated, Salk was widely accepted, and there had been no further problems with production. Understandably, there was a widespread reluctance by financiers to commit funds to a new vaccine trial, but more importantly, most children already had antibody levels that were too high for another vaccine to be tested. Sabin was fortunate in that he had retained his status as Professor at the University of Cincinnati and was thus able to accept research funds while retaining a high degree of autonomy. He had remained in close contact with colleagues within the Soviet Union, and when they asked him for a sample of his three attenuated vaccine types he agreed. No doubt he recognised the advantages of having a trial conducted within a country where the political system 'allowed government policy to be carried out with the minimum resistance from the public'.[975] There would be no double-blind trials using placebos or observation groups: all Soviet children were to be given the vaccine.

The first doses of Sabin vaccine were administered to 3000 children in Leningrad in 1957, but results were not made public until, at a conference in Washington in June 1959,[976] Sabin announced that four and a half million

Soviet children had been vaccinated with no ill effect. By September, that number had reached over six million. Delegates stood and applauded. By the beginning of 1960, a clear scientific consensus in favour of the oral, attenuated polio vaccine had emerged, a shift in position that was hardly surprising considering over seventy million Soviet citizens under the age of twenty had by then been successfully vaccinated.[977]

There are several possible reasons why the United States remained reluctant to adopt the Sabin vaccine. The NFIP was fully committed to supporting Jonas Salk and all its research funds had been focused on developing his vaccine. The NFIP would not want to admit that another vaccine was superior, especially when it was their view that the Salk vaccine had not yet been fully established. In addition, the Salk vaccine had been developed in an era that was dominated by the Cold War between the United States of America and the Soviet Union. It was probably inconceivable for politicians and government to entertain the thought that a triumph of American science could be usurped by research tested in a communist country. However, in what was a bitter blow to the NFIP, the Surgeon-General of the United States announced that the Sabin vaccine would be licensed for use in America from April 1961. In May the following year, the NHMRC in Australia recommended that Sabin's vaccine be imported as soon as possible, and within six months over one million units had arrived in the country for use in a possible emergency.

Some of the problems associated with the field trial of the Salk polio vaccine in the United States in 1955 were no doubt due to the politicisation of the research process, and the way in which the results were made public. Many findings were not published in peer-reviewed scientific journals where they could be challenged by other researchers in the field, but in public forums to which members of the media had been invited in a calculated move by the NFIP to generate intense public interest and debate.[978] On the other hand, researchers *were* working at a new frontier of virus research with all the associated pitfalls and risks associated with pioneering scientific endeavour; ostensibly, the greatest risk to the public was the decision to allow in-house review of quality control by the pharmaceutical companies.[979] With the disasters surrounding previous vaccines still fresh in the minds of researchers and the public, surely it would have been wiser to err on the side of caution and give drug companies time to fully evaluate their production process before launching a national vaccination campaign.

By the end of the 1950s, the debate on the merits of Salk versus Sabin had moved from that of a scientifically motivated debate into one involving a class-based social distinction. The highest vaccination rate with Salk occurred in white, middle- to upper-class neighbourhoods with easy, affordable access to the paediatricians who dispensed the vaccine, while in poorer areas of the country, African Americans, Puerto Ricans and some Native Americans simply could not afford to pay for the full course of three injections plus a booster. The alternative, a single twenty-seven cent dose of Sabin vaccine, was all that was needed to give protection against polio.[980] Sabin's vaccine was not entirely risk-free, for a small, but definite chance existed that, given the right conditions, the attenuated Sabin virus used in the vaccine could regain its virulence.

The fact remains that the Salk vaccine had done its job well, but with the development of Sabin's vaccine, an easier, more natural and efficient method had become available.[981] If the 1950s had belonged to Salk, the 1960s would belong to Sabin. Although Jonas Salk never wavered in his belief that his killed-virus vaccine offered the best hope for eradicating polio, by the mid-1960s the battle for supremacy was over. Albert Sabin was the new victor and the new polio hero. The development of the Salk and Sabin vaccines and their introduction and use in Australia to prevent further epidemics of polio occurring have been crucially important for the people's health. However, those immunisation levels must be maintained to prevent another outbreak. The epidemic that occurred in the 1960s was a warning that vigilance on the part of authorities is essential.[982]

For those who have never suffered from the disease, polio has been consigned to the history books. Amid the victories and bitter controversies that accompanied the search for a vaccine to prevent polio, the lives of those who were affected by contracting the disease and their families has sometimes been forgotten.

For the survivors of polio, that story needed to be told.

Chapter 9

POLIO: RETROSPECT AND PROSPECT

In the excitement generated by the discovery by Jonas Salk of a vaccine to prevent polio, memories of Elizabeth Kenny and her controversial method of treating polio paralysis gradually faded. Because of the relationship and interaction between the conflicting principles of treatment, it is difficult to evaluate how widespread the use of the Kenny treatment became in the United States. Many hospitals incorporated selected aspects of the Kenny treatment — for example, the use of hot packs in the early, acute phase of the disease, but rejected others. Some used modified splinting, but never to the extent of the full body plaster cases of the 1930s.

Traditional orthopaedic treatment for those affected by polio in the 1930s and '40s recommended bed rest with the muscles kept in a neutral position, 'a point midway between the extremes of movement', by the use of extensive splinting.[983] Treatment in Australia up to the mid-1950s remained largely unchanged, with a period of immobilisation of 'two to six months for mild cases, and up to twenty-two months for the more severe ones'.[984]

Dr Jean Macnamara of Victoria was acknowledged as the authority on polio treatment in Australia, and she was convinced that maintaining the conventional treatment was the only way to prevent deformities developing. Adults were to be kept in the 'optimum posture position' by plaster of Paris splints and wood or wire outlines, and she believed that the natural activity of children was better 'controlled' or 'rationed' by the double Thomas splint. Uppermost in her mind were two factors. The first was the need to rescue children from entering the 'cripple factory' by treating childhood 'chassis' problems like knock-knees, flat feet and curved backs with corrective splints. Secondly, she believed that 'the salvage of the potential cripple' would be expedited if a physiotherapist were to treat children as soon as the problem was detected.

Macnamara believed that the American surgeon Robert Lovett had been correct when he published his views in 1917 about the treatment of polio, and that his judgement remained valid thirty years later: 'The number of cases in which recovery is to be obtained is very greatly extended by keeping the patients from walking during the first year, and in many cases during the second year'.[985]

Sister Elizabeth Kenny challenged the conventional rehabilitation approach and taught that treatment should be introduced during the acute phase of polio, and that splinting was to be avoided. She believed that the practice of immobilising muscles increased contractures and paralysis by 'alienating' or isolating muscles from the thought process. Kenny maintained that if a patient could neither feel nor see a limb they would forget about it and how to move it.[986] In her later years, Kenny refused to draw a distinction between her treatment method and her theory of the aetiology of polio. Kenny maintained that flaccid muscles were normal and that those affected by the poliovirus experienced spasm that caused them to shorten and pull the affected limb or part into an unnatural and deformed position. For Kenny, acceptance of her treatment had to signal acceptance of her theory, and she refused to accede to the requests of many of her supporters that she separate the two.

Italy ceased the use of plaster casts in 1940, and in France patients were supported in bed by sandbags. In 1952, Dr Douglas Galbraith of Victoria declared that he 'deplored the previous custom of confining a child to a frame for long periods' and that, in his opinion, such immobilisation produced not only 'deformities of the body but also of the mind'.[987] By 1954, Canada, New Zealand, Scandinavia and the United States of America used either Kenny's or a combination of both forms of treatment. In 1954, Professor Zanoli summed up what he saw as the then current position on polio treatment:

> Moist heat as used in the method employed by Sister Kenny should be started in the acute, febrile stage and before any passive exercise is commenced. Because contractures occur very early, it is necessary to commence passive movements of limbs four or five days after the onset of the disease. Patients should not be immobilized but supported in bed by sandbags or similar and their position should be changed frequently throughout the day including lying prone in an anterior or posterior position.[988]

Despite this, practitioners in Australia, Brazil and Puerto Rico continued to immobilise patients with polio, a treatment that was later described in the

Journal of the American Medical Association as 'an abuse of rest'.[989] Not one patient in the 1937–38 epidemic in Australia was treated with hot packs in the acute stage of the disease and, even as late as 1954, medical practitioners continued to advocate complete bed rest:

> All active or passive muscular movement should not only be avoided but forbidden for up to six weeks, and the patient not allowed to lift even a finger to do anything for himself. This must be stressed on patients, sisters and nurses. Morphia, phenobarbital, potassium bromide, or chloral should be given — if necessary all of them, or combinations of the same for up to six weeks.[990]

In 1993, the American orthopaedic surgeon Leonard Peltier concluded, in contrast, that Kenny's method of treatment remained 'the best available today'.[991]

Some thirty to forty years after they first contracted polio, some survivors have experienced muscle pain, tiredness and increasing weakness of previously paralysed limbs. The condition, known as post-polio syndrome (PPS), appears more common in females than males, with the hips and back being the parts of the body most commonly affected. Many have had to be refitted for braces, or use a cane for walking; some have had to resort to using a wheelchair again, or a motorised scooter. Many survivors have been frustrated by the attitude of their medical practitioners, especially a tendency 'to discount the reality of their symptoms', glossing over them with patronising explanations like, 'empty nest syndrome, laziness, sexual frustration, nerves, boredom, all in your mind'.[992] The sheer numbers of polio survivors requiring braces or crutches, or who are dependent on wheelchairs, has encouraged the development of lighter, more effective and manoeuvrable devices. New rehabilitation techniques have evolved to strengthen muscles and restore function. Two of the major changes over the past seventy years have been society's more enlightened attitude to the disabled, and the social class of those affected by the disease. The polio survivor today is more likely to be poor and socially disadvantaged than was the case in the twentieth century.

The impact of medical science in the first half of the twentieth century was prodigious; diphtheria immunisation with toxoid in the 1920s, sulphonamides in 1933, and antimalarials and penicillin in the 1940s. Many years passed before scientists discovered the mode of transmission of polio: the epidemiological pattern was complex, and communication with other researchers working in the same field was slow. Today, we live in a world of rapid communication and exchange of ideas, along with unparalleled access to information. It is difficult to imagine a time when important discoveries or clues to the mode of transmission of the poliovirus could lie hidden on a researcher's desk or locked away in a filing cabinet, or of a period when postal services were frustratingly slow, and letters and items were often lost or misplaced. An age when libraries used card catalogues that had to be painstakingly flicked through, the checking of cross-references and bibliographic details for papers was tedious and time-consuming, and scientific and medical journals containing published results from other workers in the polio field took many weeks to make the journey to and from Australia. In 1948, epidemiologists continued to remain sceptical about their ability to state exactly how the poliovirus was transmitted from person to person, but believed they had narrowed it down to three possibilities: that polio spread by direct contact between people; by faecal contamination of food, milk or water; or by insects.[993] Five years later, the epidemiology of polio was clearer, and scientists had concluded that the disease spread from person to person through traces of faecal contamination remaining on hands or fingers. They were also aware that countries with higher standards of living were experiencing epidemics of increasing frequency and severity, and that the disease was now more prevalent in older age groups than in children under five.[994]

The discovery in 1952 that there was a transient, viraemic stage when the poliovirus was present in the circulating bloodstream signalled to scientists that development of a vaccine was possible. From 1911 to 1963, 30,977 cases of paralytic polio were notified to public health authorities in Australia. Experts have calculated that the ratio of carriers or asymptomatic cases of polio to those who developed paralytic polio varies between 100:1 to 1000:1.[995] Extrapolating this to 1951 (Australia's worst year for polio) when 4940 cases of paralytic polio were notified to authorities, means that, in a population of approximately eight million Australians, there may have been up to 494,000 carriers of poliovirus.[996] This changed in 1956, when the introduction of the Salk polio vaccine into Australia led to a dramatic reduction in the number of people with the disease. Between them, the Salk and Sabin vaccines have eliminated polio caused by wild poliovirus, which no longer circulates within the Australian population.[997]

The story that had begun with the isolation of the poliovirus by Landsteiner and Popper in 1908 was expected to conclude with the global eradication of polio in the year 2000. Unfortunately, although the Western Hemisphere was certified free of wild poliovirus in the late 1980s, the virus remains endemic in areas of South Asia and Sub-Saharan Africa. It is imperative that high levels of immunity within the population be maintained by vaccination with the inactivated polio vaccine (IPV), because it is impossible to eliminate wild poliovirus importation, especially by 'carrier' or asymptomatic members of the population. Vaccination of infants and children is the only way to establish and maintain population immunity against polio.[998] Because polio has been eliminated in many Western countries, many in the population have become complacent about immunisation, evidenced by an increasing number of parents who choose not to have themselves or their children vaccinated against polio and other diseases.[999]

Why does the idea of vaccinating their children trigger such anxiety in many people? Australians no longer have first-hand experience of polio, and some in the community now focus on the alleged dangers of the vaccines themselves rather than on the diseases they prevent. Vaccine production is one of our more rigorously regulated industries, but vaccines have been blamed for causing everything from allergies to autism: 'A low incidence of polio in a population (caused in large part by successful vaccination programs) makes the maintenance of high vaccination levels difficult, especially in the face of questioning or negative media attention'.[1000]

Periodically, the anti-vaccination lobbyists gain centre stage in the media and their often misguided views and conspiracy theories reach a wide selection of the community, thus playing on public fears. Vaccine-induced paralysis has occurred, and has been devastating for those affected, but the incidence has been very low with the OPV (Sabin) vaccine — just one in 750,000.[1001]

The problem is viewed so seriously that, in 2008, authorities in Belgium fined and jailed two sets of parents for failing to vaccinate their children against polio.[1002] Scare campaigns can have lasting effects. Whooping cough vaccination was halted in Japan in the mid-1970s because of 'public concerns over adverse neurological effects'[1003] and, in 1979, an epidemic appeared, with over 13,000 cases reported and forty-one deaths. In Nigeria in 2003, vaccinations with Sabin vaccine came to a halt when Sharia government officials claimed that the vaccine was spreading HIV and was a Western plot to sterilise and kill Muslims. As a consequence, an epidemic of polio erupted within Nigeria and spread rapidly into neighbouring countries.[1004]

The concept of herd immunity is a complex issue. The simple definition is the proportion of individuals with immunity in a given population. Herd immunity extends the protection imparted by an immunisation program beyond the vaccinated, to unvaccinated individuals. However, herd immunity is not the same as the immunological immunity acquired by vaccination. Individuals protected by indirect herd immunity remain fully susceptible to infection should they be exposed to the poliovirus.

Preventing an outbreak of epidemic polio depends on maintaining a high level of immunity within the population. If that level drops, and there is an accumulation of susceptible individuals in the population, then the threat of an outbreak from importation of wild poliovirus becomes a distinct possibility. Asymptomatic carriers of poliovirus can shed the virus in faeces for weeks after infection and are considered the primary source in an epidemic.

A 2003 NSW Public Health report concluded that although there had been an improvement in immunisation coverage, in an area in northern New South Wales around Lismore and Byron Bay the level of conscientious objection to immunisation was high enough to allow outbreaks of disease (e.g. measles) to occur.[1005] In March 2007, a 22-year-old Pakistani studying in Australia returned to his home for a holiday. While in Pakistan he became ill with nausea and flu-like symptoms, and noticed some weakness in one of his legs. Despite not feeling well, he boarded Thai Airways flight TG999 and arrived back in Melbourne via Bangkok on 2 July. The following day he felt increasing pain and weakness in his lower limbs and was admitted to Box Hill Hospital in eastern Melbourne on 6 July. Initially, polio was not suspected because of his age and the fact that he had received three doses of Sabin vaccine as a child, but he had not received a booster polio vaccination before travelling to his homeland where polio is endemic. Polio was diagnosed after Magnetic Resonance Imaging (MRI) scan revealed the classic changes of the disease in the anterior horn region of his spinal cord, and the patient was isolated and moved to a single room.[1006] Half the passengers on flight TG999 have been traced and given booster shots of polio vaccine, but over one hundred could not be contacted. Those airline passengers have indeed been fortunate to not contract polio, for the student on board with them was infectious, and spreading wild poliovirus.[1007]

Polio was indeed the most feared of the childhood diseases. The unpredictability of the epidemic outbreaks, the suddenness with which the disease struck, the severe and painful symptoms, and the possibility of long-lasting paralysis and disability increased levels of anxiety within communities, particularly among parents. Thousands died in the worldwide polio epidemics, and thousands more were left with permanent paralysis. It is difficult to estimate the recovery rate of those paralysed with the virus but, in the United States, Donald Neumann proposed: 'Roughly 10% to 40%

of persons recovered full muscle strength; the remaining 60% to 90% were left with varying degrees of residual paralysis, typically ranging from near total paralysis and subsequent death to only isolated paralysis of selected muscles'.[1008]

The student from Pakistan was fortunate; his exposure to the poliovirus left him with no paralysis. If he had suffered respiratory paralysis, then the treatment would have been exactly the same as forty years ago: he would have been placed in a respirator. There remains no cure for polio. The polio epidemics of the twentieth century have led to improvements in rehabilitative medicine and in the care of the acutely ill patient suffering from respiratory distress. Iron lungs have evolved into smaller, more efficient ventilation devices, and biochemists have developed diagnostic tests to monitor potentially life-threatening changes in body chemistry.

The transformation of Australian society by the influx of postwar immigrants, the counterculture movements of the 1960s and resistance to all forms of authority, including medical, introduced Australians to alternative health therapies. By the 1980s, a visit to the acupuncturist, chiropractor, osteopath or herbal or Chinese medicine provider was no longer viewed as unusual, and bolstered confidence in other members of the population to reject the view of those who advocated Western medicine as the only option. Today, many orthodox-trained medical practitioners are not opposed to alternative medicine, rather they are sympathetic and receptive to developing a discourse about the two forms of therapy, and appreciate the potential for the combined use of the two forms of healing. Patients themselves have done much to initiate the process because of their choice to seek advice and care from both orthodox and non-orthodox medicine.

Mainstream practitioners in the 1930s and '40s criticised Elizabeth Kenny's approach to diagnosis as haphazard; however, she based her diagnosis on observed signs and symptoms, albeit ones that did not fall within the acknowledged orthodox framework. Kenny believed that the paralysis that sometimes followed polio was as a result of 'mental alienation' and she called her treatment 'muscle re-education'. None of these terms appeared in the medical texts of the day. The history of medicine had traditionally neglected the experience of the patient, who was viewed with increasing objectivity, and the disease process in the body was separated from the sentient being. Kenny encouraged her patients to remain autonomous, to retain agency over their bodies, to work with her and her staff to help train muscles to respond and be retrained. This relationship was far removed from accepted medical practice of the time where the active care-giver delivered medical treatment to the passive care-receiver. Kenny's methods of treatment evolved through trial and error, and they were modified and improved from working with her patients. Her treatment methods were an example of evidence-based medicine.

For Elizabeth Kenny, the relationship between mind and body was paramount. She responded not only to the effects of the poliovirus on the paralysed body but also to the experience of the illness on the sufferer's life and what gave that life meaning. Orthodox medicine, in contrast, tended to be autocratic and draconian. Images of individuals encased in plaster casts and strapped to frames or papoose boards gave the impression that medicine was in control of the wayward body.

Elizabeth Kenny was a true reformer, pursuing her goal of revolutionising polio care with tenacity and strength of purpose. Largely self-taught, she readily absorbed medical facts about muscle development and function, and craved recognition of her newly acquired prowess. However, she was, at times, her own worst enemy. During her lifetime, Kenny managed to conceal everything she wished to conceal, and allowed her own history to begin with her enlistment in the First World War but, following her death, not all her secrets remained secrets. In contrast to the marginalisation of women in the early twentieth century within mainstream medicine, women were a dominant force in the field of physiotherapy. Kenny's alienation of physiotherapists was a grave error of judgement, for the physiotherapist gained professional recognition and respect in the male-dominated world of medicine far earlier than nurses. Many physicians readily accepted the value of physiotherapy in treating paralysis, yet hotly contested the relevance of Kenny's method. According to Jean Macnamara, Kenny's greatest contribution to poliomyelitis treatment was that:

> Miss [sic] Kenny has been able to use the power of the Press as no doctor would have been allowed to do, to make governments and public realize that an epidemic of poliomyelitis calls for the expenditure of public money … all paralysed people and those caring for them are greatly indebted to Miss Kenny.[1009]

Macnamara also credited 'Miss Kenny' with 'drawing attention to the harm which follows the practice of confining patients in splints', but added the rider, 'in institutions which, through staff difficulties, could not arrange for movements to be carried out at intervals short enough to ensure first attainment and then maintenance of a normal range of joint movements'.[1010] In my opinion, physiotherapists could have proved to be her greatest ally in the struggle to gain accreditation for her method of treatment, if only she had been less defensive and more open to questions about her method. In her obituary of Kenny in the *Physical Therapy Review*, Mildred Elson recalled Kenny as a 'very warm person' with a 'mischievous sense of humour', as someone patients loved for 'her kindness, reassuring manner, and skilful hands'. In her opinion, Kenny's treatment had 'stimulated everyone to do a better job' of treating polio patients and, because of this, the patient had benefitted.[1011]

During the polio epidemics, the entrenched political and cultural power of organised, mainstream medicine denied Australian citizens the right to choose how their paralysed bodies were treated. There were good people on both sides of the debate of how best to treat the body paralysed by the poliovirus. They happened to believe different things, and some of them made mistakes. In the end the advocates of new methods and those who opposed them both conceded some ground. Kenny's concept of treatment was not fully integrated with the mainstream but rather the two treatment methods began to complement each other rather than their proponents engaging in a war for supremacy. Regrettably, the armistice came too late for most Australian polio survivors.

ANNEX

Table 1. Median poliomyelitis incidence per 100,000 population

Country	1926–1930	1931–1935	1936–1940	1941–1945	1946–1950	1951–1953
Australia	3.70	5.70	14.10	4.60	15.30	32.30
Asia	0	0	0	0	0.75	0.75
Canada	6.60	6.40	9.90	6.70	14.30	35.90
Denmark	2.40	30.40	10.70	25.00	16.90	59.90
France	1.10	1.20	1.00	2.20	3.50	3.90
Latin America	0	0	0	0	1.70	4.10
Sweden	8.00	5.80	23.90	27.20	20.70	28.50
Switzerland	3.60	4.90	0	19.80	14.30	15.50
UK	3.90	1.60	2.40	1.60	11.10	8.90
USA	4.90	6.90	5.00	8.80	19.10	26.00

Source: World Health Organization, in *Proceedings of the Third International Poliomyelitis Conference*, Rome, 1954

Annex

Table 2. Cases of poliomyelitis reported by state and territory of Australia

Year	NSW	Vic	Qld	SA	WA	Tas	ACT	NT	Australia
1911	0	0	0	0	0	0	0	0	0
1912	0	0	5	0	0	3	0	0	8
1913	47	0	38	0	8	4	0	0	97
1914	79	0	6	0	0	0	0	0	85
1915	63	0	332	0	0	0	0	0	395
1916	311	76	27	0	19	3	0	0	436
1917	16	32	37	0	2	3	0	0	90
1918	50	303	13	0	4	14	0	0	384
1919	8	2	119	0	2	5	0	0	136
1920	45	5	17	0	8	1	0	0	76
1921	184	27	35	0	1	1	0	0	248
1922	33	23	25	47	0	1	0	0	129
1923	104	7	1	17	8	3	0	0	140
1924	108	12	112	0	3	3	0	0	238
1925	50	139	39	13	19	1	0	0	261
1926	78	31	42	2	13	3	0	0	169
1930	30	86	5	15	4	129	1		270
1931	87	269	34	37	0	9	0		436
1932	380	25	275	19	2	4	1	0	706
1933	16	16	12	14	3	1	0	0	62
1934	91	178	19	4	5	32	0	0	329
1935	181	64	22	18	7	8	1	0	301
1936	24	7	11	6	4	0	0	0	52
1937	70	1469	20	85	6	331	0	0	1981
1938	692	742	159	284	5	704	3	1	2590
1939	31	43	25	4	5	0	0	0	108
1940	11	19	44	63	2	0	0	0	139
1941	90	56	87	1	6	2	0		242
1942	42	27	9	3	18	8	0	0	107

Year	NSW	Vic	Qld	SA	WA	Tas	ACT	NT	Australia
1943	25	13	8	3	16	1	0	0	66
1944	14	9	7	2	4	4	0	0	40
1945	668	238	299	9	5	4	3	0	1226
1946	656	247	149	62	2	98	5	0	1219
1947	83	126	19	55	2	1	2	0	288
1948	91	56	37	89	311	7	1	1	593
1949	197	759	28	582	62	34	5	0	1667
1950	789	202	106	972	59	51	27	0	2206
1951	1608	430	1108	1488	100	177	10	19	4940
1952	394	306	166	721	41	97	1	12	1738
1953	630	284	207	398	44	112	1	1	1677
1954	555	569	134	176	436	10	26	0	1906
1955	222	235	190	182	33	7	1	4	874
1956	240	251	112	122	401	55	13	0	1194
1957	58	13	24	16	8	6	0	0	125
1958	23	60	5	10	2	0	0	0	100
1959	16	30	6	1	3	0	0	0	56
1960	9	24	5	10	4	36	0	17	105
1961	201	50	141	44	2	11	0	1	450
1962	177	20	38	17	4	0	2	1	259
1963	2	19	1	7	4	0	0	0	33
Total	9579	7599	4360	5598	1697	1984	103	57	30977

Source: Compiled by the author from Reports of the Director General of Health, Commonwealth of Australia for the years 1915–1963

NOTES

Chapter 1

1. See, for example, J.R. Paul, *A History of Poliomyelitis*; J.H.L. Cumpston, *Health and Disease in Australia: A History*; F. Fenner, *History of Microbiology in Australia*; J.S. Smith, *Patenting the Sun: Polio and the Salk Vaccine*; S. Benison, *Tom Rivers: Reflections on a Life in Medicine*; T.M. Rivers, 'The Story of Research on Poliomyelitis', *Proceedings of the American Philosophical Society*, pp.250–54; A.H. Brogan, *Committed to Saving Lives: A History of the Commonwealth Serum Laboratories*; F. Macfarlane Burnet, *Changing Patterns: An Atypical Autobiography*; F. Macfarlane Burnet and D.O. White, *Natural History of Infectious Disease*; F. Macfarlane Burnet, 'A Review of Poliomyelitis', *Medical Journal of Australia*, vol.2, no.14 (1952) p.482.

2. Some exceptions include works by F.B. Smith, 'The Victorian Poliomyelitis Epidemic 1937–1938' (Paper); J.H. Smith, 'Fear, Frustation and the Will to Overcome' (PhD thesis); J.R. Wilson, *Through Kenny's Eyes*; A. Killalea, *The Great Scourge*; A.J.G. Buxton, 'Poliomyelitis in South Australia 1937–1956' (BA Hons thesis); and K. Highley, 'For want of a Cake of Soap and a Towel' (BA Hons thesis); with chapters in larger works by P. Martyr, 'The Professional Development of Rehabilitation in Australia 1870–1981' (PhD thesis); and C. Thame, 'Health and the State' (PhD thesis).

3. E. Ford, *Bibliography of Australian Medicine 1790–1900*; J.H.L. Cumpston, 'Anterior Poliomyelitis', in *Health and Disease in Australia*; AGPS, Canberra, 1989, pp.326–328.

4. See Commissioner of Health reports for the years 1914–1961, for example, Department of Public Health Queensland, 'Annual Statement of Notifiable Diseases During Calendar Year'; Department of Public Health New South Wales, 'Notification of Infectious Diseases'; Commonwealth of Australia, 'Public Health and Related Institutions'; A. Killalea, *The Great Scourge*, p.134. The WHO believed that the incidence rates reported that included non-paralytic cases of polio were not polio but another disease.

5. A.M. Payne, 'Poliomyelitis as a World Problem' (Paper), pp.397–99.

6. Dr Marcia Falconer, a Canadian virologist, has estimated that between one and two million Australians were infected with the poliovirus between 1930 and 1960. Paralytic cases were approximately 1-5% and the number of subclinical cases estimated between four and eight million. M. Falconer, 'Spectrum of Polio Infection Effects in Australian Population', *Post-Polio Network (NSW) Inc. Network News*, p.5.

7. W.W.C. Topley, et al, *Principles of Bacteriology, Virology and Immunity*; F. Fenner, *History of Microbiology in Australia*; F. Macfarlane Burnet and D.O. White, *Natural History of Infectious Disease*; J.A. Anderson, 'Diagnosis and Treatment of Poliomyelitis

in the Early Stage' (Paper); W.T. Greene, 'The Management of Poliomyelitis' (Paper); I. McQuarrie, 'The Evolution of Signs and Symptoms of Poliomyelitis' (Paper).

8   Several histories of Australia's specialist hospitals were read during the writing of this book. Most apposite were W.K. Anderson, *Fever Hospital: A History of Fairfield Infectious Diseases Hospital*; P. Yule, *The Royal Children's Hospital: A History of Faith, Science and Love*; A. Gregory, *The Ever Open Door: A History of the Royal Melbourne Hospital 1848–1998*; and J. McCalman, *Sex and Suffering: Women's Health and a Women's Hospital: The Royal Women's Hospital, Melbourne*.

9   Defined as 'Various social, economic and cultural forces, and scientific and technical events (from antibiotics to open-heart surgery) that have operated to effect the partial suppression of medical pluralism, both actual and historical.' R. Cooter and Society for the Social History of Medicine, *Studies in the History of Alternative Medicine*, pxiii.

10 J. Templeton, *Prince Henry's: The Evolution of a Melbourne Hospital 1869–1969*.

11 R. Numbers, 'Physicians, Community and the Qualified Ascent of the American Medical Profession', in *Major Problems in the History of American Medicine and Public Health*, eds J.H. Warner and J.A. Tighe, p.302.

12 E. Willis, *Medical Dominance*, p.73.

13 See, for example, J.R. Wilson, *Through Kenny's Eyes*, p.12; C. Thame, 'Health and the State' (PhD thesis), p.205; E. Willis, 'Sister Elizabeth Kenny and the Evolution of the Occupational Division of Labour in Health Care', *Australian and New Zealand Journal of Sociology*, pp.30–38; P. Martyr, 'A Small Price to Pay for Peace', *Australian Historical Studies*, pp.47–65; M. Denton, 'Further Comments on the Elizabeth Kenny Controversy', *Australian Historical Studies*, pp.152–58.

14 Poliomyelitis has been known by several names, but all versions are associated with a disease that manifests as a flaccid, or drooping, paralysis of the limbs. Scientists use poliomyelitis to refer to the invasion of the grey matter of the spinal cord by the poliovirus. The disease primarily affected young children in the nineteenth century and was known as infantile paralysis, while 'polio' became the more common term used in the twentieth century.

15 N. Rogers, *Dirt and Disease*.

16 A.M. Payne, 'Poliomyelitis as a World Problem' (Paper), p.396.

17 F. Macfarlane Burnet, 'The Epidemiology of Poliomyelitis with Special Reference to the Victorian Epidemic of 1937–1938', *Medical Journal of Australia*, pp.325–35.

18 F.B. Smith, *Florence Nightingale*, p.160.

19 See, for example, N. Rogers, *Dirt and Disease*, chapter 1; J.R. Paul, *A History of Poliomyelitis*, chapters 15 and 21.

20 A.D. King, *Buildings and Society*, p.78.

21 Some general works on the epidemiology of polio are: P. Lépine, 'Epidemiology and Pathogenesis of Poliomyelitis: Present State of the Problem' (Paper); J.R. Paul, 'Future Prospects' (Paper); A.M. Payne, 'Poliomyelitis as a World Problem' (Paper); J.R. Paul, *A History of Poliomyelitis*. Miasma theories are covered in, among others: F.B. Smith, *Florence Nightingale*; and C.E. Rosenberg, 'Florence Nightingale on Contagion', in *Healing and History*, ed. C.E. Rosenberg.

22 E. Willis, *Medical Dominance*.

23 W. Anderson, *The Cultivation of Whiteness*, p.168; G.R. Searle, 'Eugenics and Politics in Britain in the 1930s"; *Annals of Science*, pp.159–69; P.M. Bachelard, 'Can We Diagnose Feeble-Mindedness in Children?' *Australasian Journal of Philosophy*, pp.120–30; H.T. Lovell, 'The Tasmanian Mental Deficiency Act', *Australasian Journal of Philosophy*, pp.285–89; G. Jones, 'Eugenics and Social Policy between the Wars',

The Historical Journal, pp.717–28; M. Cawte, 'Craniometry and Eugenics in Australia: R.J.A. Berry and the Quest for Social Efficiency'; *Historical Studies*, pp.35–53.

24 The most valuable for the American and British context were D.J. Wilson, *Living with Polio*; J. Silver and D.J. Wilson, eds, *Polio Voices;* and T. Gould, *A Summer Plague*.

25 Elizabeth Kenny Papers, Minnesota Historical Society, St Paul.

26 A. Portelli maintained, 'Oral narrators have within their culture certain aids to memory. Many stories are told over and over, or discussed with members of community; formalised narrative, even meter, may help preserve a textual version of an event'. A. Portelli, 'What Makes Oral History Different', in *The Oral History Reader*, eds R. Perks and A. Thomson, p.69.

27 Examples of the printed polio narratives consulted for this book are: M. Liethof, *Your Stories* (Polio Perspectives); and *Post-Polio Post* at www.post-polionetwork.org.au/news/ppn48.html; C.L. Mee, *A Nearly Normal Life*; A. Marshall, *I Can Jump Puddles*; N. Lawes-Gilvear, *Living with Polio*; T. Gould, *A Summer Plague*; A. Finger, *Elegy for a Disease*; K. Black, *In the Shadow of Polio*; V. Overheu, *It Helps to Be Stubborn*; J. Clarke, *All on One Good Dancing Leg*.

Chapter 2

28 Nita Lawes-Gilvear, *Living with Polio*, pp.20–24.

29 B. Nicholls, 'Polio Days', *Time Frame*, ABC Radio.

30 Richard Owen. D.J. Wilson, *Living with Polio*, p.21.

31 G. Buchanan, 'I Used to Jump Puddles', *Polio NSW*, no. 7, pp.2-5 www.polionsw.org.au/wp-content/uploads/2012/01/Gary-Buchanan-I-used-to-Jump-Puddles.pdf

32 Katherine Pappas. J. Silver and D.J. Wilson, eds, *Polio Voices*, p.22.

33 P. Solomon, 'Living in a Country Town', no. 8, *Member Stories* (Post-Polio Network). http://www.post-polionetwork.org.au/stories/coonabrabran.html

34 C. Bernstein, 'Mazzy Meets the Dragon', no. 3, *Member Stories* (Post-Polio Network). http://www.post-polionetwork.org.au/stories/dragon.html

35 J.C. Ross, 'A History of Poliomyelitis in New Zealand' (MA thesis), pp.36–37.

36 Malnutrition was common, especially in poorer areas, and if a child survived its first four years, it had a good chance of reaching adulthood. www.aihw.gov.au/publications/phe/motca/motca.pdf. Accessed 3 March 2009.

37 Dr Jeffreys Wood quoted in P. Yule, *The Royal Children's Hospital*, p.114.

38 Interview William Wesson (Fairfield Hospital Archives).

39 Pseudonym. Patient interview (Fairfield Hospital Archives).

40 Unfortunately, the mother's medical history has been removed from the Fairfield Hospital Archives. (Author's observation.)

41 Interview Geoff Golding (Fairfield Hospital Archives). Although polio survivors in North America, Canada and the United Kingdom refer to the respirator as the 'iron lung', in Australia the more common usage was either the 'tank' or the 'box'.

42 Sulphonamide tablets made by May and Baker.

43 Interview Vern Draffin (Fairfield Hospital Archives).

44 A raised temperature. J.H. Smith, 'Fear, Frustration and the Will to Overcome' (PhD thesis), p.363.

45 Interview Ron Gillam (Fairfield Hospital Archives).

46 In the 1930s, serum treatment advocated by Dr Jean Macnamara was based on an interpretation of the results of the examination of spinal fluid. A raised count of

leucocytes (white cells) was interpreted as a positive diagnosis for polio, despite the fact that other infections, e.g., bacterial meningitis gave similar results.

47   Interview B., J.H. Smith, 'Fear, Frustration and the Will to Overcome' (PhD thesis), pp.363–64.
48   Interview K., J.H. Smith, 'Fear, Frustration and the Will to Overcome' (PhD thesis), p.365.
49   Interview H., J.H. Smith, 'Fear, Frustration and the Will to Overcome' (PhD thesis), p.365.
50   Interview H., J.H. Smith, 'Fear, Frustration and the Will to Overcome' (PhD thesis), p.365.
51   J. Silver and D.J. Wilson, eds, *Polio Voices*, p.54.
52   Kenny Institute 50th Anniversary, Patient Letters, 1991–1992, Elizabeth Kenny Papers, Minnesota Historical Society, St Paul, Minnesota (hereafter MHS-K).
53   A. Marshall, *I Can Jump Puddles*, p.2.
54   D.J. Wilson, *Living with Polio*, p.20.
55   David Widgery. T. Gould, *A Summer Plague*, p.229.
56   Mary McInerney to Sister Kenny (n.d), Complimentary letters and parents' appreciation, undated and 1942–1949, MHS-K.
57   F.B. Smith, 'The Victorian Poliomyelitis Epidemic 1937–1938' (Paper), p.8.
58   R. Aronowitz, 'From Myalgic Encephalitis to Yuppie Flu', in *Framing Disease*, eds C.E. Rosenberg and J. Golden, p.159.
59   Interview D., J.H. Smith, 'Fear, Frustration and the Will to Overcome' (PhD thesis), p.388
60   Interview D., J.H. Smith, 'Fear, Frustration and the Will to Overcome' (PhD thesis), p.388.
61   A. Killalea, *The Great Scourge*, p.98.
62   A.J.G. Buxton, 'Poliomyelitis in South Australia 1937–1956' (BA Hons thesis), p.27; A. Killalea, *The Great Scourge*, pp.98.
63   T. Gould, *A Summer Plague*, pp.20–21.
64   See chapter 8.
65   Mrs C. Boag, Bundaberg to Earle Page (n.d.). Correspondence Relating to Diseases – Poliomyelitis, General. Inquiries and Ministerial Representations 1955–1957, A1658/1, 259/1/2 Part 2 (National Archives of Australia).
66   For historical studies dealing with the history of polio in Australia see, for example, A.J.G. Buxton, 'Poliomyelitis in South Australia 1937–1956' (BA Hons thesis); R.G.B. Cameron, 'Observations on Poliomyelitis of Epidemiological Interest', *Medical Journal of Australia*, p.705; J.H.L. Cumpston, *Health and Disease in Australia*; D.G. Galbraith, 'A Review of Poliomyelitis', *Medical Journal of Australia*, vol.2, no.14 (1952) p.483; K. Highley, 'For Want of a Cake of Soap and a Towel (BA Hons thesis); J. Macnamara, 'Treatment of Poliomyelitis During the Acute and Convalescent Phase', *Medical Journal of Australia* II, No.9, 1928. J. Macnamara, 'The Care of the Paralysis of Poliomyelitis', *Medical Journal of Australia*, pp.577–80; F.B. Smith, 'The Victorian Poliomyelitis Epidemic 1937–1938' (Paper); J.H. Smith, 'Fear, Frustration and the Will to Overcome' (PhD thesis); C. Thame, 'Health and the State' (PhD thesis).
67   F. Macfarlane Burnet, *Changing Patterns*, p.171.
68   A. Marshall, *I Can Jump Puddles*, p.9.
69   Kenny Institute 50th Anniversary, Patient Letters, 1991–1992. MHS-K.

70 M. Ashton, 'Polio Revisited after Half a Century of Peace', 2006. www.paraquad.asn.au/services/info/Polio/Vol15No4.pdf Accessed March 2007.
71 F. Davis, *Passage through Crisis*, pp.29–30.
72 J.M. Swann, *Your Stories*, Polio Network of Victoria, Autumn 2002, p.10.
73 Kenny Institute 50th Anniversary, Patient Letters, 1991–1992. MHS-K
74 G. Buchanan, 'I Used to Jump Puddles', no. 7, *Personal Polio Stories*, Post-Polio Network (NSW).
75 F. Davis, *Passage through Crisis*, pp.30–32.
76 Interview Geoff Golding (Fairfield Hospital Archives).
77 Interview of the parents of Elaine Theodore (Fairfield Hospital Archives).
78 Dr Robert Blute. J. Silver and D.J. Wilson, eds, *Polio Voices*, p.87.
79 Pseudonym. Patient interview (Fairfield Hospital Archives).
80 Interview J., J.H. Smith, 'Fear, Frustration and the Will to Overcome' (PhD thesis), p.389.
81 J. Silver and D.J. Wilson, eds, *Polio Voices*. p.27.
82 J. Silver and D.J. Wilson, eds, *Polio Voices*, p.26.
83 Judith Willemy. J. Silver and D.J. Wilson, eds, *Polio Voices*, p.26.
84 Leonard Kriegel. D.J. Wilson, *Living with Polio*, p.31.
85 L. Medlyn-White, *Your Stories*, Polio Network of Victoria, Summer 2005, p.11.
86 G. Thomas ed., 'A Story to Break the Silence', no. 45, Post-Polio Newsletter, Post-Polio Network (NSW). www.post-polionetwork.org.au/news/ppn45.html
87 N.G. Seavey, et al, *A Paralyzing Fear*, p.119.
88 C.L. Mee, *A Nearly Normal Life*, p.17.
89 C.L. Mee, *A Nearly Normal Life*, p.18.
90 N. Lawes-Gilvear, *Living with Polio*, p.24.
91 M.W.R. Davis, F.C. Robbins and T.M. Daniel, *Polio*, p.28.
92 N. Rogers, 'Silence Has Its Own Stories: Elizabeth Kenny, Polio and the Culture of Medicine', *Social History of Medicine*, Vol. 21, No.1, p.147.
93 Emily Donohue, New York State. J. Silver and D.J. Wilson, eds, *Polio Voices*, p.69.
94 Val Heath, *Your Stories*, Post-Polio Network of Victoria, Winter 2006, p.10.
95 G. Buchanan, 'I Used to Jump Puddles', no. 7, *Personal Polio Stories*, Post-Polio Network (NSW).

Chapter 3

96 Gillian Thomas ed., 'A Story to Break the Silence', Post-Polio Network, No. 45. www.post-polionetwork.org.au/news/ppn45.html
97 A. Gregory, *The Ever Open Door*, p.87.
98 M. Foucault, *The Birth of the Clinic*, pp.54–55.
99 B.S. Turner, *Medical Power and Social Knowledge*, p.209.
100 For readings on Australia's hospitals, see, for example, K. Inglis, *Hospital and Community: A History of the Royal Melbourne Hospital*; A. Gregory, *The Ever Open Door: A History of the Royal Melbourne Hospital 1848–1998*; J. McCalman, *Sex and Suffering: Women's Health and a Women's Hospital: The Royal Women's Hospital, Melbourne*; W.K. Anderson, *Fever Hospital: A History of Fairfield Infectious Diseases Hospital*; A. Hyslop, *Sovereign Remedies: A History of Ballarat Base Hospital, 1850s*

to 1980s; C.R. Boughton, *A Coast Chronicle: The History of the Prince Henry Hospital*; A.M. Mitchell and Alfred Hospital Melbourne, *The Hospital South of the Yarra: A History of Alfred Hospital Melbourne from Foundation to the Nineteen-Forties*; P. Yule, *The Royal Children's Hospital: A History of Faith, Science and Love*.

101 Performed by passing a long needle through the spinal vertebrae into the lumbar space that enclosed the spinal cord. Cerebrospinal fluid (CSF) was then removed for diagnostic studies.
102 C.L. Mee, *A Nearly Normal Life*, p.15.
103 H.R. Gillan, *Your Stories*, Polio Network of Victoria, 2008, p.10.
104 Robert Hudson. D.J. Wilson, *Living with Polio*, p.41.
105 Interview Geoff Golding (Fairfield Hospital Archives).
106 T. Daniel, 'Polio and the Making of a Doctor', in T.M. Daniel and F.C. Robbins, eds, *Polio*, p.82.
107 Anon. J. Silver and D.J. Wilson, eds, *Polio Voices*, p.32.
108 C. Pugleasa. N.G. Seavey, et al, *A Paralyzing Fear*, p.123.
109 Maureen O'Sullivan. T. Gould, *A Summer Plague*, p.231.
110 L. Medlyn-White, *Your Stories*, Polio Network of Victoria, Summer 2005, p.11.
111 G. Thomas, ed., 'A Story to Break the Silence', no. 45, Post-Polio Newsletter, Post-Polio Network (NSW)
112 J.M. Swann, *Your Stories*, Polio Network of Victoria, Autumn 2002, p.10.
113 G. Thomas, ed., 'A Story to Break the Silence', no. 45, Post-Polio Newsletter, Post-Polio Network (NSW)
114 David Widgery. T. Gould, *A Summer Plague*, p.230.
115 P. Kerr, Interview with Dr Woodruff, author of *Two Million South Australians*, Canberra, 1988. Personal collection, Dr Anthea Hyslop, ANU.
116 A nine-year-old girl from rural Victoria who had been ill for four days. She died ten days later. Report Book (No. 13) of the Medical Superintendent, Dr J.V. Scholes (Fairfield Hospital Archives).
117 Report Book (No. 13) of the Medical Superintendent, Dr J.V. Scholes (Fairfield Hospital Archives).
118 Medical Superintendent of Fairfield Hospital to Dr J.H.L. Cumpston. General Research into Particular Subjects – Poliomyelitis, A1658/616/5/2 (NAA).
119 Sisters and senior nurses from Sydney's Royal Alexandra Hospital for Children, the Royal North Shore Hospital and Prince Henry all attended Fairfield Hospital. Report Book (No. 13) of the Medical Superintendent, Dr J.V. Scholes (Fairfield Hospital Archives).
120 Report Book (No. 13) of the Medical Superintendent, Dr J.V. Scholes (Fairfield Hospital Archives).
121 Report Book (No. 13) of the Medical Superintendent, Dr J.V. Scholes (Fairfield Hospital Archives).
122 A. Killalea, *The Great Scourge*, pp.87–91.
123 A. Killalea, *The Great Scourge*, p.91.
124 Elizabeth Kenny decided in 1932 that nurses trained in her method would abandon the traditional white and instead wear a cornflower-blue uniform. She felt it was not as frightening for the children. A. Steele, L. Cooper and M. Barron. Matron Barron, Letters on Sister Kenny, TR1829/1/16 (State Library of Queensland).

Notes

125 Simon Parritt. T. Gould, *A Summer Plague*, p.235.
126 S. Barnett, 'Member Stories', no. 7, Post-Polio Network NSW www.post-polionetwork.org.au/news/stories/
127 G. Thomas, ed., 'A Story to Break the Silence', no. 45, Post-Polio Newsletter, Post-Polio Network (NSW)
128 Interview J., J.H. Smith, 'Fear, Frustration and the Will to Overcome' (PhD thesis), p.393.
129 G. Buchanan, 'I Used to Jump Puddles', no. 7, *Personal Polio Stories*, Post-Polio Network (NSW). www.polionsw.org.au/wp-content/uploads/2012/01/Gary-Buchanan-I-used-to-jump-puddles.pdf
130 A. Greuber quoted in A. Killalea, *The Great Scourge*, p.89.
131 Richard Alldritch, Resident at the University of Minnesota Hospital 1948–1949. N.G. Seavey, et al, *A Paralyzing Fear*, p.115.
132 Dr Greenberg. J. Silver and D.J. Wilson, eds, *Polio Voices*, p.56.
133 William Berenberg. J. Silver and D.J. Wilson, eds, *Polio Voices*, p.31.
134 A. Killalea, *The Great Scourge*, p.39; Anon., 'The "Iron Lung" in Australia', *The Hammer: Newsletter of the Health and Medicine Museums*, 2003, p.20.
135 T. Gould, *A Summer Plague*, pp.309–10.
136 The respirator or iron lung worked by negative pressure ventilation, created in a chamber enclosing the body of the patient except for the head. A motor blew air into the enclosure, forcing the chest wall and the lungs to collapse. When the air was sucked out of the chamber, the air pressure around the patient's face was now higher than the pressure around the chest, and air was forced into the lungs. The rhythmic breathing normally produced by a person's chest and lungs was now generated by the machine. Developed by Philip Drinker, an engineer at the Harvard School of Public Health. T.M. Daniel and F.C. Robbins, eds, *Polio*, p.10.
137 Interview Geoff Golding (Fairfield Hospital Archives).
138 Larry Alexander. D.J. Wilson, *Living with Polio*, p.44.
139 Interview Anon. (Fairfield Hospital Archives).
140 Regina Brown. J. Silver and D.J. Wilson, eds, *Polio Voices*, p.55.
141 J. Vickers-Willis, 'Footprint: From the Iron Lung' http://vickers-willis.com/html/homefromtheironlung.htm.
142 Richard Rosenwald and Regina Brown. J. Silver and D.J. Wilson, eds, *Polio Voices*, p.48; J. Vickers-Willis, 'Footprint: From the Iron Lung'. http://vickers-willis.com/html/homefromtheironlung.htm
143 Interview B., J. Smith, 'Fear, Frustration and the Will to Overcome' (PhD thesis), pp.403–04.
144 G. Buchanan, 'I Used to Jump Puddles', no. 7, *Personal Polio Stories*, Post-Polio Network (NSW).
145 Interview F., J.H. Smith, 'Fear, Frustration and the Will to Overcome' (PhD thesis), p.404.
146 K. Black, *In the Shadow of Polio*, p.14.
147 K. Black, *In the Shadow of Polio*, p.64.
148 N. Lawes-Gilvear, *Living with Polio*, p.29.
149 Edward B., J. Silver and D.J. Wilson, eds, *Polio Voices*, p.50.
150 B. Serotte, 'Contagious', *Fourth Genre*, p.129.

151 Lorenzo Milam. D.J. Wilson, *Living with Polio*, p.51.
152 A.R. Beisser, *Flying without Wings*, p.18.
153 A.R. Beisser, *Flying without Wings*, p.23.
154 Lawrence Becker. T. Gould, *A Summer Plague*, p.290.
155 Interview F., J.H. Smith, 'Fear, Frustration and the Will to Overcome' (PhD thesis), p.404.
156 *Australian News Bulletin*, 5 February 1947, newspaper cutting in Report Book (No. 13) of the Medical Superintendent, Dr J.V. Scholes (Fairfield Hospital Archives).
157 G. Thomas, ed., 'A Story to Break the Silence', no. 45, Post-Polio Newsletter, Post-Polio Network (NSW)
158 Kenny Institute 50th Anniversary: Patient letters, 1991-1992, MHS-K
159 Interview H., J.H. Smith, 'Fear, Frustration and the Will to Overcome' (PhD thesis), pp.371–75.
160 J.H. Smith, 'Fear, Frustration and the Will to Overcome' (PhD thesis), p.377.
161 C. Thame, 'Health and the State' (PhD thesis), p.344.
162 A married man with tuberculosis received £6/10/- per week with nine shillings for each child under sixteen years, while the polio survivor collected £2/5/- per week plus five shillings for each dependent child. Correspondence Relating to Diseases – Poliomyelitis, General, 1948–1956, A1658/1 (NAA).
163 H.L. Anthony to East Torrens Board of Health, 22 August 1951. Correspondence Relating to Diseases – Poliomyelitis, General. Inquiries and Ministerial Representations, 1957–1962, A1658/1259/1/1 Part 1 (NAA).
164 F. Macfarlane Burnet, 'A Review of Poliomyelitis', *Medical Journal of Australia*, vol.2, no.14 (1952) p.482.
165 C.S. Keefer, 'Social Aspects of Poliomyelitis: United States' (Paper).
166 Anon., 'Insurance against Polio', *The Sydney Morning Herald*, 13 September 1949.
167 D.J. Wilson, *Living with Polio*, p.60.
168 F. Davis, *Passage through Crisis*, pp.68–69.
169 A. Killalea, *The Great Scourge*, p.109.
170 S. Sherson, *Being There*, p.36.
171 Interview Brian Caulfield, 16 May 1995 (Fairfield Hospital Archives).
172 Interview D., J. Smith, 'Fear, Frustration and the Will to Overcome' (PhD thesis), p.387.
173 Interview Geoff Golding (Fairfield Hospital Archives).
174 Interview Geoff Golding (Fairfield Hospital Archives).
175 Shirley M, quoted in 'Testimonials for Sister Kenny' (n.d).
176 Margaret Considine. N.G. Seavey, et al, *A Paralyzing Fear*, p.128.
177 Charlene Pugleasa. N.G. Seavey, et al, *A Paralyzing Fear*, p.128.
178 Simon Parritt. T. Gould, *A Summer Plague*, p.236.
179 Beatrice Nail. J. Silver and D.J. Wilson, eds, *Polio Voices*, p.47.
180 Convalescent home in Victoria.
181 E. Murray, *Your Stories*, Polio Network of Victoria, Summer 2006, p.10.
182 Originally known as the Coast Hospital, Prince Henry was designated as an infectious diseases hospital in 1881.
183 L. Ellis, 'Post-Polio Post', Post-Polio Network (NSW) No. 37. www.post-polionetwork.org.au/news/ppn37.html Accessed March 2008.

184 Interview William Wesson (Fairfield Hospital Archives).
185 Gloria Smothers. J. Silver and D.J. Wilson, eds, *Polio Voices*, p.54.
186 Interview Valda Millie Heath (Fairfield Hospital Archives).
187 J.M. Swann, *Your Stories*, Polio Network of Victoria, Autumn 2002, p.10.
188 G. Thomas, ed., 'A Story to Break the Silence', no. 45, Post-Polio Newsletter, Post-Polio Network (NSW).
189 P. Bazley, *Your Stories*, Polio Network of Victoria, Autumn 2008, p.10
190 B. Watson, *Your Stories*, no. 72, Polio Network of Victoria, p.10.
191 Interview William Wesson (Fairfield Hospital Archives).
192 N. Lawes-Gilvear, *Living with Polio*, pp.31–32.
193 A. Killalea, *The Great Scourge*, p.106.
194 Interview Brian Caulfield (Fairfield Hospital Archives).
195 Interview Edna Thilby (Fairfield Hospital Archives).
196 J.M. Swann, *Your Stories*, Polio Network of Victoria, Autumn 2002, p.10
197 Interview Anon. (Fairfield Hospital Archives).
198 Interview Valda Millie Heath (Fairfield Hospital Archives).
199 Ian Dury. T. Gould, *A Summer Plague*, p.230.
200 Anon. D.J. Wilson, *Living with Polio*, p.122.
201 G. O'Reilly, 'Post-Polio Post', Post-Polio Network (NSW) no 48.
202 G. O'Reilly, 'Post-Polio Post', Post-Polio Network (NSW) no 48.
203 Mike Pierce. J. Silver and D.J. Wilson, eds, *Polio Voices*, p.45.
204 N. Spurr, *Spurr of the Moment*. http://hometown.aol.com.au/noelspurr/myhomepage/club.html. Accessed March 2008.
205 Interview Edna Thilby (Fairfield Hospital Archives).
206 David Olsen. D.J. Wilson, *Living with Polio*, p.117.
207 Interview F., J.H. Smith, 'Fear, Frustration and the Will to Overcome' (PhD thesis), pp.402-403.
208 A. Fairchild, 'The Polio Narratives', *Bulletin of the History of Medicine*, pp.488–524.
209 June had been an in-patient, first in Fairfield and then in the Austin Hospital, Melbourne, for almost sixty years. June died in October 2009. Interview June Middleton (Fairfield Hospital Archives).
210 Glossopharyngeal breathing. Canadian polio survivor Gary McPherson described the technique: 'You take a breath through your nose or your mouth, then hold your breath and add to it with gulps of air. I start by taking a neck breath with my accessory muscles. I get about 150cc of air in my lungs and then I hold it. Next I open my mouth and draw my tongue and throat muscles down to allow air to enter my throat. Then I close my mouth and force the air down my throat with my tongue and throat muscles while I hold my breath.' www.ventusers.org/edu/valnews/val10-1a.html.

Chapter 4

211 A.J. Metcalfe, Director General of Health. A.J. Metcalfe, Interstate Committee on Poliomyelitis, 1951, A1658 617/1/17 (NAA).
212 Normal flora is a microbiological term used to describe the more or less permanent residents of the human body and its environment. Sometimes called indigenous flora, it is native to a particular place or country. The so-called 'traveller's tummy'

is often a response by the body to encountering a new set of indigenous flora. (Author's note.)
213 P. Lépine, 'Epidemiology and Pathogenesis of Poliomyelitis' (Paper).
214 E. Ford, *Bibliography of Australian Medicine 1790–1900*, p.21
215 E. Casely, 'Physiotherapy in South Australia', *The Australian Journal of Physiotherapy*, pp.164–69.
216 Cumpston cites Cleland and Ferguson in J.H.L. Cumpston, *Health and Disease in Australia*, p.326.
217 Later studies within the Aboriginal population in the Northern Territory bore this out. J. Miles, 'Observations on Serum from Aborigines in the Northern Territory of Australia', *Medical Journal of Australia*, pp.773–76; J. Stokes, 'Observations on Serum from Aborigines in the Northern Territory of Australia', *Medical Journal of Australia*, pp.433–38.
218 Data were published in the *Medical Journal of Australia* from 1917–1922; in *Health*, the journal of the former Commonwealth Department of Health from 1924 to the Second World War; and after the war in the *Commonwealth Year Book*. www.health.gov.au/internet/main/publishing.nsf.
219 Poliomyelitis first became notifiable in Tasmania in 1911, and by 1922 was a requirement in all states and territories. Notifiable diseases surveillance, 1917 to 1991. www.health.gov.au/internet/main/Publishing.nsf/. Accessed March 2008.
220 Department of Public Health New South Wales, 'Notification of Infectious Diseases', Report of the Director General of Public Health, 1915–1918 and 1919–1921.
221 Later scientific study revealed that polioviruses are highly resistant to environmental changes, and can survive for long periods in faecal matter and sewage.
222 Epidemics recorded in Broken Hill in 1916 and 1917. Department of Public Health New South Wales, 'Notification of Infectious Diseases', Report of the Director General of Public Health.
223 New York Department of Health, *A Monograph on the Epidemic of Poliomyelitis (Infantile Paralysis) in New York City in 1916*.
224 N. Rogers, *Dirt and Disease*.
225 N. Rogers, *Dirt and Disease*, p.1.
226 R. Aronowitz, 'From Myalgic Encephalitis to Yuppie Flu', in *Framing Disease*, eds C.E. Rosenberg and J. Golden, p.159.
227 F. Cox, *A Review of Recent Literature on Typhoid Fever and Acute Anterior Poliomyelitis*.
228 R.V. Southcott, N.D. Crosby and N.S. Stenhouse, 'Studies on the epidemiology of the 1947–1948 epidemic of poliomyelitis in South Australia', *Medical Journal of Australia*, pp.481–96.
229 A. Marshall, *I Can Jump Puddles*, p.2.
230 H.T. Parker, *Crippled Children in Tasmania*, p.13.
231 J.H.L. Cumpston, *Health and Disease in Australia*, p.326.
232 Department of Public Health Queensland, 'Anterior Poliomyelitis', Annual Report on the health and medical services of the State of Queensland, vol. 1, 1935–1938.
233 J.H.L. Cumpston, *Health and Disease in Australia* and 'Poliomyelitis Notifications' in *Commonwealth Year Books* 1931–1964.
234 Polio notifications per state 1947–1956: New South Wales 4742; Victoria 3222; Queensland 1996; South Australia 4723; Western Australia 1477; Tasmania 550; Northern Territory 14 and Australian Capital Territory 94. Tasmania reported 2176

Notes

cases in the prewar period and 550 postwar. J. White, Commonwealth of Australia, 'Public Health and Related Institutions', Reports of the Director General of Health, 1947–1958.

235 Department of Public Health N.S.W., 'Notification of Infectious Diseases', Report of the Director General of Public Health, 1930–1933.

236 Western Australia's first major epidemic was in 1948, and in 1954 notified 436 cases of polio.

237 Medical Officer, Department of Health, Melbourne City Council. H.W. Bull, 'Poliomyelitis in the City of Melbourne 1937–1938', *Medical Journal of Australia*, pp.809–12.

238 H.W. Bull, 'Poliomyelitis in the City of Melbourne 1937–1938, *Medical Journal of Australia*, pp.809–12. The Infectious Disease Regulations for Victoria in 1932 stated that 'every person suffering from poliomyelitis was to be isolated and detained in isolation until the MO of Health is satisfied that such a person is no longer liable to convey infection ... all contacts attending school were to be isolated for 21 days ... other contacts were to be kept under surveillance'. VPRS/8971/P001, Infectious Disease Regulations 1932 /76 (PROV).

239 All of Sandringham and most of Caulfield, Oakleigh, Mordialloc and Moorabin, portions of Brighton and Malvern and a small section of the Mulgrave Shire. Anon., 'Closing of All Schools in Wide Area Is Advised', *The Sun*, 24 July 1937.

240 F.B. Smith, 'The Victorian Poliomyelitis Epidemic 1937–1938' (Paper), p.2

241 Medical Officer of Health for the City of Melbourne and later Chairman of the Joint State and Municipal Committee for Combating Infantile Paralysis. J. Dale, 'The Epidemiology of Poliomyelitis', *Medical Journal of Australia*, pp.258–62.

242 There are many articles in Melbourne and Sydney newspapers during the period. In A. Killalea, *The Great Scourge*, Killalea quotes an impressive number of newspaper references to support her epidemiological evidence on the spread of the epidemic in 1937–1938 in Tasmania.

243 A. Killalea, *The Great Scourge*, p.53.

244 Anon., 'Cats Killed in Paralysis Fear', *The New York Times*, 26 July 1916.

245 F.B. Smith, 'The Victorian Poliomyelitis Epidemic 1937–1938' (Paper), p.8.

246 Poliomyelitis: Sister Kenny's Treatment. Papers Returned by the Hon. W.M. Hughes Ex Minister for Health, A1928/1/ 802/17/1 (NAA).

247 A.J.G. Buxton, 'Poliomyelitis in South Australia 1937–1956' (BA Hons thesis).

248 Anon., 'Closing of All Schools in Wide Area Is Advised', *The Sun*, 24 July 1937.

249 299 cases were reported. Department of Public Health Queensland, 'Annual Statement of Notifiable Diseases During Calendar Year', Annual Report of the Commissioner of Public Health, 1925 and 1932.

250 Department of Public Health Queensland, 'Anterior Poliomyelitis', Annual Report on the health and medical services of the State of Queensland. In line with the south, schools were closed if a case occurred, and theatres and swimming pools closed, but only for children under sixteen. 160 cases were reported in 1937–38 in Queensland.

251 The Parliament of the Commonwealth of Australia, 'Report of the Administration of the Northern Territory', Report of the District Officer, Alice Springs, 1937–1938–1939, p.18.

252 A.J. Metcalfe, Director General of Health to Secretary, Department of Territories, 7 May 1952. Poliomyelitis in Aborigines, National Health and Medical Research Council, A452/1952/179 (NAA).

253 J. Miles, 'Observations on Serum from Aborigines in the Northern Territory of Australia', *Medical Journal of Australia*, pp.773–76. Blood was taken from both nomadic and settlement dwellers, and indicated that contact with white settlers made no difference to antibody levels.
254 Type I, Brunhilde and Type III, Leon.
255 Eight cases reported. Commonwealth of Australia, 'Public Health and Related Institutions', Reports of the Director General of Health.
256 An elderly man near Alice Springs with a history suggestive of polio in 1925. He had residual paralysis of one upper limb. J. Stokes, 'Observations on Serum from Aborigines in the Northern Territory of Australia', *Medical Journal of Australia*, pp.433–38.
257 J. Stokes, 'Observations on Serum from Aborigines in the Northern Territory of Australia, *Medical Journal of Australia*, pp.433–38.
258 The first Americans arrived in Brisbane on 22 December 1941, and by mid-1943 the number in Australia had risen to 150,000 with the largest concentrations in Queensland near Brisbane, Rockhampton, and Townsville. www.awm.gov.au/encyclopedia/homefront/us_forces.asp.
259 Department of Public Health Queensland, 'Anterior Poliomyelitis', Annual Report on the health and medical services of the State of Queensland, vol. 2, 1939–1945. Other states amalgamated their reports for the war years into one volume.
260 F. Macfarlane Burnet, 'The Epidemiology of Poliomyelitis with Special Reference to the Victorian Epidemic of 1937–1938'. *The Medical Journal of Australia*, pp.325–35.
261 Macnamara graduated in March 1922 as MBBS (Honours). She gained a First in Anatomy, Medicine, Obstetrics, Gynaecology and Surgery, and a Second in Physiology.
262 D. Zwar, *The Dame: The Life and Times of Dame Jean Macnamara, Medical Pioneer*, p.1.
263 J. Macnamara, Correspondence 1923–1968, Papers of Jean Macnamara, MS2399 1/18d/79f (National Library of Australia).
264 For details on Jean Macnamara's early life see D. Zwar, *The Dame*, pp.1–8.
265 A. Gregory, *The Ever Open Door*, p.198.
266 W. Nichol, 'The Medical Profession in New South Wales', *Australian Economic History Review*, pp.115–16; D. Dyason, 'The Medical Profession in Colonial Victoria, 1834–1901', in *Disease, Medicine, and Empire*, eds R.M. MacLeod and M.J. Lewis, p.198.
267 W. Nichol, 'The Medical Profession in New South Wales', *Australian Economic History Review*, pp.115–16.
268 The Victorian Branch of the BMA was formed in 1879, and was seen as being more representative of different categories of medical practitioners than the Medical Society of Victoria, which had been criticised for representing 'only the elite of the profession' and not the 'rank and file of general practitioners'. E. Willis, *Medical Dominance*, p.144.
269 T.S. Pensabene, *The Rise of the Medical Practitioner in Victoria*; J.A. Gillespie, 'Medical Markets and Australian Medical Politics', *Labour History*, no 54, pp.30–46
270 E. Willis, *Medical Dominance*, p.33.
271 B. Gandevia, 'Medicine in the Local Newspaper: The Early Australian Gazettes', in *New Countries and Old Medicine*, eds L. Bryder and D. Dow, p.181; G. Davison, et al, *The Outcasts of Melbourne*, pp.140–60.
272 F.L. Apperly, A Guide to Rockefeller Foundation records, projects RG1.1, Series 410/1/4, Rockefeller Archive Centre, Tarrytown, New York, NY (hereafter RAC). See also W.S. Carter, RG1.1, Series 410/1/3, RAC.

Notes

273 G.J. Carmichael, *Hospital Children*, p.71.
274 P. Yule, 'The Doctors 1900–1923', in *The Royal Children's Hospital*, p.59. For example, a medical report from May 1889 quoted by Yule details one Henry Owens who while 'under treatment for Typhoid developed Diphtheria ... and was removed to the Pavilion and died'. Another child admitted 'suffering from Diabetes' also 'developed Diphtheria and died'.
275 At that time the hospital was known as the Melbourne Hospital for Sick Children.
276 P. Yule, *The Royal Children's Hospital*, p.78.
277 G.J. Carmichael, *Hospital Children*, p.73.
278 By 1897, £16,000 had been raised. W.K. Anderson, *Fever Hospital*, p.24.
279 W.K. Anderson, *Fever Hospital*, p.23.
280 W.K. Anderson, *Fever Hospital*, p.88.
281 P. Yule, *The Royal Children's Hospital*, p.122.
282 A.K. McMurtrie, 'Nursing Care of Crippled Children in the United States', *The American Journal of Nursing*, pp.115–18; J. Macnamara, 'After-Care of Poliomyelitis', *Medical Journal of Australia*, pp.616–17; J. Macnamara, 'The Early Treatment of Poliomyelitis', *Medical Journal of Australia*, pp.374–77; M. Parson, 'The Nursing Care of Orthopedic Children', *The American Journal of Nursing*, pp.135–37; J.R. Paul, *A History of Poliomyelitis*; J.L. Stevenson, 'After-Care of Infantile Paralysis', *The American Journal of Nursing*, pp.729–33; W.C. Mackenzie, 'Section on Diseases in Children', *Medical Journal of Australia*, p.285.
283 L.F. Peltier, *Orthopaedics*, p.23.
284 J. Bourke, 'Mutilating', in *Dismembering the Male*, p.51.
285 S. Koven, 'Remembering and Dismemberment', *The American Historical Review*, pp.1167–1202.
286 B.S. Turner, *Medical Power and Social Knowledge*, p.209.
287 H. Barry, *Orthopaedics in Australia*, p.50.
288 Born of Welsh parents in 1857, Sir Robert Jones specialised in treating crippled children. With Dame Agnes Hunt he developed an open-air hospital for crippled children in Oswestry, Shropshire. Over the years, many Australian orthopaedic surgeons trained there, and Jean Macnamara visited it in 1931.
289 In 1920 MacKenzie said that limbs were to be placed in a 'zero' position (muscles at anatomical rest) and a plaster of Paris cast applied immediately. At that stage he believed that the value of massage was exaggerated. W.C. MacKenzie, 'Section on Diseases in Children', *Medical Journal of Australia*, p.285.
290 P. Bentley and D. Dunstan, 'Muscle Re-Education', in *The Path to Professionalism*, p.91.
291 Gradual exercises of muscles to regain strength.
292 Known as 'rubbers' in nineteenth century Britain, the term changed to 'masseuse' or massage specialist early in the twentieth century. Later, physiotherapist was used (physical therapist in the United States).
293 J. Macnamara, 'Treatment of Poliomyelitis During the Acute and Convalescent Phase', *Medical Journal of Australia*, Vol.II, no.9.
294 Heliotherapy was first provided at 'Edgecliffe' in Beach Road, Hampton, Victoria. In 1926 a property at Frankston (now Mt Eliza) was acquired by the Committee of the RCH and the new Orthopaedic section was opened on 3 March 1930.
295 P. Yule, *The Royal Children's Hospital*, p.208.

296 P. Yule, *The Royal Children's Hospital*, p.194.
297 J.H. Wicksteed, *The Growth of a Profession*.
298 J.H. Wicksteed, *The Growth of a Profession*, p.25.
299 P. Bentley and D. Dunstan, *The Path to Professionalism*, p.19.
300 Australasian Massage Association, 'Special General Meeting of the Queensland Branch to Consider the Matter of Miss Kenny', *The Australasian Nurses' Journal*, p.203.
301 Emil von Behring and Shibasabura Kitasato in 1890 at the Institute for Infectious Diseases in Berlin. The following year, serum was used on a child suffering from diphtheria. The French took up large-scale production of diphtheria antitoxin serum using horses, and Lister introduced the serum into Britain in 1895. R. Porter, 'From Pasteur to Penicillin', in *The Greatest Benefit to Mankind*, pp.438–39.
302 F. Macfarlane Burnet, 'A Review of Poliomyelitis', *The Medical Journal of Australia*, vol.2, no.14 (1952) pp.481–84; F. Macfarlane Burnet and D.O. White, *Natural History of Infectious Disease*; F. Macfarlane Burnet, 'Immunological Recognition of Self', *Science*, pp.307–11.
303 S. Flexner, 'A Note on the Serum Treatment of Poliomyelitis (Infantile Paralysis)', *Science*, pp.259–61.
304 S. Flexner and H.L. Amoss, 'The Relation of the Meninges and Choroid Plexus to Poliomyelitic Infection', *Journal of Experimental Medicine*, pp.525–37.
305 The Joint State and Municipal Committee for Combating Infantile Paralysis in Victoria was formed as a result of a conference of state and metropolitan authorities. Its purpose was to provide serum following consultation with a polio specialist. The state agreed to fund serum for the 'poor and indigent' to a maximum of 10/6d by paying the medical practitioner on receipt of proof of service provided. Public Records of Victoria (hereafter PROV),VPRS/6345/327/279, General Correspondence.
306 Some councils were in favour of the scheme, while others like St Kilda, Oakleigh, Richmond and Fitzroy were against it. Malvern and Sandringham agreed to contribute up to £20, but no more.
307 G. Spencely, 'The Minister for Starvation', *Labour History*, p.144.
308 T.H. Kewley, *Social Security in Australia*, p.85.
309 VPRS/3183/P0000/70, Poliomyelitis Council of Victoria, 1930–1932. (PROV)
310 Her initial salary from the Committee was £7 per week plus 9d a mile expenses. For the financial year ending June 1926, the costs of the campaign were £638/11/0, and Macnamara's fees totalled £420/2/0, approximately £8 per week. That sum was equal to the yearly wage paid to the Medical Superintendent of the Children's Hospital (A. Gregory, *Ever Open Door*, p.198), and in 1925, the basic wage was £4/4/0 for a 44-hour week. In addition, Macnamara would have been receiving fees from her private practice in Little Collins Street. VPRS/3183/P0000/71. Poliomyelitis Council of Victoria Minute Books, 1931–1938 (PROV).
311 Department of Public Health N.S.W., 'Notification of Infectious Diseases', Report of the Director General of Public Health, 1926–1929; Department of Public Health Queensland, 'Annual Statement of Notifiable Diseases During Calendar Year'.
312 F. Morgan, 'The Preparation of Serum from Human Donors Recovered from Poliomyelitis', *Medical Journal of Australia*, pp.264–67.
313 Through the spinal column.
314 R. Webster, 'Anterior Poliomyelitis', *Medical Journal of Australia*, p.124.
315 P. Yule, *The Royal Children's Hospital*, p.195.
316 J. Macnamara, Series 11, Notes for Articles, MS 2399 (NLA).

Notes

317 Guillain-Barré syndrome is an uncommon inflammatory disorder in which the body's immune system attacks the nerves, typically causing severe weakness and numbness that usually starts in the extremities and quickly worsens. Whole-of-body paralysis can eventuate. Recent research has proposed that President Franklin D. Roosevelt was a victim of this disease and not poliomyelitis. www.mayoclinic.com/ health/ guillain-barre-syndrome/DS00413.

318 W.C. MacKenzie, 'Section on Diseases in Children', *Medical Journal of Australia*, p.285; R. Webster, 'Anterior Poliomyelitis', *Medical Journal of Australia*, p.293.

319 J.H. Warner, 'The History of Science and the Sciences of Medicine', *Osiris*, pp.164–93.

320 C.E. Rosenberg, 'Framing Disease', in *Explaining Epidemics and Other Studies in the History of Medicine*, p.313.

321 Letters from Thelma C., Thomas K., Mrs Finch, Letters to Jean Macnamara, 23 October 1929, 18 November 1930, 25 November 1930. J. Macnamara, Series 7, Notebooks, 1925-1966, MS 2399 (NLA). In 1929, Jean Macnamara was paid £1/1/- per hour by the Council for taking blood. VPRS 3183/P000/000071, Minutes, Polio Committee (PROV).

322 Professor F.B. Smith's opinion was that a 'good family history' would be one where there was no TB, venereal disease or alcoholism within the family (personal communication). Dr Greenham, Corryong to Macnamara, 8 July 1931. J. Macnamara, Series 7, Notebooks, 1925–1966, MS2399 (NLA).

323 For example, Haemophilia (a sex-linked clotting defect passed from mother to son) and Thallassaemia (Mediterranean disease, anaemia caused by a defect in the haemoglobin molecule) and AIDS.

324 Hepatitis A and AIDS for example.

325 M. Cawte, 'Craniometry and Eugenics in Australia', *Historical Studies*, pp.35–53.

326 J. Macnamara, Series 1, Correspondence, 1923-1968, MS 2399 (NLA).

327 P. Yule, *The Royal Children's Hospital*, p.200.

328 Isobel Hodge to Macnamara, Hodge, I., J. Macnamara, Series 1, Correspondence 1923–1968, MS 2399 (NLA).

329 F. Macfarlane Burnet and J. Macnamara, 'The Activity of Stored Antipolymyelitic Serum in Experimental Poliomyelitis', *Medical Journal of Australia*, Vol. 2, no. 5 (1929).

330 In 1917 Flexner had reported that his experiments using serum on monkeys were 'very promising'. F. Cox, *A Review of Recent Literature on Typhoid Fever and Acute Anterior Poliomyelitis*, p.62.

331 Flexner to Macnamara, June 1929, Simon Flexner Papers, RG 1/1.2 Reel 70 RAC.

332 Dean Rusk, President, the Rockefeller Foundation, 1954, Series 200/1/1 RAC. See also J. Macnamara, Series 1, Correspondence 1923–1968, MS 2399 (NLA).

333 A 'Virgin soil' epidemic. The disease was said to have spread from nearby Solomon Islands.

334 Reprint of letter from F.E. Cox, Chief Quarantine Officer, Victoria, 10 February 1929; Simon Flexner Papers, RG 1/1.2 Reel 70 RAC.

335 Macnamara to Flexner, 2 March 1930 Simon Flexner Papers, RG 1/1.2 Reel 70 RAC.

336 Macnamara to Flexner, Simon Flexner Papers, RG 1/1.2 Reel 70 RAC.

337 Macnamara to Flexner, 11 March 1931, Simon Flexner Papers, RG 1/1.2 Reel 70 RAC.

338 Editorial, 'Poliomyelitis', *Medical Journal of Australia*, pp.257–58.

339 Lyons would be voted leader of the United Australia Party in May 1931, and elected Prime Minister in January 1932. K. White, *Joseph Lyons*.

340 Ever conscious of the advantages of having powerful and influential friends, in 1932 Macnamara asked her mother to insert a notice in the social pages of *The Argus* to inform readers that she was convalescing from her appendectomy at Eastnor Castle as the guest of Lady Somers. J. Macnamara, Series 1, Correspondence 1923–1968, MS 2399 (NLA).

341 Estimated at £34,000. *The Mercury*, Hobart, 30 June 1931. J. Macnamara, Series 4, Newspaper cuttings, 1933–1964, MS2399 (NLA).

342 Anon., 'Poliomyelitis in Hobart', *The Australasian Nurses' Journal*, Vol. 29 (1932)

343 M. Brodie, 'A Comparison between Convalescent Serum and Non-Convalescent Serum in Poliomyelitis', *Journal of Experimental Medicine*, pp.507–19.

344 M. Brodie, 'The Role of Convalescent Serum in Preparalytic Poliomyelitis', *Journal of Immunology*, pp.353–61.

345 S. Benison, *Tom Rivers*, p.70.

346 W. Park, 'Serum Treatment in Poliomyelitis', *Public Health*, pp.284–86.

347 Medical Officer to the Infantile Paralysis Committee. Department of Public Health N.S.W., 'Notification of Infectious Diseases', Report of the Director General of Public Health, 1934–1937.

348 *Medical Journal of Australia*, Vol 1, 1933, p.43.

349 Mostyn Powell was appointed as Medical Officer to the Committee in December 1936, and reported his findings that he doubted whether serum was of any use, but it was harmless and probably gave comfort to sufferers and their families. VPRS 3183/P0000/71, Minutes, Polio Committee (PROV).

350 R. Southby, 'Treatment of Acute Anterior Poliomyelitis in the Early Stages', *Medical Journal of Australia*, pp.367–73.

351 Walshe was against the use of serum in any form, it was a 'rosy possibility that had not been fulfilled' and was useless. VPRS 3183 P0000/71, Serum donors (PROV).

352 VPRS 3183 P0000/72, Papers, Files re Polio Committee 1927–1939 (PROV).

353 VPRS 3183/P0000/71, Interview with Frank Macfarlane Burnet (PROV).

354 J. Paul, *A History of Poliomyelitis*, p.198.

355 F. Macfarlane Burnet, *Changing Patterns*, p.158.

356 S. Benison, 'Poliomyelitis and the Rockefeller Institute', *Journal of the History of Medicine*, pp.74–93.

357 F.B. Smith, 'The Victorian Polio Epidemic 1937–1938 (Paper), p.4.

358 S. Benison, *Tom Rivers*, p.167.

359 F. Macfarlane Burnet, *Changing Patterns*, p.158.

360 A.J.G. Buxton, 'Poliomyelitis in South Australia 1937–1956' (BA Hons thesis), p.26.

361 Department of Public Health Queensland, 'Anterior Poliomyelitis', Annual Report on the health and medical services of the State of Queensland, 1938.

362 VPRS/3183/P0000/71, Jean Macnamara, Fellowship (PROV).

363 J. Macnamara, Series 1, Correspondence, 1923-1968, MS 2399 (NLA).

364 D.P. O'Brien, Rockefeller Foundation Paris, RG6, SG1, RAC. The International Health Board of the Rockefeller Foundation maintained an office in Paris from 1917 as the headquarters for the work of the Commission for the Prevention of Tuberculosis in France.

365 She did confide to her family that she felt 'events were moving too fast'. J. Macnamara, Series 1, Correspondence, 1923-1968, MS 2399 (NLA)

366 J. Macnamara, Series 1, Correspondence, 1923-1968, MS 2399 (NLA).

367 J. Macnamara, Series 1, Correspondence, 1923-1968, MS 2399 (NLA).
368 Ralph Crisp and Dr Cuthbert from Perth, Western Australia. J. Macnamara, Series 1, Correspondence, 1923-1968, MS 2399 (NLA).
369 J. Macnamara, Series 1, Correspondence, 1923-1968, MS 2399 (NLA).
370 Her relief at not having to go to the United States was evident from her letters home. She went over O'Brien's head and wrote directly to Dr Carter in New York asking his permission to stay in England. A few weeks later she wrote that 'this little old appendix has allowed me to get my own way' to 'defeat O'Brien'. J. Macnamara, Series 1, Correspondence, 1923-1968, MS 2399 (NLA).
371 The Foundation supported her travels around the United States and Canada to visit various orthopaedic hospitals where she met Jessie Stevenson, the most 'critical, careful and practical worker in polio in the United States'. J. Macnamara, Series 1, Correspondence, 1923-1968, MS 2399 (NLA).
372 J. Macnamara, Series 1, Correspondence, 1923-1968, MS 2399 (NLA).
373 'Wild horses would not drag me back to serum therapy … perhaps I'll do some veterinary work with sheep'. J. Macnamara, Series 1, Correspondence, 1923-1968, MS 2399 (NLA).
374 J. Macnamara, Series 11, Notes for Articles, MS 2399 (NLA).
375 J. Macnamara, Series 7, Notebooks, 1925–1966, MS 2399 (NLA).
376 J. Macnamara, Series 7, Notebooks, 1925–1966, MS 2399 (NLA).
377 D. Zwar, *The Dame*, p.107.
378 J. Macnamara, Series 7, Notebooks, 1925–1966, MS 2399 (NLA).
379 Dr Shields (UAP) addressing Parliament in November, 1937. J. Macnamara, Series 4, Newspaper cuttings, 1933-1964, MS2399 (NLA).
380 J. Macnamara, Series 11, Notes for Articles, MS2399 (NLA).
381 P. Colville, 'Reports of Official Delegates: Australia' (Paper), p.28.
382 E. Riska and K. Wegar, eds, *Gender, Work and Medicine*, p.3.
383 S. Williams, "Obituary–Annie Jean Macnamara", *Medical Journal of Australia*, p.473.
384 D. Zwar, *The Dame*, pp.94–97.
385 Jean Macnamara was made a Dame Commander of the Order of the British Empire in 1935 for her services in the field of poliomyelitis. Zwar, *The Dame*.

Chapter 5

386 The term 'disabled' is currently preferred, but during the early to mid-twentieth century in Australia, 'crippled' was the predominant social identity for those with a physical disability. For that reason, 'crippled' has been used in context.
387 C.E. Rosenberg, 'Florence Nightingale on Contagion', in C.E. Rosenberg, ed., *Healing and History*; A. Hyslop, *Sovereign Remedies*; A. Gregory, *The Ever Open Door*, p.93.
388 A. Strauss, 'The Structure and Ideology of American Nursing', in *The Nursing Profession*, ed., F. Davis, p.102.
389 R. Bingham, 'The Kenny Treatment for Infantile Paralysis', *The Journal of Bone and Joint Surgery*, pp.647–50.
390 J. Pohl to Cohn, May 1953. Victor Cohn Papers in Elizabeth Kenny Papers, MHS-K.
391 In 1952, the treatment at the Kenny Institute in Minneapolis was 'hot packs eight hours per day and changed every hour. In the acute stage packing was for twelve hours and if acute pain was present, patients were packed for twenty four hours.' Interview of Vivian Hannan. Victor Cohn Papers in Elizabeth Kenny Papers, MHS-K.

392 J.R. Wilson, *Through Kenny's Eyes*, p.12; E. Willis, 'Sister Elizabeth Kenny and the Evolution of the Occupational Division of Labour in Health Care', *Australian and New Zealand Journal of Sociology*, p.204.

393 C. Thame, 'Health and the State' (PhD thesis), p.205.

394 'Sister Kenny', *The Sydney Telegraph*, 1 December 1952, p.3.

395 A bibliography of science and medical literature published in 1951 by the National Foundation for Infantile Paralysis in the United States of America listed 123 references to the Kenny method for the treatment of polio paralysis. M. Fishbein, et al, eds, *A Bibliography of Infantile Paralysis, 1789–1949*.

396 R. Bingham, 'The Kenny Treatment for Infantile Paralysis', *The Journal of Bone and Joint Surgery*, p.650. At the time the paper was published, Dr Bingham was working at the New York Orthopaedic Hospital.

397 Dr Reginald McKellar Hall, an orthopaedic surgeon at the Children's Hospital in Perth in the 1950s was one of the few who followed Kenny's method. R.D. McKellar Hall, *Reflections of an Orthopaedic Surgeon*.

398 Joan was a patient in Hampton Hospital in Victoria in 1952, and was under the care of Dr Jean Macnamara. Joan Smith, *Your Stories*, Polio Network of Victoria, Summer 2007, p.11.

399 J.C. Ross, 'A History of Poliomyelitis in New Zealand' (MA thesis), p.71.

400 Third International Poliomyelitis Conference, Rome 1954. *Poliomyelitis: Papers and Discussions Presented at the Third International Poliomyelitis Conference*.

401 The exceptions were the Royal Children's Hospital in Perth and the Royal Newcastle Hospital where treatment in the acute phase was bed rest without the use of restraining splints, hot packs and stretching exercises. E. Byrne and A. Roberts, 'Polio Epidemic of 1950–51 in the Newcastle Area', *Medical Journal of Australia*, pp.10–12.

402 J.R. Wilson, *Through Kenny's Eyes: An Exploration of Sister Elizabeth Kenny's Views About Nursing*; Wade Alexander, *Sister Elizabeth Kenny: Maverick Heroine of the Polio Treatment Controversy*; V. Cohn, *Sister Kenny: The Woman Who Challenged the Doctors*; E. Bigland, *The True Story About Sister Kenny*.

403 E. Crofford, *Healing Warrior: A Story About Sister Elizabeth Kenny*; H. Thomas, *Sister Elizabeth Kenny, Lives to Remember*; M. Colbeck, *Sister Kenny of the Outback*; H. Levine, *I Knew Sister Kenny: A Story of a Great Lady and Little People*; E.W. Docker, *Sister Kenny*.

404 Sisters Ella Morphett and Pattie Kirton to Cohn. Victor Cohn Papers, Interviews and other sources, A-W, 1940s-1970s, MHS-K.

405 R. Numbers, 'Physicians, Community and the Qualified Ascent of the American Medical Profession', in *Major Problems in the History of American Medicine and Public Health*, eds J.H. Warner and J.A. Tighe, p.302. In November 1932 Jean Macnamara was in the United States on a Rockefeller Scholarship. She wrote to her family 'The whole standard of medical education here is very low, so no wonder christian scientists [sic] and the chiropractors etc flourish'. J. Macnamara, Series 1, Correspondence 1923-1968, MS 2399 (NLA).

406 See, for example, P. Martyr, *Paradise of Quacks*.

407 E. Willis, *Medical Dominance*, p.73.

408 Aikens to Cohn. Victor Cohn Papers, Interviews and other sources, A-W, 1940s-1970s, MHS-K.

409 Birth certificate for Elizabeth Kenny. Correspondence Relating to Sister Kenny Foundation, 16/2 (University of Queensland) hereafter UQ.

410 Anne Walters, Millicent Woodward and the three sisters who survived Elizabeth Kenny: Julia Farquharson, Mary Scotney and Margaret Scotney. Victor Cohn Papers, Interviews and other sources, A-W, 1940s-1970s, MHS-K.

Notes

411 Farquharson and Scotney. Victor Cohn Papers, Interviews and other sources, A-W, 1940s-1970s, MHS-K.
412 Millicent Woodward. Victor Cohn Papers, Interviews and other sources, A-W, 1940s-1970s, MHS-K.
413 Anne Walters. Victor Cohn Papers, Interviews and other sources, A-W, 1940s-1970s, MHS-K.
414 Millicent Woodward. Victor Cohn Papers, Interviews and other sources, A-W, 1940s-1970s, MHS-K.
415 Millicent Woodward. Victor Cohn Papers, Interviews and other sources, A-W, 1940s-1970s, MHS-K.
416 'Westbrook Head Station', *Toowoomba Chronicle* 1896.
417 Millicent Woodward. Victor Cohn Papers, Interviews and other sources, A-W, 1940s-1970s, MHS-K.
418 Farquharson and Scotney. Victor Cohn Papers, Interviews and other sources, A-W, 1940s-1970s, MHS-K.
419 Victor Cohn visited the site in 1955.
420 E. Kenny and M. Ostenso, *And They Shall Walk*, p.17.
421 Farquharson and Scotney. Victor Cohn Papers, Interviews and other sources, A-W, 1940s-1970s, MHS-K.
422 E. Sandow, *The Construction and Reconstruction of the Human Body*.
423 E. Sandow, *The Construction and Reconstruction of the Human Body*, p.3.
424 W.G. Wright, *Muscle Training in the Treatment of Infantile Paralysis*, p.1.
425 Anne Walters confirmed that Kenny was living with the 'almost blind' Granny Moore in 1908. Anne Walters. Victor Cohn Papers, Interviews and other sources, A-W, 1940s-1970s, MHS-K.
426 Minnie Bell was the daughter of Richard Moore.
427 'Great Northern Bakery, JH Bell, Baker and Confectioner'. Advertisement in *The Guyra Argus*, 12 March 1908.
428 Minnie Bell. Victor Cohn Papers, Interviews and other sources, A-W, 1940s-1970s, MHS-K.
429 'T.E. Sole, Auctioneer, Stock, Station and General commission Agent, North Guyra. Cash buyer of all kinds of farm produce'. *The Guyra Argus*, 26 January 1906.
430 Reg McAllister, Chemist, Guyra. Victor Cohn Papers, Interviews and other sources, A-W, 1940s-1970s, MHS-K .
431 *The Guyra Argus*, March 1911.
432 Patience Moore to Alexander. Wade Alexander Papers, undated and 1862–1951, 2001' MHS-K.
433 See, for example, V. Cohn, *Sister Kenny*; J.R. Wilson, *Through Kenny's Eyes*; W.K. Alexander, *Sister Elizabeth Kenny*.
434 The Sydney Norland Institute, Lower Forth Street, Woollahra, Sydney.
435 'Sydney's Premier Nursing School.' *The Guyra Argus*, p.3.
436 On several occasions Kenny quoted that figure as the amount she paid for nursing tuition in Sydney.
437 Millicent Woodward states that Kenny left Guyra in January 1911 after selling potatoes for three or four years. Victor Cohn Papers, Interviews and other sources, A-W, 1940s-1970s, MHS-K.

438 Eleanor MacKinnon to W.M. Hughes, 14 February 1935. Poliomyelitis: Sister Kenny's Treatment. Papers Returned by the Hon. W.M. Hughes Ex Minister for Health, A1928/1, 802/17/1 (NAA).
439 Certificate awarded by The Sydney Norland Institute to those who completed the training course.
440 Kenny was photographed in that uniform, which closely resembled the one worn by volunteer collectors for the 'Saturday Hospital Fund'. Millicent Woodward. Victor Cohn Papers, Interviews and other sources, A-W, 1940s-1970s, MHS-K.
441 Proceeds from her potato selling days in Guyra.
442 'Starting a Hospital', *The Australasian Nurses' Journal*, 15 March 1913, p.80.
443 Jack Kenny, nephew, quoted in J.R. Wilson, 'The Findings', in *Through Kenny's Eyes*, p.34.
444 The Queensland Bush Nursing Association was not formed until 1914, and before then, no organised attempt had been made to supply nurses in outback districts. When the NSW Bush Nurses Association advertised for bush nurses, it stipulated that applicants must be members of the ATNA or the RVTNA and have general and obstetric certificates. *Australasian Nurses' Journal*, 15 October 1914. It was not until 1920 when the Bush Nursing Association received £15,000 from the British Red Cross that local communities in outback districts erected several small cottages with a surgery attached.
445 Named after the patron saint of County Kilkenny in Ireland.
446 'The lad, Sam Healy, who was severely injured in a riding accident on 23 February was in a much improved condition in Nurse Kenny's hospital', *Clifton Courier*, 10 March 1914.
447 Eileen Donohue. Victor Cohn Papers, Interviews and other sources, A-W, 1940s-1970s, MHS-K.
448 Thomas Thompson, *Stanthorpe Border Post* to Cohn. Victor Cohn Papers, Interviews and other sources, A-W, 1940s-1970s, MHS-K.
449 Anon., 'Health Act Amendment Act of 1911, Queensland', *The Australasian Nurses' Journal*, p.42.
450 The formation of a Nurses' Association had first been considered in Sydney in 1892, but, until 1899, the women had been unable to agree on what constituted a trained nurse. That changed when the Australasian Trained Nurses Association (ATNA) was formed. Victoria was the first state to form its own association (RVTNA) and local councils were established in Queensland, South Australia, Western Australia and Tasmania. The Associations agreed that nurses would be trained for three, four or five years in an accredited hospital. The length of training required to complete the degree depended on the number of beds, and forty beds were considered the minimum for accreditation as a teaching hospital.
451 Anon., 'Nursing Legislation in Queensland', *The Australasian Nurses' Journal*, p.1.
452 From January to December 1912.
453 Anon., 'State Registration', *The Australasian Nurses' Journal*, pp.110-111
454 W. Madsen, 'Early 20th Century Untrained Nursing Staff in the Rockhampton District', *Journal of Advanced Nursing*, pp.308–09.
455 'The Minister may dispense with such of the certificates, examinations, or other conditions for the registration of Nurses under this Act as to him may seem just in favour of any person who, during the three years immediately preceding the first day of January, one thousand nine hundred and twelve, has been employed in the calling of Nurse'. 'Health Act Amendment Act of 1911, Queensland', *The Australasian Nurses' Journal*, p.42.

Notes

456 A copy of her Attestation Paper held in the National Archives of Australia is not complete and bears no official signature. The question on qualifications on the front page has been completed in Kenny's handwriting; her date of enlistment is given as 30 May 1915, and her age as thirty-one years when she was in fact thirty-four. Her statement of service, which is signed, lists her embarkation date as 19 December 1916 from Sydney on the P&O *Orontes* and her arrival in Plymouth as 17 February 1917. The nominal roll for the First World War held at the Australian War Memorial has her enlistment as 30 May 1916. Elizabeth Kenny Collection, Attestation Paper, NAA 1928/802/17/1.

457 William Henry Harold Kenny, DCM, Medaille Militaire. www.lighthorse.org.au/Perhist/kenny.htm. Accessed 2007.

458 In October 1915, the *Clifton Courier* advised that St Canice had been sold and was now known as Allies Private Hospital.

459 Any nurse trained in a hospital of over fifty beds and with good credentials would have no difficulty finding employment by the War Office. *ATNA Journal*, 15 April 1915, p.142.

460 Registration, *The British Journal of Nursing*, 10 July 1915.

461 V. Cohn, 'War Nurse', in *Sister Kenny*; J.R. Wilson, *Through Kenny's Eyes*; W. Alexander, *Sister Elizabeth Kenny*.

462 The battles took place in April and May of 1915, and Kenny did not arrive in Marseilles until 2nd August. See V. Cohn, *Sister Kenny*, p.54; J.R. Wilson, *Through Kenny's Eyes*, p.37; J. Pearn, *Pioneer Medicine in Australia*. Alexander says she was wounded at Ypres 'later in the year' but adds that 'whether or not Kenny was wounded by enemy action' cannot be determined for certain. W.K. Alexander, *Sister Elizabeth Kenny*, p.32.

463 'Clifton Patriots', *Toowoomba Chronicle*, 5 June 1915. Over the following week, Kenny was guest of honour at 'an enjoyable afternoon tea at Tullymore, Spring Creek', and was presented with a 'handsome travelling rug' by the Red Cross Society in Clifton. See 'Nurse Entertained', *Toowoomba Chronicle*, 24 June 1915, and 'Red Cross Clifton', *Toowoomba Chronicle*, 20 June 1915.

464 'Personal', *Sydney Morning Herald*, 25 June 1915.

465 I. Martin, 'When Needs Must', *Health and History*, p.91.

466 Alice Perrott. Victor Cohn Papers, Interviews and other sources, A-W, 1940s-1970s, MHS-K.

467 The State Library of Queensland cites the source as unknown and the date given is 4 August 1915. I have not been able to find the original in a search of Queensland newspapers around that date. http://hdl.handle.net/10462/deriv/127933.

468 See medal card of Kenny, Elizabeth WO 372/23. www.nationalarchives.gov.uk. Examination of this card revealed that Kenny was not awarded any medal by the British War Office, nor does any service record exist. The acronym AANS was identical to that for the Australian Army Nursing Service and may have initiated the confusion that exists about when and where Kenny enlisted.

469 A pencilled entry on her Australian service record states 'all her service was between Australia and the UK on transports and at no time is she recorded as being in France'.

470 Michael Kenny to Cohn, 8 March 1955. When Kenny visited her relatives in 1915 she was not in uniform.

471 The French Flag Nursing Corps, *The British Journal of Nursing*, 17 July 1915.

472 'Nobby', *Toowoomba Chronicle*, 11 December 1915.

473 Elizabeth Kenny Collection, Attestation Paper, NAA 1928/802/17/1.

474 Sister Kirton. Victor Cohn Papers, Interviews and other sources, A-W, 1940s-1970s, MHS-K.
475 L.E. Armstrong, 'Massage in English War Hospitals', *The Australasian Nurses' Journal*, pp.46–47.
476 Once in England, the wounded were further assessed and if it was believed that the injury was liable to keep them out of action for more than six months they were transported back home. A.G. Butler, *The Official History of the Australian Army Medical Services in the War of 1914–1918*.
477 J. Bassett, *Guns and Brooches*, p.71.
478 J. Bassett, *Guns and Brooches*, p.70.
479 W. Vinicombe to Cohn. Victor Cohn Papers, Interviews and other sources, A-W, 1940s-1970s, MHS-K.
480 Kenny's insistence that her heart was in poor health was a source of conflict between her and staff at the Townsville clinic in 1934. Dr Jay Davis to Cohn. Victor Cohn Papers, Interviews and other sources, A-W, 1940s-1970s, MHS-K.
481 Elizabeth Sterne (Warwick President of the Country Women's Association (CWA) in 1925) was adamant Kenny did not treat any polio cases until the 1920s. Both Ella Morphett and Patty Kirton agree that it was after the First World War.
482 S. Kuhn to Cohn. Victor Cohn Papers, Interviews and other sources, A-W, 1940s-1970s, MHS-K.
483 See, for example, V. Cohn, *Sister Kenny*; J.R. Wilson, *Through Kenny's Eyes*; J. Pearn, *Pioneer Medicine in Australia*; and others.
484 The CWA gave her 'every assistance' to promote her stretcher through Queensland and New South Wales, 12 January 1955. Elizabeth Sterne to Cohn. Victor Cohn Papers, Interviews and other sources, A-W, 1940s-1970s, MHS-K.
485 Daphne's mother was an Avery and knew Elizabeth Kenny from her days as a governess to the family. Kenny helped Amelia Avery dress for her wedding to William in July 1910.
486 William Cregan to Cohn. Victor Cohn Papers, Interviews and other sources, A-W, 1940s-1970s, MHS-K.
487 Cregan to Cohn. Victor Cohn Papers, Interviews and other sources, A-W, 1940s-1970s, MHS-K.
488 Sam Rooney to Cohn. Victor Cohn Papers, Interviews and other sources, A-W, 1940s-1970s, MHS-K.
489 William Cregan. Victor Cohn Papers, Interviews and other sources, A-W, 1940s-1970s, MHS-K.
490 Wade Alexander gave details on Kenny during the early 1930s in W.K. Alexander, *Sister Elizabeth Kenny*, pp.50–53.
491 At that time, Charles Edward Chuter was Assistant Under-Secretary in the Home Secretary's Department in the Queensland State Government and a member of the Brisbane and South Coast Hospitals Board. In 1935, Chuter became Under-Secretary of the newly formed Department of Health and Home Affairs. www.adb.online.anu.edu.au/biogs/A130469b.htm.
492 Under her scheme, nurses would provide mothercraft and infant welfare services, visit children in primary schools and teach first-aid classes with the help of the St John's Ambulance Brigade.
493 Charles Edward Chuter Papers, OM 65/17/33 (Oxley Library, State Library of Queensland) hereafter Oxley-SLQ.

Notes

494 Kenny to Chuter, 27 January 1932. 'Have just returned from Warwick, Goondawindi and Singleton'. Charles Edward Chuter Papers, OM 65/17/35 Oxley -SLQ.

495 Charles Edward Chuter Papers, OM 65/17/33, Oxley -SLQ.

496 Allen Sewell to Cohen. Victor Cohn Papers, Interviews and other sources, A-W, 1940s-1970s, MHS-K. See also, R. Patrick, *A History of Health & Medicine in Queensland 1824–1960*, p.103.

497 R. Patrick, *A History of Health & Medicine in Queensland 1824–1960*, p.103.

498 www.goldencasket.com/corporate.

499 www.adb.online.anu.edu.au/biogs/A130469b.htm.

500 British Medical Association, Queensland Branch. Queensland State Archives.

501 Arthur Fadden (Prime Minister 1941), a member of the party and a former Alderman on the Townsville City Council, was elected to the Queensland Legislative Assembly for the seat of Kennedy in 1932. He was a firm supporter of Elizabeth Kenny. www.primeministers.naa.gov.au.

502 Edward (Ned) Hanlon was home secretary from 1932-1935 when he became secretary for health and home affairs. http://adb.anu.edu.au/biography/hanlon-edward-michael-ned-10411.

503 R. Patrick, *A History of Health & Medicine in Queensland 1824–1960*, p.76.

504 Betty Jorgensen, Kathleen Holloway and Sheila Bradley. Charles Edward Chuter Papers, OM 65/17/35 Oxley -SLQ.

505 Elizabeth Sterne to Cohn. Victor Cohn Papers, Interviews and other sources, A-W, 1940s-1970s, MHS-K.

506 The Love Estate was administered by Arthur Fadden, who was an active supporter of the Townsville clinic. George Kenyatta to Cohn. Victor Cohn Papers, Interviews and other sources, A-W, 1940s-1970s, MHS-K.

507 Julia Farquharson to Cohn. Victor Cohn Papers, Interviews and other sources, A-W, 1940s-1970s, MHS-K.

508 F.G. Fisher, *Raphael Cilento: A Biography*, p.20.

509 The AITM was established in 1909. It was charged with investigating and developing methods to maintain the health of whites working in the tropics. At that time, it was viewed as essential to demonstrate that Australians of European origin could work and prosper north of the Tropic of Capricorn. The economic wellbeing of the new nation of Australia was at stake. See W.K. Anderson, 'No Place for a White Man', in *The Cultivation of Whiteness: Science, Health and Racial Destiny in Australia*.

510 F.G. Fisher, *Raphael Cilento*, p.74.

511 Cilento was now Director, Division of Tropical Hygiene and Chief Quarantine Officer for North Queensland (1928–1933). In September 1933, the Division was abolished and Cilento transferred to Canberra as Senior Medical Officer in the Commonwealth Department of Health, a position he loathed and which led to a worsening relationship with J.H.L. Cumpston. www.asap.unimelb.edu.au /bsparcs/biogs/P001138b.htm.

512 F.G. Fisher, *Raphael Cilento*, p.69.

513 F.G. Fisher, *Raphael Cilento*, p.80.

514 Some of her critics had suggested that the power of Kenny's personality played a major role in her treatment and because of this, it would be impossible to teach others to apply her method. Rae W Dungan collection, Letters and Correspondence, Fryer Library, UQ.

515 Cilento to Steele. Matron Barron Letters on Sister Kenny, Series 1, TR 1829, SLQ.
516 Cooper to Barron, Matron Barron Letters on Sister Kenny, Series 1, TR 1829, SLQ.
517 Kenny to Chuter, 3 July 1934. Charles Edward Chuter Papers, OM65/17/38 SLQ.
518 By the end of July, Sisters Eales and Groth had joined the staff at the Townsville Clinic, and Sisters Shaw and Gillespie arrived in December 1934. Matron Barron Letters on Sister Kenny, Series 1, TR 1829, SLQ.
519 Barron to Steele. Matron Barron Letters on Sister Kenny, Series 1, TR 1829, SLQ.
520 Steele to Barron, Matron Barron Letters on Sister Kenny, Series 1, TR 1829, SLQ.
521 Steele to Barron, Matron Barron Letters on Sister Kenny, Series 1, TR 1829, SLQ.
522 The Goodna Hospital for the Insane near Brisbane was a State run facility and under the auspices of the Health and Home Affairs Department from 1935-1963. Steele to Barron. Matron Barron Letters on Sister Kenny, Series 1, TR 1829, SLQ.
523 Chuter to Kenny. Charles Edward Chuter Papers, OM65/17 Oxley-SLQ.
524 F.G. Fisher, *Raphael Cilento*, p.78.
525 Steele to Barron. Matron Barron Letters on Sister Kenny, Series 1, TR 1829, SLQ.
526 Steele to Barron. Matron Barron Letters on Sister Kenny, Series 1, TR 1829, SLQ.
527 Kenny to Chuter. Charles Edward Chuter Papers, OM65/17/37 Oxley-SLQ.
528 R. Cilento, 'Report on the Muscle Re-Education Clinic, Townsville'. Rae W Dungan Collection, UQFL354, UQ.
529 Letter from Mrs T.L. Rheuben, *Townsville Daily Bulletin*, 5 April 1935.
530 R. Cilento, 'Report on the Muscle Re-Education Clinic, Townsville', 9 August 1934. Rae W Dungan Collection, UQFL354, UQ.
531 Kenny replied to Cilento's report in a scornful letter to E.M. Hanlon on 5 September 1934. She replied to each one of his criticisms paragraph by paragraph and made no attempt to hide her disdain for his findings, especially his views on pensions for polio sufferers. However, soon after receiving Kenny's letter, Hanlon offered Cilento the post of Director General of Health and Medical Services for the State of Queensland.
532 Aikens to Cohn. Victor Cohn Papers, Interviews and other sources, A-W, 1940s-1970s, MHS-K.
533 Fisher wrote that Cilento was 'deeply wounded' at being 'subjected to the most violent public and private vilification'. F.G. Fisher, *Raphael Cilento*, p.81.
534 Kenny to Mann. Charles Edward Chuter Papers, OM 65/17/37 Oxley-SLQ.
535 Dr James Guinane. Victor Cohn Papers, Interviews and other sources, A-W, 1940s-1970s, MHS-K.
536 *The Townsville Bulletin*, 1 April 1935.
537 Also known as Billy Hughes, he was Prime Minister of Australia from October 1915 until 1922. He became minister for health in 1934 in the Lyons government.
538 A friend to Elizabeth Kenny. Previously at the Norland Institute, and now a member of the Hospitals Commission of NSW, she had shown Hughes a film of Kenny administering treatment at the clinic in Townsville. Mackinnon to Hughes. Poliomyelitis: Sister Kenny's Activities, A1928/1/802/17/1 (NAA).
539 A1928/1/802/17/1 (NAA).
540 Director General of Health, Commonwealth of Australia.
541 Cumpston to Hughes. Poliomyelitis: Sister Kenny's Activities. A1928/1/802/17/1 (NAA).

Notes

542 Commonwealth Department of Health, 1936, 'Report of the Australian Conference on Crippled Children'. Rae W Dungan Collection, UQFL 354, UQ.

543 Dr Douglas Galbraith, Medical Superintendent of the Orthopaedic Section of the Children's Hospital at Frankston.

544 Galbraith to Hughes. The Children's Hospital Committee in Melbourne wrote to Hughes on 30 May offering facilities for Kenny to carry out the treatment, but Cumpston believed that because the relationship between Kenny and Queensland had deteriorated, he was doubtful whether a clinic would be established. A1928/1/802/17/1 (NAA).

545 Honorary Surgeon to the Orthopaedic Section, Frankston.

546 Galbraith and Whitaker to W.M. Hughes, 30 March 1935. A1928/1/802/17/1 (NAA).

547 In the electorate of W.M. Hughes.

548 Minister H.P. Fitzsimons to W.M. Hughes, 15 May 1935. A1928/1/802/17/1 (NAA).

549 Mary Kenny, Photographs and Papers, TR 2931 SLQ.

550 Chuter to Kenny, 17 May 1935. Charles Edward Chuter Papers, OM 65/17/37 Oxley-SLQ.

551 Charles Edward Chuter Papers OM 65/17/34 Oxley-SLQ.

552 'Sister Kenny to Continue Townsville Clinic', *Townsville Daily Bulletin*, 20 May 1935. 'Sister Kenny Clinic Opened at Brisbane', *Townsville Daily Bulletin*, 11 June 1935.

553 Until 1938.

554 'Fed up with Doctors Freezing out Sister Kenny', *The Truth*, 13 November 1937.

555 D.H. Borchardt, 'Part V Queensland', Checklist of Royal Commissions: select committees and boards of inquiry (Brisbane: 1970). Drs Thelander, McDonnell, Nye, Lahz, Paterson, Duhig, Gibson and Bostock were appointed as Commissioners. They were given three years to investigate Kenny's claims.

556 Now Dame Jean Connor, Physician-in-charge, Physiotherapy Clinic, Children's Hospital, Melbourne. Report of the Australian Conference of Crippled Children. Rae W Dungan Collection, UQFL 354, UQ.

557 Sister Elizabeth Kenny, no affiliation given, 'The treatment of the cripple'. Report of the Australian Conference of Crippled Children. Rae W Dungan Collection, UQFL 354, UQ.

558 J.G. Norris, Honorary Secretary, Victorian Society for Crippled Children. Report of the Australian Conference of Crippled Children. Rae W Dungan Collection, UQFL 354, UQ.

559 Crawford represented the BMA (QLD) and was Chairman of the Queensland Branch of the Australasian Massage Association. Rae W. Dungan collection, UQFL 354, UQ.

560 Report of the Australian Conference of Crippled Children. Rae W Dungan Collection, UQFL 354, UQ.

561 R.D. McKellar Hall, *Reflections of an Orthopaedic Surgeon*, p.41.

562 R.D. McKellar Hall, *Reflections of an Orthopaedic Surgeon*, p.47.

563 The treatment methods described by Kenny in her first book bear little resemblance to those in her later works. For example, she advocated hydrotherapy, but made no distinction between therapy in large communal pools (which she denounced) and individual treatment in a bath. The language is convoluted, difficult to understand

and unsophisticated. The impression given is that she was searching for words to adequately explain the symptoms she was observing. E. Kenny, *Infantile Paralysis and Cerebral Diplegia, Methods Used for the Restoration of Function*.

564 Several letters were published in newspapers supporting Kenny. See, for example, James Ferguson, 'Sister Kenny', *The Sunday Mail*, March 1987. 'Fed up with Doctors Freezing out Sister Kenny' and 'Tiny Child Is Pathetic Pawn to Challenge BMA', *Smith's Weekly*, 20 November 1937.

565 Kenny to Dungan, 15 February 1937. Rae W. Dungan collection, UQFL 354, UQ.

566 W.M. Hughes to Cabinet, 1937, A6006/1937/12/31 (NAA).

567 Chief Medical Officer of Health, London County Council.

568 The London City Council gave her thirty cases (including eleven early paralysis cases) wards, equipment and nursing staff. Interview Dr Richard Metcalfe. Victor Cohn Papers, Interviews and other sources, A-W, 1940s-1970s, MHS-K.

569 Interview Dr Richard Metcalfe. Victor Cohn Papers, Interviews and other sources, A-W, 1940s-1970s, MHS-K.

570 Interviews with Lawson, Reardon, Reynolds and Metcalfe, staff of Queen Mary's Carshalton. Victor Cohn Papers, Interviews and other sources, A-W, 1940s-1970s, MHS-K.

571 Dr F.H. Mills to Ministry of Health, London, 6 September 1937. Treatment of Poliomyelitis at Queen Mary's Hospital for Children, Carshalton, 28 October 1937. Charles Edward Chuter Papers papers, OM 65/17/38. Oxley-SLQ.

572 Dr Shields (UAP) addressing Parliament in November, 1937. J. Macnamara, Series 4, Newspaper cuttings, 1933-1964, MS2399 (NLA).

573 Charles Edward Chuter Papers, OM 65/17/38 Oxley-SLQ.

574 See Cases 2, 3, 8, 29 and 30 in the Report of the Royal Commission. For example, 'Will walk with one or two sticks without crutches or callipers in two years with consistent clinic treatment. Would expect her to walk sufficiently well to assist with housework and walk to the tram.' Charles Edward Chuter Papers, OM 65/17/37 Oxley-SLQ.

575 The cost for the clinic with a medical officer and eight assistants was estimated at £3000pa with an average of 160 patients per day. Chuter to Minister of Health. Charles Edward Chuter Papers, OM 65/17/37 Oxley-SLQ.

576 Kenny to Chuter. Charles Edward Chuter Papers, OM 65/17/38 Oxley-SLQ.

577 Sister Mary Luddy. Scrapbook, Charles Edward Chuter Papers, OM 65/17/2/3 Oxley-SLQ.

578 Kenny to Chuter, 24 April 1939. Charles Edward Chuter Papers, OM 65/17/34 Oxley-SLQ.

579 Aubrey Pye, 31 January 1940. Victor Cohn Papers, Interviews and other sources, A-W, 1940s-1970s, MHS-K.

580 Pye to Chuter. Charles Edward Chuter Papers, OM 65/17/34 Oxley-SLQ

581 Interview with Fryberg. Victor Cohn Papers, Interviews and other sources, A-W, 1940s-1970s, MHS-K.

582 Dr Jarvis Nye to Cohn. Victor Cohn Papers, Interviews and other sources, A-W, 1940s-1970s, MHS-K.

583 W. Forster and E. Price, 'An Investigation of 23 Cases of Poliomyelitis Treated by the Kenny Method at the Children's Hospital Hampton, Victoria', 1939. Rae W. Dungan collection, UQ 354/15, UQ.

584 Drs Nye, Arden, Pye, Lee, Fryberg and Professor Wilkinson signed the letter to Basil O'Connor of the NFIP. Charles Edward Chuter Papers, OM 65/17/38 Oxley-SLQ.
585 Interview with Fryberg. Victor Cohn Papers, Interviews and other sources, A-W, 1940s-1970s, MHS-K.

Chapter 6

586 Details on her time in America and Canada from Wade Alexander Papers, MHS-K and W.K. Alexander, 'Sent to the United States', in *Sister Elizabeth Kenny*. In 2014, Naomi Rogers published her extensive study of Kenny's years in America, *'Polio Wars: Sister Kenny and the Golden Age of American Medicine.'*
587 Former law partner of President Franklin Roosevelt and close associate.
588 Forgan Smith to O'Connor. National Foundation for Infantile Paralysis, O'Connor, Basil 1940-1947, MHS-K.
589 Commonwealth Fund Archives, Harkness Report-Sister Elizabeth Kenny Foundation. SG1, Series 2/24/210 RAC.
590 Miland Knapp was Chief of the Department of Physical Medicine at Minneapolis General Hospital and Wallace Cole was Chief of the Department of Orthopaedics at the University of Minnesota. Interview Miland Knapp. Victor Cohn Papers, Interviews and other sources, A-W, 1940s-1970s, MHS-K.
591 In 1942, The Exchange Club of Minneapolis started the Sister Kenny Endowment and Education Fund, a nonprofit organisation that paid Kenny $416 per month 'until the day she died'. Kenny could not accept donations directly as she was on a visitor's visa and, as such, was forbidden from accepting charity. Jim Interview Jim Henry. Victor Cohn Papers, Interviews and other sources, A-W, 1940s-1970s, MHS-K.
592 Macnamara to Carter, June 1933. J. Macnamara, Series 1, Correspondence 1923–1968, MS 2399.
593 Elizabeth Kenny. Victor Cohn Papers, Sister Elizabeth Kenny Foundation Records, Elizabeth Kenny Correspondence MHS-K.
594 A.L. Plastridge, Report: Trip to observe work of Sister Kenny, 15 March 1941. Elizabeth Kenny Polio Treatment, Reports and Paper on (Others), MHS-K.
595 Robert L. Bennett, MD, Warm Springs to Dr Frank Krusen, 6 August 1942. Victor Cohn Papers, Dr Frank Krusen's Elizabeth Kenny File, MHS-K.
596 For a detailed discussion and assessment of the Kendall's visit to Minneapolis in 1941, see N. Rogers, *Polio Wars*, pp.44-49.
597 Kenny to Chuter, 4 October 1940. Charles Edward Chuter Papers, OM 65/17/33 Oxley-SLQ.
598 Kenny to Chuter, May 1942. Charles Edward Chuter Papers, OM 65/17/33 Oxley-SLQ.
599 Gudakunst to Dr Knowlton, 22 January 1942. Victor Cohn Papers, Interviews and other sources, A-W, 1940s-1970s, MHS-K.
600 1800 Chicago Avenue, Minneapolis. Initially accommodated around 180 patients but was expanded in 1951.
601 William Stewart, Director State Crippled Children's Service University of Missouri; Associate Professor Washburn, University of Wisconsin; H.A. Smart, M.D., Virginia; F.L. McNaughton, McGill University Department of Neurology and Neurosurgery. Correspondence, Incoming for the Period 1942–1947. Elizabeth Kenny Collection, UQFL16/1/2, UQ.
602 Able to receive tax-exempt donations from corporations and the general public. In 1943 the proposed grant of $139,000 was rejected by the NFIP. Inventory: Journal Articles, Papers and Letters In 'Kenny's Brown Bag' MHS-K.

603 'Changing Clinical Care' in N. Rogers, *Polio Wars*, p.87.
604 The AMA sponsored the report. R. Ghormley, et al, 'Evaluation of the Kenny Treatment of Infantile Paralysis', *Journal of the American Medical Association*, pp.406–09.
605 'American Physicians Claim Paralysis Not Cured by Kenny', *Ottawa Evening Journal*, June 1944.
606 US $845,000 for a period of three years. Marvin Kline, Kenny Institute to Basil O'Connor, 18 July 1944. MHS 143.E.10.4f.
607 All the letters written to FDR were forwarded to the NFIP. Roosevelt, Franklin D: Papers as President, President's Secretary's File, Letters of support for Sister Elizabeth Kenny February 1944–1945, Franklin D Roosevelt Library.
608 National Research Council. Report of Special Committee. Series K, 15/118, RAC.
609 The NIB was a non-profit membership corporation for the protection of contributors and philanthropic agencies. National Information Bureau, 8 December 1947. Series K, 14/114, RAC.
610 J.D. Rockefeller to A.W. Packard, 6 January 1942. Polio - National Foundation for Infantile Paralysis/National Foundation, 1937-1949. Series K, 14/114, RAC.
611 National Information Bureau, Series K, 14/114, RAC.
612 It stated that the Foundation needed to raise $40 million in 1949 if the program was not to be curtailed. It had already raised almost $26 million that year. The official estimate for likely polio cases in 1949 was between 33,000 and 38,000. National Foundation for Infantile Paralysis, Series K, 14/114, RAC.
613 Dr Hart Van Riper, 8 January 1948. Harkness Report and Sister Elizabeth Kenny Foundation, SG1 Series 2, 24/210 RAC.
614 In 1948 there were 27,908 cases of polio in the USA. The Foundation spent $7 million on medical care, distributed 600 respirators and employed an extra 2400 nurses, 153 physical therapists and thirty-five doctors. No figures were available for 1948, but in 1947, $18 million was raised. The subsidy per patient in 1948 was $250. 'Polio Drains a Treasury', *The New York Times*, 7 October 1949.
615 Professor and Chairman of the Department of Bone and Joint Surgery, Northwestern University Medical School, Chicago. Lewin to Cohn, 19 October 1954. Victor Cohn Papers, Interviews and other sources, A-W, 1940s-1970s, MHS-K.
616 For an analysis on how Sister Kenny used her position as the 'people's choice' to further her claim for equal footing with the medical establishment to access and conduct laboratory research into the aetiology and prevention of polio, see N. Rogers, 'Sister Kenny Goes to Washington: Polio, Populism and Medical Politics in Postwar America', in *The Politics of Healing*, ed. R.D. Johnston, pp.97-116.
617 H. Spencer Jordan, California, to Kenny 28 October 1944. Complimentary letters and parents' appreciation, undated and 1942–1949. MHS-K.
618 William Ballard, Hollywood, 9 March 1945. Complimentary letters and parents' appreciation, undated and 1942–1949. MHS-K.
619 Edward Smythe to Kenny. Complimentary letters and parents' appreciation, undated and 1942–1949. MHS-K.
620 Edward Smythe to Kenny. Complimentary letters and parents' appreciation, undated and 1942–1949. MHS-K.
621 Edward Smythe to Kenny. Complimentary letters and parents' appreciation, undated and 1942–1949. MHS-K.
622 J. Hall to Kenny. Complimentary letters and parents' appreciation, undated and 1942–1949. MHS-K.

623 Mrs Roberts to Kenny. Complimentary letters and parents' appreciation, undated and 1942–1949. MHS-K.
624 Cosette Dexter to Kenny. 2 February 1944. Complimentary letters and parents' appreciation, undated and 1942–1949. MHS-K.
625 Mrs Bonnell to Kenny. Complimentary letters and parents' appreciation, undated and 1942–1949. MHS-K.
626 R. Ghormley, et al, 'Evaluation of the Kenny Treatment of Infantile Paralysis', *Journal of the American Medical Association*. M.G. Brown and Mrs Rich to Kenny. Complimentary letters and parents' appreciation, undated and 1942–1949. MHS-K.
627 Mrs V. Houben, San Francisco; Loretta Pierce, New York. A five million dollar nationwide fundraising campaign to support the newly-established Kenny Foundation was launched in November 1945. Known as 'Pennies for Kenny' it was promoted by Bing Crosby.
628 My deduction from letters on file is that 89 staff were paid $40,724 in 1945 and travelling expenses totalled $2680. That left the sum paid to Kenny approximately $6431 or $178 per month. Victor Cohn papers, Sister Elizabeth Kenny Foundation Records, Elizabeth Kenny Correspondence, MHS-K.
629 Charles Chuter to Kenny, 2 June 1942. Chuter had been moved from the Department of Health to that of Local Affairs after Cilento 'had made serious charges' against him. Charles Edward Chuter Papers, OM 65/17/33 Oxley-SLQ.
630 Hanlon defended his decision by declaring that the whole of the medical profession had been won over to the Kenny treatment. That was obviously untrue. 'Minister Defends Policy on Kenny Treatment', *The Telegraph*, 9 September 1942.
631 K.W. Starr to A. Pye. 4 July 1939. Elizabeth Kenny Collection, Correspondence, UQFL16, UQ.
632 Charles Edward Chuter Papers OM 65/17/34 Oxley-SLQ.
633 Professor E.J. Goddard of Queensland University. Charles Edward Chuter Papers OM 65/17/34 Oxley-SLQ.
634 P. Lewin, 'The Kenny Treatment of Infantile Paralysis During the Acute Stage', *Illinois Medical Journal*, Vol. 81, pp.281–296.
635 Letter E. Kenny to J. Henry, 15 June 1945. Henry, James. Personal Correspondence and Related papers, undated and 1943-1976. MHS-K.
636 'Celluloid', in N. Rogers, *Polio Wars*, pp.265–66.
637 Charles Edward Chuter Papers, OM 65/17/38 Oxley-SLQ.
638 Charles Edward Chuter Papers, OM 65/17/38 Oxley-SLQ
639 Supply of Scientific and Agricultural Information. Elizabeth Kenny Institute, A1067/A46/2/7/2 (NAA).
640 R.D. McKellar Hall, *Reflections of an Orthopaedic Surgeon* pp.46-47.
641 Macnamara was made a Dame of the British Empire in the King's Birthday Honours list in 1935 in recognition of her orthopaedic work with crippled children.
642 J. Macnamara, 'Preventative Orthopaedics and the Physiotherapist', *Medical Journal of Australia*, p.296.
643 J. Macnamara, 'The Prevention of Crippling following Poliomyelitis', *Medical Journal of Australia*, p.4.
644 R.W. Lovett, 'Fatigue and exercise in the treatment of infantile paralysis', paper cited in J. Macnamara, 'The Care of the Paralysis of Poliomyelitis', *Medical Journal of Australia*, p.578.

645 F. Macfarlane Burnet, 'Health Bulletin of Department of Health Victoria, January–June 1945', cited in J. Macnamara, 'The Care of the Paralysis of Poliomyelitis', *Medical Journal of Australia*, p.577.
646 R.D. McKellar Hall, *Reflections of an Orthopaedic Surgeon*, p.47.
647 Shirley Wister, physiotherapist. P. Bentley and D. Dunstan, 'Muscle Re-Education', in *The Path to Professionalism*, p.111.
648 E. Kenny, 'Evidence Concerning My Seven Years Activities in the United States of America', Elizabeth Kenny Collection, UQFL16/1/3.
649 Memorandum, circulars, letters, etc re Kenny Clinic, 1937–1943. Charles Edward Chuter Papers, OM 65/17/38 Oxley-SLQ.
650 Letters, Memorandums, Cuttings Relating to Sister Kenny, 1943–1945, Charles Edward Chuter Papers: 1940–1950, OM 65/17/33 Oxley-SLQ.
651 Kenny to Huenekens. Administration, Huenekens, Dr E.J., 1947-1949, MHS-K.
652 Kenny to James Henry, 13 November 1952. J. Henry, Personal Correspondence and Related Papers, 1942–1951. Elizabeth Kenny papers, MHS-K.
653 USA vs Koolish, 340 F.2d 513 (8th Circuit 1965).
654 R. Metcalfe, 'A Critical Evaluation of the Kenny Treatment', *The Medical Press and Journal*, pp.477–80.
655 Canberra, Sir Earle Page to Parliament, 23 October 1952. Newspaper and Magazine Articles Regarding Elizabeth Kenny, Australia Undated and 1916-1952 MHS-K
656 F. Macfarlane Burnet, *Changing Patterns*, pp.167–68.
657 J.R. Paul, *A History of Poliomyelitis*, p.344.
658 Hart E. Van Riper to Committee on Interstate and Foreign Commerce of the United States House of Representatives, May 13, 1948. Victor Cohn papers, Additional Research Correspondence, MHS-K.
659 For example, Dr Catherine Worthingham, Director of Physical Education at the NFIP and Florence and Henry Kendall of the Baltimore Children's Hospital.
660 P. Bentley and D. Dunstan, 'Muscle Re-Education', in *The Path to Professionalism*, p.101.
661 Jim Porteous and Simon Porritt. T. Gould, *A Summer Plague*, p.235.

Chapter 7
662 D. Widgery. T. Gould, *A Summer Plague*, p.230.
663 J.M. Swann, Your Stories, Polio Network of Victoria, Autumn 2002, p.10.
664 Franklin Delano Roosevelt, 1945. http://amhistory.si.edu/polio/howpolio/fdr.htm
665 J. Vickers-Willis, 'From the Iron Lung', 11 March 1954. http://vickers-willis.com/html/homefromtheironlung.htm. Accessed March 2008.
666 E. Kübler-Ross, *On Death and Dying*.
667 See, for example, D.J. Wilson, *Living with Polio*; N.G. Seavey, et al, *A Paralyzing Fear*; Various interviews by Barbara Rossall-Wynne, Austin Hospital, Melbourne, The Bryan Richard Speed Infectious Diseases Collection, Fairfield Hospital, 1904–1996.
668 C.L. Mee, *A Nearly Normal Life*, p.70.
669 V. Overheu, *It Helps to Be Stubborn*, p.21.
670 T. Gould, *A Summer Plague*, p.317.
671 H. Gallagher, *Black Bird Fly Away*, p.88.
672 D.J. Wilson, *Living with Polio*, pp.50–51.

Notes

673 Clem Tomson, 'Respirator Ward', Fairfield Hospital Ward 12. http://hometown.aol.com.au/noelspurr/myhomepage/club.html. Accessed January 2008.
674 B. Watson, Post Polio Network of Victoria, Autumn 2008.
675 L. Ellis, Post-Polio Post', No 37, Post-Polio Network (NSW).
676 L. Ellis, Post-Polio Post', No 37, Post-Polio Network (NSW).
677 Interview J., J.H. Smith, 'Fear, Frustration and the Will to Overcome' (PhD thesis), p.373.
678 Interview D., J.H. Smith, 'Fear, Frustration and the Will to Overcome' (PhD thesis), p.374.
679 A. Killalea, *The Great Scourge*, p.108.
680 Arvid Schwartz. D.J. Wilson, *Living with Polio*, p.125.
681 J.H. Smith, 'Fear, Frustration and the Will to Overcome' (PhD thesis), p.371.
682 Interview A., J.H. Smith, 'Fear, Frustration and the Will to Overcome' (PhD thesis), p.371.
683 P. Solomon, 'Living in a Country Town', Member Stories, no. 8, Post-Polio Network (NSW); Interview Geoff Golding (Fairfield Hospital Archives).
684 Dr Sandiland, Chair of Medical Staff, Fairfield Hospital. W.K. Anderson, *Fever Hospital*, p.121.
685 Interview with Mr and Mrs Parker, parents of Elaine Theodore (Fairfield Hospital Archives).
686 A. Killalea, *The Great Scourge*, p.109.
687 Sylvia Barker, Nursing Supervisor in the 1950s. J. Silver and D.J. Wilson, eds, *Polio Voices*, p.30.
688 Pseudonym. (Fairfield Hospital Archives).
689 Michael Davis. D.J. Wilson, *Living with Polio*, p.118.
690 A. Finger, *Elegy for a Disease*, p.6.
691 The rocking bed was like a large seesaw and used gravity with the shifting weight of the abdominal organs against the diaphragm to force air in and out of the lungs. The chest respirator was a shell that used pressure to force the chest down to expel air from the lungs and then released it.
692 Jim Marugg. D.J. Wilson, *Living with Polio*, p.128.
693 Louis Sternburg. D.J. Wilson, *Living with Polio*, p.93.
694 D.J. Wilson, 'Braces, Wheelchairs, and Iron Lungs', *Journal of Medical Humanities* 26, pp.188-190.
695 J. Vickers-Willis, 'From the Iron Lung'. http://vickers-willis.com/html/homefromtheironlung.htm.
696 Fairfield Hospital, 1950s. N. Spurr, *Spurr of the Moment*. Formerly available from: http://hometown.aol.com/noelspurr/myhomepage/club.html.
697 H. Gallagher, *FDR's Splendid Deception*.
698 H. Gallagher, *FDR's Splendid Deception*, pp.34–44; D.M. Oshinsky, 'Warm Springs', in *Polio*, pp.24–42.
699 I.K. Zola, *Missing Pieces*, p.205.
700 Extensive efforts were made by Roosevelt and his supporters to hide the full extent of the President's disability from the American public and the press supported those efforts. See Gallagher, *FDR's Splendid Deception*, and J. Duffy, 'Franklin Roosevelt: Ambiguous Symbol for Disabled Americans', *Midwest Quarterly*, pp.113–35.

701 In the early twentieth century, 'massage' described the treatment given by providers known as 'masseurs' or 'masseuses'. (In the United States 'physical therapists'.)
702 P. Bentley and D. Dunstan, *The Path to Professionalism*.
703 B. Linker, 'The Business of Ethics', *Journal of the History of Medicine and Allied Sciences*, pp.320–54.
704 R. Cooter, 'The Cause of the Crippled Child', in *Surgery and Society in Peace and War*.
705 P. Bentley and D. Dunstan, 'Consolidating the Gains – the 1950s', in *The Path to Professionalism*, p.129.
706 In-patient Hampton Hospital, Victoria, 1952. J. Smith, 'Your Stories – Joan's Journey', *Personal Polio Stories*, Vol. 19/4 (Polio Perspectives), p.11.
707 Gary Buchanan, Polio NSW, Summer 2012, p.2.
708 Ruthanne Werner, Pennsylvania, 1952. J. Silver and D.J. Wilson, eds, *Polio Voices*, p.70.
709 Beatrice Nau, Kentucky, 1943. J. Silver and D.J. Wilson, eds, *Polio Voices*, p.46.
710 Edward O'Connor, Bronx, NYC, 1955. J. Silver and D.J. Wilson, eds, *Polio Voices* p.49.
711 Ian Dury, England. T. Gould, *A Summer Plague*, p.231.
712 C. Mee, *A Nearly Normal Life*, p.64.
713 Michael Davis. T.M. Daniel and F.C. Robbins, eds, '1944 Kentucky Polio Epidemic', in *Polio*, p.34.
714 Jim Porteous. T. Gould, *A Summer Plague*, p.238.
715 Administration, Complimentary letters and parents' appreciation, undated and 1942–1949. MHS-K.
716 Janice Platt, Rochester, NY, 1942. Administration, Kenny Institute 50th Anniversary, Patient Letters, 1991–1992. MHS-K.
717 Sylvia Barker, New York. In J. Silver and D.J. Wilson, eds, *Polio Voices*, p.29.
718 For example, Minnesota Historical Society, St Paul, Minnesota, and Franklin Delano Roosevelt Library, Hyde Park, New York.
719 Mrs Danielson, Minneapolis, 1944. Administration, Kenny Institute 50th Anniversary, Patient Letters, 1991–1992. MHS-K.
720 Mrs Beckton, Washington DC, 1945. Administration, Kenny Institute 50th Anniversary, Patient Letters, 1991–1992. MHS-K.
721 Rose Fitterer, Washington Park Hospital, Chicago. Administration, Kenny Institute 50th Anniversary, Patient Letters, 1991–1992. MHS-K.
722 Michael Davis. T.M. Daniel and F.C. Robbins, eds, '1944 Kentucky Polio Epidemic', in *Polio*, p.31.
723 The source was not identified. A. Finger, *Elegy for a Disease*, p.118.
724 C. Mee, *A Nearly Normal Life*, p.67.
725 Kenny to Dryden, Duncan Hospital in Wanganui, 10 January 1948. Biographers Research Papers, Elizabeth Kenny, reports and other papers, undated and 1941–1951. MHS-K.
726 Mr Parker, father of Elaine aged sixteen months in 1936. Interview with Mr and Mrs Parker, parents of Elaine Theodore (Fairfield Hospital Archives).
727 A. Killalea, *The Great Scourge*, p.114.
728 Shirley made a complete recovery, and when her parents took her back to the original specialist some months later, his only comment was that 'it was a miracle that she could walk'. In S. Barnett, Member Stories Broadway', no. 7, Post-Polio Network (NSW).

Notes

729 D.J. Wilson, *Living with Polio*, p.126.
730 T. Gould, *A Summer Plague*, p.236.
731 Brigadier Metcalfe was a consultant orthopaedic surgeon to the Army during the Second World War and later worked at Carshalton. Jim Porteous. T. Gould, *A Summer Plague*, p.238.
732 Metcalfe to Cohn, 29 August 1955. Biographers' Research Papers, Victor Cohn's Elizabeth Kenny Research Notes, Transcriptions, Correspondence and Other Papers; J. Brand, *The History of the National Foundation for Infantile Paralysis*. Biographers' Research Papers, Victor Cohn's Elizabeth Kenny Research Notes, Transcriptions, Correspondence and Other Papers, MHS-K.
733 George Durr, New York State, 1936. J. Silver and D.J. Wilson, eds, *Polio Voices*, p.65.
734 Invercargill in 1937, Christchurch and Dunedin in 1942, and the Duncan Hospital in Upper Hutt in 1945. J.C. Ross, 'A History of Poliomyelitis in New Zealand' (MA thesis), pp.58–59.
735 J.C. Ross, 'A History of Poliomyelitis in New Zealand' (MA thesis), p.62.
736 J.C. Ross, 'A History of Poliomyelitis in New Zealand' (MA thesis), p.62.
737 G. Buchanan, 'I Used to Jump Puddles', no. 7, *Personal Polio Stories*, Post-Polio Network (NSW).
738 B. Watson, 'Polio Story', in M. Liethof, ed., *Stories* (Polio Perspectives).
739 G. Stock, 'Prima Ballerina', *The Weekend Australian*, 2006.
740 Interview Les Corneille (Fairfield Hospital Archives).
741 Interview Una White (Fairfield Hospital Archives).
742 Anon., 'Respirator Ward', Fairfield Hospital Ward 12.
743 G. Thomas, ed., 'A Story to Break the Silence', no. 45, Post-Polio Newsletter, Post-Polio Network (NSW)
744 D.G. Pritchard, 'The Development of Schools for Handicapped Children in England During the Nineteenth Century', *History of Education Quarterly*, pp.215–222.
745 H.H. Kessler, *The Crippled and the Disabled*; S. Koven, 'Remembering and Dismemberment', *The American Historical Review*, pp.1167–202.
746 W. Vickers, 'Report on the Education and Treatment of Cripples in the United States of America', *Medical Journal of Australia*, pp.9–10.
747 A. Curtis, 'The Crippled Childrens' School', *The American Journal of Nursing*, pp.427–28.
748 See M.L. Ingram, 'Trends in Education of Crippled Children', *Journal of Educational Sociology*, pp.339–47; H.H. Kessler, *The Crippled and the Disabled*; E.C. Scofield, 'Schools for Segregation of Crippled Children', *The American Journal of Nursing*, pp.469–70.
749 E.T. Honesty, 'The Handicapped Child', *The Journal of Negro Education*, pp.304–24.
750 M.V. Kennedy and H.C.D. Somerset, 'Bringing up Crippled Children' (Report).
751 Formerly available from: www.yooralla.com.au/history.php. Accessed 3 July 2005.
752 J.C. Ross, 'A History of Poliomyelitis in New Zealand' (MA thesis), p.42.
753 K.F. Coles, *The History of the New South Wales Society for Crippled Children*, p.2.
754 The suburbs were Carlton, Fitzroy, Collingwood and North Melbourne. B. Gleeson, 'Domestic Space and Disability in Nineteenth-Century Melbourne, Australia', *Journal of Historical Geography*, pp.223–40.
755 K.F. Coles, *The History of the New South Wales Society for Crippled Children*, p.2.

756 K.F. Coles, *The History of the New South Wales Society for Crippled Children*, p.2.
757 In six months Rotarians traced more than 800 children in Sydney and, in 1932, surgeons examined 1153 children. K.F. Coles, *The History of the New South Wales Society for Crippled Children*, p.39.
758 K.F. Coles, 'Sir Lorimer Dodds', in *The History of the New South Wales Society for Crippled Children*.
759 A.M. Norris, ed., *The Society*, p.42.
760 Freeman described how women beggars displayed their crippled children on street corners. J. Freeman, *Lights and Shadows of Melbourne Life*.
761 See, for example, Vagabond and M. Cannon, *The Vagabond Papers*.
762 K.F. Coles, *The History of the New South Wales Society for Crippled Children*, p.39.
763 J. Macnamara, 'After-Care of Poliomyelitis', *Medical Journal of Australia*, pp.616–17.
764 J. Macnamara, Series 7, Notebooks, 1925–1966. MS2399 (NLA).
765 J. Macnamara, Series 7, Notebooks, 1925–1966. MS2399 (NLA).
766 Methodist missionary and founder of Yooralla Hospital School in Melbourne.
767 N. Marshall, *The Yooralla Story*, p.3.
768 K.F. Coles, *The History of the New South Wales Society for Crippled Children*, p.15.
769 K.F. Coles, *The History of the New South Wales Society for Crippled Children*, p.15.
770 K.F. Coles, *The History of the New South Wales Society for Crippled Children*, p.17.
771 In 1929, the Committee of the Children's Hospital bought an old home with eight hectares of land and a beach frontage at Mt Eliza and built an orthopaedic unit of forty beds. It was closed in 1970 after demand for its services dwindled following the discovery of antibiotics and the Salk vaccine.
772 G.J. Carmichael, *Hospital Children*, pp.49–50.
773 P. Yule, 'The Beginnings of the Allied Health Professions', in *The Royal Children's Hospital*, p.196.
774 J. Macnamara, Series 1, Correspondence 1923–1968. MS2399 (NLA).
775 Interview of the parents of Elaine Theodore, 13 November 1992 (Fairfield Hospital Archives).
776 K.F. Coles, *The History of the New South Wales Society for Crippled Children*, p.39.
777 J. Macnamara, Series 1, Correspondence 1923–1968. MS2399 (NLA).
778 P. Bentley and D. Dunstan, 'Muscle Re-Education', in *The Path to Professionalism*, p.92.
779 P. Bentley and D. Dunstan, *The Path to Professionalism*, p.98.
780 The situation in the other states improved from around 1937. A full-time massage therapist was appointed at the Adelaide Children's Hospital in 1938, and there were three therapists in Hobart, Devon and Launceston in 1937. P. Bentley and D. Dunstan, *The Path to Professionalism*, pp.98–99. In Queensland and New South Wales both Societies for Crippled Children began campaigns in the early 1930s to raise funds to build homes to provide accommodation and treatment for children.
781 P. Yule, *The Royal Children's Hospital*. Frankston accommodated eighty-eight patients and was almost always full. In 1936 a further twelve beds were made available at Brighton Convalescent Hospital for infantile paralysis cases.
782 Tasmanian Society for the Care of Crippled Children, Annual Report, 1939, Parliamentary Papers.
783 Swann Road, Taringa. Queensland Society for Crippled Children, *Souvenir of Government House Fete in Aid of Qld Society for Crippled Children*, p.45.

Notes

784 Coles, K.F. *The History of the New South Wales Society for Crippled Children*.

785 Reverend S.G. Drummond, 'Country Surveys, and the Work of the Far West Children's Health Scheme' (Report), p.19.

786 In 1925 a survey in New York State revealed that crippled children made up around seven per cent of the population, with fifty per cent under sixteen years. The ratio of crippled children averaged around 2.5 to 3 per thousand. M.L. Ingram, 'Trends in Education of Crippled Children', *Journal of Educational Sociology*, pp.339–47. Extrapolating those results to New South Wales would give an estimated 14,000 crippled children with around 7000 eligible for a pension. A report in 1925 showed 17,514 persons drawing a pension in New South Wales at an annual cost of £780,000. W. Vickers, 'Report on the Education and Treatment of Cripples in the United States of America', *Medical Journal of Australia*, pp.9–10.

787 *Documenting a Democracy-Victoria* www.foundingdocs.gov.au/area-aid-8.html

788 See, for example, A.M. Norris, ed., *The Society: Being Some Account of the Victorian Society for Crippled Children and Adults*; Royal Children's Hospital, Collected Papers of the Royal Children's Hospital and Paediatric Society of Victoria, 1935.1960 (NLA); K.F. Coles, *The History of the New South Wales Society for Crippled Children*; N. Marshall, *The Yooralla Story: A History of the Yooralla Hospital School for Crippled Children, 1918–1977*; Almoner's report, 1939, Tasmanian Society for the Care of Crippled Children, Parliamentary Papers; H.T. Parker, *Crippled Children in Tasmania*.

789 J.H. Smith, 'Fear, Frustration and the Will to Overcome' (PhD thesis), p.406.

790 N. Marshall, *The Yooralla Story*; Almoner's report, 1939, Tasmanian Society for Crippled Children.

791 K.F. Coles, *The History of the New South Wales Society for Crippled Children*, p.16.

792 Pat Featherstone, Member stories, No.4, Post-Polio Network (NSW).

793 Twenty five per cent of children were paralysed following infantile paralysis. H.T. Parker, *Crippled Children in Tasmania*.

794 100 savings accounts were opened at the Hobart Savings Bank. Almoner's report, 1939, Tasmanian Society for Crippled Children.

795 One to a bootmaker and the other to a dressmaker. Almoner's report, 1939, Tasmanian Society for Crippled Children.

796 Almoner's report, 1939, Tasmanian Society for Crippled Children.

797 G. Buchanan, 'I Used to Jump Puddles', no. 7, *Personal Polio Stories*, Post-Polio Network (NSW).

798 Almoner's report, 1939, Tasmanian Society for Crippled Children.

799 N. Marshall, *The Yooralla Story*; A.M. Norris, ed., *The Society*; R.D. McKellar Hall, *Reflections of an Orthopaedic Surgeon*.

800 H. Gallagher, *FDR's Splendid Deception*, p.28.

801 Rick Spalsbury, Oklahoma City. J. Silver and D.J. Wilson, eds, *Polio Voices*, p.67.

802 Interview C., J.H. Smith, 'Fear, Frustration and the Will to Overcome' (PhD thesis), p.406.

803 Interview A., J.H. Smith, 'Fear, Frustration and the Will to Overcome' (PhD thesis).

804 Interview A., J.H. Smith, 'Fear, Frustration and the Will to Overcome' (PhD thesis).

805 B. Watson, *Your Stories*, Polio Network of Victoria.

806 Interview Valda Millie Heath, 12 November 1992 (Fairfield Hospital Archives).

807 Interview A., J.H. Smith, 'Fear, Frustration and the Will to Overcome' (PhD thesis), p.394.

808 Interview June Middleton, 3 September 1992 (Fairfield Hospital Archives).
809 'Melbourne woman has spent 60 years in iron lung', *Herald Sun*, 5 April 2009.
810 Mrs A. Duprey, Burlington VT to Sister Kenny, January 1943. National Foundation for Infantile Paralysis. MHS 143.E.10.4F.
811 Jean Johnson. T. Gould, *A Summer Plague*, p.278.
812 Interview Brian Caulfield, 16 May 1995 (Fairfield Hospital Archives); L. Pruscino, 'Polio Story', in M. Liethof, ed., *Stories* (Polio Perspectives); J.M. Swann, *Your Stories*, Polio Network of Victoria, Autumn 2002, p.10.
813 G. Thomas, ed., 'A Story to Break the Silence', no. 45, Post-Polio Newsletter, Post-Polio Network (NSW).
814 Interview Una White (Fairfield Hospital Archives).
815 Interview C., J.H. Smith, 'Fear, Frustration and the Will to Overcome' (PhD thesis), p.396.
816 George Durr. J. Silver and D.J. Wilson, eds., *Polio Voices*, p.65; Cindy Bernstein, 'Mazzy Meets the Dragon', no. 3, *Personal Polio Stories* Post-Polio Network (NSW).
817 G. Thomas, ed., 'A Story to Break the Silence', no. 45, Post-Polio Newsletter, Post-Polio Network (NSW).
818 G. Thomas, ed., 'A Story to Break the Silence', no. 45, Post-Polio Newsletter, Post-Polio Network (NSW).
819 Interview D., J.H. Smith, 'Fear, Frustration and the Will to Overcome' (PhD thesis), p.375.
820 H. Atkinson, 'My Story', 'Post-Polio Post', no 26, Post-Polio Network (NSW).
821 J.M. Swann, 'Polio Story', *Your Stories*, Autumn 2002, Polio Network of Victoria, p.10.
822 Royal Park (68), Queenscliff (68), Forest Hills, Caulfield (50) and Shennington. VPRS/6345/P0000/327/279, Polio Campaigns, 1930–1933, Consultative Council on Poliomyelitis (PROV).
823 The Council voted to grant a yearly sum of £1500 to the Royal Melbourne Hospital to improve the capacity of its splint workshop. The cost of the splints was divided equally between the hospital, the patient and the Hospitals and Charities Commission. VPRS/6345/P0000/392, Splint Production October 1947–August 1970, Consultative Council on Poliomyelitis (PROV).
824 A.M. Norris, ed., *The Society*, pp.45–47.
825 P. Bentley and D. Dunstan, *The Path to Professionalism*, p.104.
826 Ballarat, Geelong, Mooroopna, Mildura, Horsham, Hamilton and Bendigo. VPRS 6345/P0000/113, Accommodation and aftercare for cripples (PROV).
827 VPRS 6345/P0000/112, Training of physiotherapists, treatment of paralysis (PROV).
828 VPRS 6345/P0000/113, 1949 epidemic (PROV).
829 A. Killalea, *The Great Scourge*, p.113.
830 A Sister Andrews. Interview Valda Millie Heath (Fairfield Hospital Archives).
831 Alice Farnham, an American osteopath in Melbourne. Louis Pruscino, *Your Stories*, Autumn 2007, p.10.
832 E. Willis, 'Sister Elizabeth Kenny and the Evolution of the Occupational Division of Labour in Health Care', *Australian and New Zealand Journal of Sociology*, pp.30–38.
833 From 1945 till 1952. Interview Valda Millie Heath (Fairfield Hospital Archives).

834 In 1952.
835 Interview Valda Millie Heath (Fairfield Hospital Archives).
836 Interview Una White (Fairfield Hospital Archives).
837 D.J. Wilson, *Living with Polio*, p.159.
838 G. Buchanan, 'I Used to Jump Puddles', no. 7, *Personal Polio Stories*, Post-Polio Network (NSW).
839 Charles Mee. D.J.Wilson, *Living with Polio*, p.161.
840 Anon in G. Thomas, ed., 'A Story to Break the Silence', no. 45, Post-Polio Newsletter, Post-Polio Network (NSW).
841 J.M. Swann, *Your Stories*, Polio Network of Victoria.
842 Interview D., J.H. Smith, 'Fear, Frustration and the Will to Overcome' (PhD thesis), p.35.
843 Interview D., J.H. Smith, 'Fear, Frustration and the Will to Overcome' (PhD thesis), p.35.
844 P. Corrigan, 'Polio Story', *Your Stories*, Polio Network of Victoria.
845 Anon. G. Thomas, ed., 'A Story to Break the Silence', no. 45, Post-Polio Newsletter, Post-Polio Network (NSW).
846 J.M. Swann, *Your Stories*, Polio Network of Victoria, Autumn 2002, p.10.

Chapter 8

847 Dr Thomas Rivers, virologist, Emeritus Member of the Rockefeller Institute for Medical Research, New York, 1926–1962. S. Benison, *Tom Rivers*, p.146.
848 T.M. Rivers, 'The Story of Research on Poliomyelitis', *Proceedings of the American Philosophical Society*, pp.250–54; S. Benison, *Tom Rivers*, p.146.
849 See, for example, W.W.C. Topley, et al, *Principles of Bacteriology, Virology and Immunity*; F. Macfarlane Burnet and D.O. White, *Natural History of Infectious Disease*; F. Fenner, *History of Microbiology in Australia*.
850 F. Macfarlane Burnet and D.O. White, *Natural History of Infectious Disease*, pp.70–88.
851 N.J. Tomes, 'American Attitudes Toward the Germ Theory of Disease', *Journal of the History of Medicine and Allied Sciences*, p.28.
852 Koch's postulates state four criteria that must be fulfilled to define a causative organism: (1) the organism must be observed in all cases of the disease; (2) it must be isolated in pure culture or on artificial media; (3) inoculation of the culture into an animal must produce the same disease; and (4) the organism had then to be recovered from the inoculated animal. J.L. Bennington, et al, eds, *Saunders Dictionary and Encyclopedia of Laboratory Medicine and Technology*, p.853.
853 Jakob von Heine from Germany and Oskar Medin from Sweden.
854 F. Robbins, 'Reminiscenses of a Virologist', T.M. Daniel and F.C. Robbins, eds, *Polio*, p.7.
855 T.M. Daniel and F.C. Robbins, eds, *Polio*, p.12.
856 A period when the virus is circulating in the bloodstream and antibodies can be detected.
857 F. Macfarlane Burnet, 'A Review of Poliomyelitis', *Medical Journal of Australia*, vol.2, no.14 (1952) p.482.
858 'Clinical Infection Poliomyelitis'. www.nlm.nih.gov/medlineplus/print/ency/article/001402.htm; T.M. Daniel and F.C. Robbins, eds, *Polio*, pp.97–119.

859 The retraining of muscle cells to take over the role of other damaged cells formed the basis of the 're-education' treatment refined by Sister Elizabeth Kenny in Townsville, Queensland.

860 'The quadriceps proximally and the anterior tibilas distally', cited in D.A. Neumann, 'Polio', *Journal of Orthopaedic and Sports Physical Therapy*, pp.479–92.

861 If the virus affected the nerve cells in the cervical spine and brain stem that controlled breathing and swallowing, then the severe 'bulbar' type of paralysis eventuated.

862 J.R. Paul, *A History of Poliomyelitis*; R. Southby, 'Acute Poliomyelitis in Victoria', *Medical Journal of Australia*, pp.9–10; J.A. Anderson, 'Diagnosis and Treatment of Poliomyelitis in the Early Stage' (Paper), pp.110–11.

863 A full-body-sized iron chamber that functioned as a mechanical bellows.

864 Formerly available from www.nlm.nih.gov/medlineplus/print/ency/article/001402.htm. Accessed 17 March 2007.

865 S. Benison, 'Poliomyelitis and the Rockefeller Institute', *Journal of the History of Medicine*, pp.74–93.

866 F. Macfarlane Burnet and D.O. White, *Natural History of Infectious Disease*, p.57.

867 S. Flexner and H.L. Amoss, 'The Relation of the Meninges and Choroid Plexus to Poliomyelitic Infection', *Journal of Experimental Medicine*, pp.525–37.

868 S. Flexner, 'Respiratory vs Gastro-Intestinal Infection in Poliomyelitis', *Journal of Experimental Medicine*, p.209.

869 S. Flexner and H. Noguchi, 'Experiments on the Cultivation of the Microorganism Causing Epidemic Poliomyelitis', *Journal of Experimental Medicine*, pp.461–85; Flexner and Amoss, 'The Relation of the Meninges and Choroid Plexus to Poliomyelitic Infection', p.25.

870 The toxin produced by the diphtheria bacillus is a classic example. When modified anti-toxin against diphtheria was introduced as a preventive measure in 1884, it proved an effective weapon in the elimination of that childhood disease.

871 S. Flexner and H. Noguchi, 'Experiments on the Cultivation of the Microorganism Causing Epidemic Poliomyelitis', *Journal of Experimental Medicine*, pp.461–85.

872 One 40,000th of a millimetre.

873 A. Kita and P. Durfee, *Dr. Noguchi's Journey*; S. Benison, *Tom Rivers*, p.110.

874 T.M. Rivers, 'The Story of Research on Poliomyelitis', *Proceedings of the American Philosophical Society*, pp.250–54.

875 McCallum and Kendall in the United States and Ledingham and Eagles in England.

876 S. Benison, *Tom Rivers*, pp.182–93.

877 R. Webster, in 'Scientific'*Medical Journal of Australia*, p.293.

878 During the Swedish epidemic of 1911, Flexner and Lewis detected the virus in mesenteric lymphatic glands, saliva, the nasopharynx and the intestine of acute cases, convalescents and apparently healthy contacts. S. Flexner and P.A. Lewis, 'Experimental Epidemic Poliomyelitis in Monkeys', *Journal of Experimental Medicine*, pp.227–55.

879 See N. Rogers, *Dirt and Disease: Polio before FDR*; H. Gallagher, *FDR's Splendid Deception*.

880 S. Benison, *Tom Rivers*, p.193.

881 S. Flexner, 'Respiratory vs Gastro-Intestinal Infection in Poliomyelitis', *Journal of Experimental Medicine*, p.209.

Notes

882 Webster was appointed as a full-time pathologist in 1913, and the laboratory was 'regarded as the best' in Victoria. P. Yule, 'The Doctors 1900–1923', in *The Royal Children's Hospital*, p.126.

883 Webster placed an advertisement in the *Argus* in March 1918, offering to buy monkeys. P. Yule, *The Royal Children's Hospital*, p.127.

884 The first polio epidemic in Victoria occurred in 1908, and in 1918, over 300 notifications were received. R. Webster, 'Anterior Poliomyelitis', *Medical Journal of Australia*.

885 R. Webster, 'Anterior Poliomyelitis', *Medical Journal of Australia*.

886 T.M. Rivers, 'The Story of Research on Poliomyelitis', *Proceedings of the American Philosophical Society*, pp.250–54.

887 Walter and Eliza Hall Institute of Research in Pathology and Medicine in Melbourne. www.adb.online.anu.edu.au/biogs/A170158b.htm. Accessed 23 May 2008.

888 F. Macfarlane Burnet, *Changing Patterns*, p.36.

889 F. Morgan, 'The Preparation of Serum from Human Donors Recovered from Poliomyelitis', *Medical Journal of Australia*, pp.264–67.

890 Macnamara to Flexner, 22 January 1929. RG301 6, Box 3, RAC.

891 Rockefeller Institute MV, a mixed virus strain that became adapted to monkeys and was neurotrophic.

892 The Rockefeller virus was eventually shown to be Type II (Lansing), and the Melbourne strain to be Type I (Brunhilde). C. Sexton, *The Seeds of Time*, p.87.

893 Flexner to Macnamara, 23 September 1929. RG301 6, Box 3, RAC.

894 F. Macfarlane Burnet, 'The Epidemiology of Poliomyelitis with Special Reference to the Victorian Epidemic of 1937–1938', *Medical Journal of Australia*, pp.325–35.

895 F. Macfarlane Burnet, *Changing Patterns*, p.79.

896 www.guardian.co.uk/footandmouth/story/0,,2215280,00.html. Accessed 30 November 2007.

897 From 86 in 1930 to 269 in 1931.

898 The allocation was US $2000pa for three years. The Commonwealth Government contributed £400pa to employ Jean Macnamara as a part-time assistant for clinical and fieldwork. Dr Kellaway to Dr Alan Gregg, Australia Hall Institute 1933–1935. 28 May 1934. RG2 1924-1951, Australia 1934, 102/803.

899 Dr Kellaway was Director of the Walter and Eliza Hall Institute from 1923 to 1944. F. Macfarlane Burnet, *Walter and Eliza Hall Institute, 1915–1965*, pp.21–32.

900 A. Sabin and P. Olitsky, 'Cultivation of the Poliomyelitis Virus in Vitro in Human Embryonic Nervous Tissue', *Proceedings of the Society of Experimental and Biological Medicine*, pp.357–59.

901 E. Robertson, 'An Examination of the Olfactory Bulbs in Fatal Cases of Poliomyelitis During the Victorian Epidemic of 1937–38', *Medical Journal of Australia*, pp.156–162.

902 J. Paul and J. Trask, 'Detection of Poliomyelitis Virus in So-Called Abortive Types of the Disease', *Journal of Experimental Medicine*, pp.319–43.

903 In 1940 a healthy monkey cost around US $10–15, but the war in the Pacific meant supply was curtailed. T. Rivers, 'The Story of Research on Poliomyelitis', *Proceedings of the American Philosophical Society*, pp.250–54.

904 F. Macfarlane Burnet, et al, 'The Use of *Macacus Cynomolgus* as an Experimental Animal', *Australian Journal of Experimental Biology and Medical Science*, pp.375–91.

905 F. Macfarlane Burnet, *Changing Patterns*, p.164.

906 Victor Hugo Wallace, 1940, 77/65, The Eugenics Society of Victoria Minute Book 2/1/3 (University of Melbourne Archives).
907 C. Sexton, *The Seeds of Time*, p.90.
908 F. Macfarlane Burnet, 'Influenza Virus Infections of the Chick Embryo Lung', *British Journal of Experimental Pathology*, p.147.
909 From the Latin *in vitro* meaning 'within glass'. Growing the virus outside a living organism under laboratory conditions.
910 S. Benison, *Tom Rivers*, p.447.
911 For their discovery of the ability of poliomyelitis viruses to grow in cultures of various types of tissue. http://nobelprize.org/nobel_prizes/medicine/laureates/1954/index.html. Accessed 24 November 2007.
912 V. Cohn, 'Deluge of Dimes Hits White House Mail', *Minneapolis Morning Tribune*, April 1945, pp.46–54.
913 F.C. Robbins, 'Reminiscenses of a Virologist', in *Polio*, eds T.M. Daniel and F.C. Robbins, p.12; R.E. Frischer, 'Waiting for Society to Catch Up', in *Polio*, eds T.M. Daniel and F.C. Robbins, p.125.
914 F. Macfarlane Burnet and D. Lush, 'Studies on Experimental Herpes Infection in Mice, Using the Chorioallantoic Technique', *The Journal of Pathology and Bacteriology*, pp.241–59.
915 Burnet to Alan Gregg, General Correspondence Australia. Rockefeller Foundation Records, International Health Board/Division records, RG 5, 410/2/15, RAC.
916 Both men worked at the New York City Department of Public Health.
917 Benison, *Tom Rivers*, p.185.
918 S. Benison, *Tom Rivers*, pp.184–90.
919 S. Benison, *Tom Rivers*, pp.184–90.
920 Macfarlane Burnet, 'The Epidemiology of Poliomyelitis with Special Reference to the Victorian Epidemic of 1937–1938', *Medical Journal of Australia*, pp.325–35.
921 J.S. Smith, *Patenting the Sun*, pp.126–28.
922 VAPP occurred in about one case for every 2.4 million doses of oral poliomyelitis vaccine (OPV) distributed. Two cases of VAPP have been notified in Australia (1986 and 1995).
923 Many detailed accounts exist on the development of the Salk and Sabin vaccines. See, for example, J.S. Smith, *Patenting the Sun: Polio and the Salk Vaccine*; J.R. Paul, *A History of Poliomyelitis*; F. Fenner, *History of Microbiology in Australia*; D.M. Oshinsky, *Polio: An American Story*; F. Macfarlane Burnet, *Changing Patterns: An Atypical Autobiography*; P. Fisher, *The Polio Story*; A.H. Brogan, *Committed to Saving Lives: A History of the Commonwealth Serum Laboratories*. Because of the risk of VAPP, inactivated (Salk) poliomyelitis vaccine (IPV) was reintroduced in November 2005 and is now used for all doses of polio vaccine in Australia. IPV cannot cause VAPP. www.immunise.health.gov.au. Accessed 2 February 2009.
924 F. Macfarlane Burnet, *Changing Patterns*, p.169.
925 Since the earliest days of virology, typing of viruses has been an important tool to characterise viral populations and to study their epidemiology. Typing provides information on the relationship among isolates within the same group, species, or genus.
926 There are three types of poliovirus, but many strains, e.g., Brunhilde, Lansing and Leon. S. Benison, *Tom Rivers*, pp.453–54.
927 'Crucial Year in the Polio Battle', *The Sydney Morning Herald*, 5 April 1953, p.8.
928 J.S. Smith, *Patenting the Sun*, pp.140–43.

Notes

929 In a double-blind clinical trial subjects are randomly allocated to receive either the active drug or a look-alike placebo. Neither the subject nor those administering or monitoring the drug are privy to which is being given. This is to nullify the 'placebo effect' or enigmatic benefit that some subjects experience merely by taking part in a clinical trial.

930 L. Dawson, 'The Salk Polio Vaccine Trial of 1954', *Clinical Trials*, pp.122–30.

931 L. Dawson, 'The Salk Polio Vaccine Trial of 1954', *Clinical Trials*, pp.122–30.

932 623,972 schoolchildren were injected with vaccine or placebo and more than a million others participated as observed controls. M. Meldrum, 'A Calculated Risk: The Salk Polio Vaccine Field Trials of 1954', *British Medical Journal*, pp.1233–36.

933 'New Polio Vaccine Launched', *The New York Times*, 13 April 1955, p.1.

934 T. Francis, et al, 'An Evaluation of the 1954 Poliomyelitis Vaccine Trials', *American Journal of Public Health*, pp.1–63.

935 B. Furman, 'US Blames Own Tests in Cutter Vaccine Incident, Inadequacy of Virus Inactivation in Plant', *The New York Times*, 26 August 1955, p.1.

936 Technical report by the US Public Health Service in 1955, cited in L. Dawson, 'The Salk Polio Vaccine Trial of 1954', *Clinical Trials*, pp.122–30.

937 D.M. Oshinsky, 'The Cutter Fiasco', in *Polio*, p.228.

938 Annie Dillard quoted in J.S. Smith, *Patenting the Sun*, p.263.

939 F. Macfarlane Burnet, 'Current Thought on the Prophylaxis of Poliomyelitis', *Medical Journal of Australia*, pp.192–94.

940 B. Furman, *The New York Times*, 1 May 1955, p.9.

941 'Crucial Year in the Polio Battle', *The Sydney Morning Herald*, 3 April 1953, p.8; 'New Polio Discovery Claimed', *The Sydney Morning Herald*, 17 April 1951, p.1; P.L. Dodds, 'Increasing Hopes for Polio Vaccine', *The Sydney Morning Herald*, 16 November 1952; D.S. Pennycuick, 'Is Polio to be Conquered at Last?' *The Sydney Morning Herald*, 11 February 1954.

942 'Crucial Year in the Polio Battle', *The Sydney Morning Herald*, 3 April 1953, p.8.

943 For example, vivisectionists and Christian Scientists. Poliomyelitis – General – Propaganda against Poliomyelitis. National Archives of Australia, Commonwealth Department of Health, A1658, 259/1/17.

944 F. Macfarlane Burnet, 'A Review of Poliomyelitis', *Medical Journal of Australia*, vol.2, no.14 (1952) pp.481–84.

945 Fifth Menzies Ministry-Minutes of Full Cabinet Meetings Held 19 October 1953 to 4 July 1954. National Archives of Australia, Commonwealth of Australia, A4907/1/3.

946 Correspondence Relating to Diseases–Poliomyelitis General 1948–1956. National Archives of Australia, Commonwealth Department of Health, NAA 1658/1.

947 Department of Trade and Customs to Mrs Ash, Queensland, 3 May 1955. Correspondence Relating to Diseases–Poliomyelitis, General. Inquiries and Ministerial Representations 1957–1962. National Archives of Australia, Commonwealth Department of Health, A1658/1/259, 1/2 Part 2.

948 DA Cameron to Dr Lange, Sydney, 27 May 1957. NAA A1658/1, 259/1/2 Part 2.

949 NAA A1658/1, 259/1/2 Part 2.

950 Children under fourteen, pregnant women, and those at high risk from contact (e.g., family members and health care workers). General Research into Particular Subjects, Poliomyelitis. National Archives of Australia, National Health and Medical Research Council, A1658/616/5/2.

951 Commonwealth of Australia, 'Reports of the Director General of Health for the Years 1954–1956'.
952 Correspondence Relating to Diseases–Poliomyelitis, General 1957–1963. National Archives of Australia, Commonwealth Department of Health, A1658/1259/1/2 Part 2.
953 Correspondence Relating to Diseases–Poliomyelitis, General 1957–1963. National Archives of Australia, Commonwealth Department of Health, A1658/1259/1/2 Part 2.
954 For an examination of one anti-vaccination campaign in Australia, see C. Hooker, 'Diphtheria, Immunisation and the Bundaberg Tragedy', *Health and History*, pp.52–78.
955 Poliomyelitis –General –Propaganda against Poliomyelitis NAA 1658/1259.
956 Warnambool City had received 4800 completed cards with 2150 parents consenting. Mordialloc City reported 2428 consents in 5350 cards, and Ferntree Gully reported that 2520 parents consented and 1420 refused. Anon., 'Anti-Polio Campaign', *The Australian Municipal Journal*, p.344.
957 In those aged between fifteen and forty-four, the response was even poorer: 16% of Victorians were immunised compared with 59% (NSW), 46% (Qld), 46% (SA), 44% (WA), and 52% in Tasmania. It is not surprising there were further outbreaks in the late 1950s and early 1960s. C.E. Cook to Prime Minister Menzies, 5 December 1956. Correspondence Relating to Diseases–Poliomyelitis, General. Inquiries and Ministerial Representations 1957–1962. NAA A1658/1, 259/1/2 Part 3. Commonwealth Statistician, 'Year Book of the Commonwealth of Australia', 1965 (Report).
958 Correspondence Relating to Diseases–Poliomyelitis, General 1957–1963. Nationa Archives of Australia, Commonwealth Department of Health, A1658/1259/1/2 Part 2.
959 Correspondence Relating to Diseases–Poliomyelitis, General 1957–1963. National Archives of Australia, Commonwealth Department of Health, A1658/1259/1/2 Part 2.
960 H.M. Wade to D.A. Cameron, 14 February 1962, A1658/1, 259/1/2 Part 3 (NAA).
961 In New South Wales, the vaccine was stored and distributed from district hospitals to local GPs. W.F. Sheahan to D.A. Cameron, 21 October 1957, A1658/1, 259/1/2 Part 2 (NAA).
962 C. Hooker, 'Diphtheria, Immunisation and the Bundaberg Tragedy', *Health and History*, pp.52–78.
963 F. Macfarlane Burnet, *Changing Patterns*, pp.63–69.
964 F. Macfarlane Burnet, *Changing Patterns*, p.63.
965 C. Hooker, 'Diphtheria, Immunisation and the Bundaberg Tragedy', *Health and History*, p.53.
966 Correspondence Relating to Diseases–Poliomyelitis, General. Inquiries and Ministerial Representations 1957–1962. NAA A1658/1, 259/1/2 Part 3.
967 W.F. Sheahan to D.A. Cameron, 21 October 1957, A1658/1, 259/1/2 Part 3 (NAA).
968 *The Sun*, 7 June 1960, p.4.
969 200,000 units of untested vaccine were imported. These had to be tested by the reference laboratories before being released. Director General of Health, 'Report, July 1 1961 to June 30 1962', p.86.
970 The Laboratory of Biological Control in the US admitted that it did not have sufficient facilities in 1955 to test every batch of the Salk vaccine produced by the pharmaceutical houses. The responsibility for testing the vaccine lay with individual manufacturers. P. Fisher, *The Polio Story*, p.76.
971 Tasmania experienced a severe epidemic in 1960–61 with a case rate higher than eight per thousand, and between May 1961 and May 1962 a major outbreak started in

the Wollongong area of New South Wales. National Health and Medical Research Council, 'Poliomyelitis in Australia', *Medical Journal of Australia*, pp.935–40.

972 National Health and Medical Research Council, 'Poliomyelitis in Australia', *Medical Journal of Australia*, pp.936.

973 It was later discovered that the Type III component in the vaccine lacked potency or the ability to provoke an immune response in the recipient. The Queensland cases were Type III. National Health and Medical Research Council, 'Poliomyelitis in Australia', *Medical Journal of Australia*, pp.935–40.

974 A. Sabin quoted in D.M. Horstmann, et al, 'The Trial Use of Sabin's Attenuated Type 1 Poliovirus Vaccine in a Village in Southern Arizona', *American Journal of Epidemiology*, pp.169–84.

975 P. Fisher, *The Polio Story*, p.76; S. Benison, *Tom Rivers*, pp.564–73.

976 First International Conference on Live Virus Vaccines, June 1959.

977 Macfarlane Burnet visited Moscow as a guest of the Academy of Medical Sciences in the summer of 1960, and by the end of that year, polio had almost disappeared from the USSR. F. Macfarlane Burnet, *Changing Patterns*, p.172.

978 'New Polio Vaccine Launched', *The New York Times*, 13 April 1955, p.1.

979 T. Francis, et al, 'An Evaluation of the 1954 Poliomyelitis Vaccine Trials', *American Journal of Public Health*, pp.1–63; L. Dawson, 'The Salk Polio Vaccine Trial of 1954', *Clinical Trials*, pp.122–30.

980 And it was, of course, far easier to administer a single dose of Sabin to the population than to give three injections of Salk vaccine. L. Dawson, 'The Salk Polio Vaccine Trial of 1954', *Clinical Trials*, pp.122–30.

981 Sabin's vaccine used a weakened poliovirus to take advantage of the natural human response to attack by the virus while Salk's method manipulated and changed the poliovirus in a way that altered the normal course of events in the human body.

982 Australian Government and Medicare Australia, 'Immunisation Register'. www1.hic.gov.au/general/acircirgacir. Accessed 24 February 2009.

Chapter 9

983 W. Kent Hughes, 'Letter to Editor', *Medical Journal of Australia*.

984 E. Casely, 'Physiotherapy in South Australia', *The Australian Journal of Physiotherapy*, pp.164–69.

985 R.W. Lovett, 'Fatigue and exercise in the treatment of infantile paralysis', cited in J. Macnamara, 'The Care of the Paralysis of Poliomyelitis', *Medical Journal of Australia*, pp.577–80.

986 A program on ABC television's 'Catalyst' (21 May 2009) appeared to support Kenny's theory. Researchers postulate that 'our brains are born with a basic map of a four limbed body outline, and that the map needs constant updating from the senses ... touch ... vision ... joint position. These send a live feed to a part of the brain known as the right parietal lobule — which integrates the feeds, and updates the body map.' www.abc.net.au/catalyst/stories/2576978.htm. Accessed 25 May 2009.

987 D. Galbraith, 'Rehabilitation in Poliomyelitis', *Medical Journal of Australia*, p.483.

988 P.R. Zanoli, 'Orthopaedics and Physical Medicine' (Paper), p.415.

989 S. Mead, 'A Century of the Abuse of Rest', *Journal of the American Medical Association*, pp.344–45.

990 A.M. Mackintosh, 'The Treatment of Acute Poliomyelitis', *Medical Journal of Australia*, p.417.

991 L.F. Peltier, *Orthopaedics*, p.174.
992 M. Westbrook, 'An Australian Survey of the Late Effects of Polio', *Polio Papers* (Paper), p.48.
993 J.A. Anderson, 'Public Health Aspects of Poliomyelitis' (Paper), p.317.
994 P. Lépine, 'Epidemiology and Pathogenesis of Poliomyelitis (Paper), pp.129–37.
995 Formerly accessible at www.cdc.gov/mmwrhtml.htm.
996 The Australian population in 1947 was 7,579,358. Commonwealth Statistician, 'Year Book of the Commonwealth of Australia', 1951 (Report), p.306.
997 The last Australian case of polio caused by wild poliovirus was in 1977.
998 The two most recent outbreaks of polio in the United States were amongst members of religious groups who object to vaccination. Inactivated Poliovirus (IPV) is advised for routine polio vaccination in countries where the wild poliovirus has been eliminated but Oral Poliovirus (OPV) remains the vaccine of choice for mass vaccination to control polio outbreaks because it produces a higher initial level of antibody, and shedding of the attenuated virus in faecal matter improves overall community protection.
999 The Australian Childhood Immunisation Register (Immunisation Register) was developed in 'response to a decline in childhood immunisation in Australia and the alarming increase in preventable childhood diseases'. Australian Government and Medicare Australia, 'Immunisation Register'. www1.hic.gov.au/general/acircirgacir.
1000 P. Fine, et al, 'Herd Immunity', *Clinical Infectious Diseases*, pp.911–16.
1001 D.A. Henderson, et al, 'Paralytic Disease Associated with Oral Polio Vaccines', *Journal of the American Medical Association*, pp.41–8.
1002 Associated Press, 'Belgium Threatens to Jail Parents Who Refuse to Vaccinate Children' (Polio Perspectives), p.5.
1003 Anon., 'No Vaccine for the Scaremongers', *Bulletin of the World Health Organization*, pp.417–496.
1004 AAP., 'Polio Outbreak in Nigeria Sparked by Vaccine, Experts Say', *Polio Perspectives*, Summer 2007, p.4; C. Kapp, 'Surge in Polio Spreads Alarm in Northern Nigeria. Rumours About Vaccine Safety in Muslim-run States Threaten WHO's Eradication Programme', *Lancet*, pp.1631–32.
1005 B. Hull and P. McIntyre, 'Mapping Immunisation Coverage and Conscientious Objectors to Immunisation in NSW', *NSW Public Health Bulletin*, pp.8–12.
1006 A.J. Stewardson, et al, 'Imported Case of Poliomyelitis, Melbourne, Australia, 2007', *Emerging Infectious Disease*. www.cdc.gov/EID/content/15/1/63.htm. Accessed 2009.
1007 The poliovirus can live in the human body for weeks: it is a truly transnational disease. R.L. Bruno, 'Thanks to One Unvaccinated Student, Australia Has Its First Case of Polio in 21 Years', *New Mobility*, p.8.
1008 D.A. Neumann, 'Polio', *Journal of Orthopaedic and Sports Physical Therapy*, pp.479–92.
1009 J. Macnamara, 'The Prevention of Crippling following Poliomyelitis,' *Medical Journal of Australia*, p.7.
1010 J. Macnamara, 'The Prevention of Crippling following Poliomyelitis,' *Medical Journal of Australia*, pp.7–8
1011 M. Elson, 'Editorial, Sister Elizabeth Kenny', *Physical Therapy Review*, p.81.

BIBLIOGRAPHY

Primary Sources

1. Australia

1.1 Archives Office of Tasmania, Hobart

Office of the Minister for Health, Semi-Private Correspondence, Reports and Addresses TA406, HSD23/1/1.

1.2 Fairfield Hospital Archives, Austin Hospital, Melbourne

1.2.1 The Bryan Richard Speed Infectious Diseases Collection: Fairfield Hospital 1904–1996

Interviews of former patients conducted by Barbara Rossall-Wynne, Archivist. Transcripts by Kerry Highley. Interviewees:

Anonymous;
Lisbeth Anderson;
Brian Caulfield, 16 May 1992;
Les Corneille, 3 April 1992;
Vern Draffin;
Dr Frank Foster, 7 March 1994;
Ron Gillam, 5 January 1994;
Geoff Golding, 1 August 1992;
Valda Millie Heath, 12 November 1992;
Neville Hogan, 13 November 1992;
Jack Irvine;
Liz Jones, 3 September 1993;
Garry Marr, 18 June 1992;
June Middleton, November 1992;
Elaine Theodore and her parents, Mr and Mrs Parker, 13 November 1992;
Edna Thilby, 16 April 1992;
William Wesson, 18 March 1992;
Una White, 5 January 1994;
and Maureen Wright, 12 November 1992.

1.2.2 Printed Archives

Record Book of Patients admitted, no. 32, 1937.
Report Book (no. 13) of the Medical Superintendent, Dr J.V. Scholes, 1937.
Photographic album created by Vern Draffin. Other photographic material.

1.3 National Archives of Australia (NAA), Canberra

1.3.1 Commonwealth Department of Health

Diseases – Poliomyelitis – Outbreaks and Cases, General. A1658/1/259/4/1
Poliomyelitis: Sister Kenny's Activities, A1928/1/802/17, Section 3.
Poliomyelitis in Australia: History and Statistics, National Archives of Australia, A1928/1/802/16.
Poliomyelitis: Sister Kenny's Treatment. Papers Returned by the Hon. W.M. Hughes Ex Minister for Health, A1928/1/802/17/1.
Correspondence Relating to Diseases – Poliomyelitis, General, 1948–1956, A1658/1/259/1/1.
Correspondence Relating to Diseases – Poliomyelitis, General, 1957–1963, A1658/1/259/1/2.
Correspondence Relating to Diseases – Poliomyelitis, General. Inquiries and Ministerial Representations 1957–1962, A1658/1/259/1/1.
Correspondence Relating to Diseases – Poliomyelitis, General. Inquiries and Ministerial Representations, 1955–1957, A1658/1/259/1/2.
Letter from Department of Trade and Customs to Mrs Ash, Queensland, A1658/1/259/1/2, Part 2.
Correspondence Relating to Diseases – Poliomyelitis, General. Inquiries and Ministerial Representations, 1957–1962, A1658/1/259/1/2 Part 3
Dr Hunter BMA, Letter to Federal Minister of Health, D.A. Cameron, 18 September 1957, A1658/1, 259/1/2, Part 3.
H.M. Wade, Letter to Federal Minister of Health, D.A. Cameron, 14 February 1962, 1957, A1658/1, 259/1/2, Part 3.
Letter from Minister for Health W.F. Sheahan to D.A. Cameron, A1658/259/1/2, Part 3.
Diseases – Poliomyelitis – Outbreaks and Cases General, A1658/1/259/4/1.
Diseases – Poliomyelitis – Outbreaks and Cases in Australia, A1658/1/259/4/2.
Poliomyelitis: Epidemiology and Preventive Measures in Western Australia, 1948, A1658/259/1/1, Part 1.
Poliomyelitis – General – Propaganda against Poliomyelitis, A1658, 259/1/17.
Metcalfe, A.J, Interstate Committee on Poliomyelitis, 1951, A1658/617/1/17.
General Research into Particular Subjects – Poliomyelitis, National Health and Medical Research Council General Research into Particular Subjects, Poliomyelitis, A1658/616/5/2.
Dr P. Bazeley – Production of Anti-Poliomyelitis Vaccine, A463/17, 197/26.
Hughes, W.M., Hughes to Cabinet, 1937, A6006/1937/12/31.
Parliamentary Papers of Western Australia, Royal Visit to Western Australia, 1954. Detailed Working Programme, PP302/1/WA30198, Part 3.

Bibliography

1.3.2 Commonwealth of Australia
Fifth Menzies Ministry–Minutes of full Cabinet Meetings held 19 October 1953 to 4 July 1954, A4907/1/3.

1.3.3 Department of Foreign Affairs and Trade
Supply of Scientific and Agricultural Information. Elizabeth Kenny Institute, A1067/A46/2/7/2

1.3.4 Elizabeth Kenny Collection
Attestation Paper, NAA 1928/802/17/1.

1.3.5 National Health and Medical Research Council
General research into particular subjects – Poliomyelitis A1658/616/5/2
Poliomyelitis in Aborigines, A452/54/1952/179
Northern Territory –NHMRC, Poliomyelitis in Aborigines, A452/54/1952/179

1.4 National Library of Australia (NLA), Canberra
Papers of Jean Macnamara, MS 2399.

1.4.1 Series 1. Correspondence, 1923–1968
Personal correspondence to and from Jean Macnamara, Items 1–523.
Items 7/5, 1/18d/79f, 1/23, 1/28, 1/36, 1/36b, 1/44, 1/41a, 1/150, 11/55, 11/60, 1/1/310-373, 1/16e, 1/18d, 1/163b, 1/1/60, 1/16/17k, 1/120, 4/1.
Hodge, I., Correspondence, 1923–1968, MS 2399, 7/5.
Stevenson, J., Letter to Jean Macnamara, 22 September 1932, 1/111.
Keogh, T., Letter from Thomas Keogh to Jean Macnamara, 11 November 1930, 7/5.

1.4.2 Series 2. Personal papers, 1915–1962
Report to Dr W.S. Carter, Rockefeller Institute on her visit to the United States of America, 1/176d.

1.4.3 Series 4. Newspaper cuttings, 1933–1964
Items 1–4.

1.4.4 Series 5. Pictorial material

1.4.5 Series 7. Notebooks, 1925–1966
23 October 1929.
11 November 1930.
18 November 1930.
25 November 1930.

1.4.6 Series 11. Notes for articles
Items 11/55, 11/60 and 11/63.

1.4.7 Royal Children's Hospital
Collected Papers of the Royal Children's Hospital and Paediatric Society of Victoria, 1935–1960.

1.5 Public Record Office Victoria (PROV), Melbourne

1.5.1 Charity, Relief and Health. Town Clerk's Correspondence Files

1.5.1.1 VPRS/3183/P0000/65
Polio Campaigns 1930–1938
Polio Papers 01/01/1925

1.5.1.2 VPRS/3183/P0000/69
Polio Campaigns, 1930–1932
Minutes, Polio Committee

1.5.1.3 VPRS/3183/P0000/70
Poliomyelitis Council of Victoria, 1930–1932
Minutes, Polio Committee

1.5.1.4 VPRS/3183/P0000/71
Poliomyelitis Council of Victoria Minute Books, 1931–1938
Minutes of Joint Government and Municipality Anti-Polio Campaign, Victoria. 1918–1931
Minute Book August 1936–November 1936
Minutes, Polio Committee
Jean Macnamara to Committee
Jean Macnamara, Fellowship
Interview with Frank Macfarlane Burnet
Minutes of Medical Committee controlling Campaign against Poliomyelitis, 1931
Serum donors: Subsidies to councils

1.5.1.5 VPRS/3183/P0000/72
Poliomyelitis, 1931–1938
Papers, Files re Polio Committee 1927–1939

1.5.2 General Correspondence Files

1.5.2.1 VPRS/6345/P0000/112
Training of physiotherapists, treatment of paralysis, 638/3.

1.5.2.2 VPRS/6345/P0000/113
Accommodation and aftercare for cripples, 638/8.
1949 epidemic, 638/11.

1.5.2.3 VPRS/6345/P0000/327
Polio Campaigns, 1930–1933, Consultative Council on Poliomyelitis, /279.

1.5.2.4 VPRS/6345/P0000/392
Lady Duggan and Red Cross Homes for cripples, /819.
Commonwealth/State relationship, /820.

Bibliography

Cost of splints, /821.

Jacket respirators, /822.

Splint production, October 1947 – August 1970, Consultative Council on Poliomyelitis, /824.

1.5.3 General Correspondence Files

1.5.3.1 VPRS 8291/P0001

Polio 1931–1938, Papers, Files of Polio Committee 1929/1939

Receipts for Campaigns from Victorian councils /119

Polio figures from Footscray Council, /119

Public Health /98

Infectious Disease Regulations 1932 /76

1.5.4 General Correspondence Files, Multiple Number System

1.5.4.1 VPRS 10430/P00001

Health/Polio. City of Brighton. Polio and Immunisation records, January 1970.

1.6 State Library of New South Wales, Sydney

1.6.1 Elizabeth Kenny – papers, 1936–1937, MSS 5855

Letter from Dunne, C.J., 1937. Papers covering the establishment of the Elizabeth Kenny Clinic in New South Wales.

1.7 State Library of Queensland, Brisbane

1.7.1 John Oxley Library, Heritage Collections

1.7.1.1 Mary Kenny, Photographs and Papers, TR2931

1.7.1.2 Matron Barron Letters on Sister Kenny, TR1829

1.7.2 John Oxley Library, Manuscript Collection

1.7.2.1 OM65-17, Charles Edward Chuter papers 1940–1950

Letters, memorandums, cuttings relating to Sister Kenny, 1943–1945, 17/33.

Letters and cuttings re Kenny Clinic, 1933–1943, 17/34.

Memorandum, circulars, letters, etc. re Kenny Clinic, 1933–1943. Report of the Royal Commission on the Investigation of Infantile Paralysis, Brisbane, December 1937, 17/35.

Memorandum, circulars, letters, etc. re Kenny Clinic, 1933–1943. Report of the Royal Commission on the Investigation of Infantile Paralysis, Brisbane, December 1937, 17/37.

Memorandum, circulars, letters, etc. re Kenny Clinic, 1937–1943, 17/38.

Memorandum, circulars, letters, etc. re Kenny Clinic. Treatment of poliomyelitis at Queen Mary's Hospital for Children, Carshalton, 28 October 1937, 17/38.

1.8 University of Queensland, Brisbane (UQ)

1.8.1 Fryer Library, Elizabeth Kenny Collection UQFL16

1.8.1.1 Box 1, Correspondence and 3 attached reviews

1.8.1.1.1 Folder 1

Correspondence, incoming and outgoing for the period 1939–1951. Includes correspondence between Hospital Superintendents and others concerning the Kenny treatment and management of the Kenny Clinics.

1.8.1.1.2 Folder 2

Correspondence, incoming for the period 1942–1947. Mainly letters of appreciation from doctors and others in the US and Canada who attended or visited the Kenny Clinic in Minneapolis, Minnesota.

Washburn, A., Letter to Elizabeth Kenny, 22 October 1942

1.8.1.1.3 Folder 3

Kenny, E., 'Evidence Concerning My Seven Years Activities in the United States of America', Report dated 14 October 1947 to Hon. E. M. Hanlon, MLA, Premier of Queensland.

1.8.1.1.4 Folder 4

Kenny, E., 'My Report on Conference with the Medical Profession in Fourteen Foreign Countries', 1947.

1.8.1.2 Box 2, Correspondence relating to Sister Kenny Foundation

1.8.1.3 Box 4, Papers, 1934–2001

Correspondence of Mary and Stewart McCracken.

1.8.1.4 Box 5, Papers 1940–2000

Correspondence of Mary and Stewart McCracken, 1993–2000.
Papers, 1992–1998.
Correspondence of Mary and Stewart McCracken.

1.8.2 Fryer Library, Rae W. Dungan Collection UQFL 354

1.8.2.1 Box 1

Letter to Dr Dungan from Sir Raphael Cilento, 11 May 1939.
Notes, treatment of patients in acute stage of poliomyelitis.
Thesis extracts and letters from the *Medical Journal of Australia*, 1938.
Starr, K., A report to the Minister for Health, NSW on Sister Kenny's method of treatment of infantile paralysis, May 1939.
Various correspondence concerning Sister Kenny's treatment.
Letters and reports from Sister Kenny to various correspondents.
Commonwealth Department of Health, Report of the Australian Conference of Crippled Children, 1936.

Bibliography

Dungan, R.W., Various sets of typewritten notes concerning Sister Kenny's work, method, procedures and recommendations.

Notes and letters from Dr Dungan's practice and Sister Kenny's reports to Dr Dungan.

Letters. C. Chuter to R. Dungan, Guinane to Chuter, Hanlon to Krieger, 1934–1935.

Letters and correspondence.

Reports to various people regarding Sister Kenny's work.

Letters and correspondence.

Cilento, R., 'Report on the Muscle Re-Education Clinic, Townsville', 12 December 1934.

Foster, W. and Price, E., 'An investigation of 23 cases of poliomyelitis treated by the Kenny Method at the Children's Hospital Hampton, Victoria', 1939.

1.9 University of Melbourne Archives, Melbourne

Burnet, Macfarlane, Sir, 1880–1985, 89/34. Personal correspondence between Linda Burnet and family, 1931–1933.

Derham, Alfred Plumley, 1897–1962, 63/24. Material relating to work at the Children's Hospital.

Murphy, Leonard J.T., 1984–1985, 91/114. Photocopy of Professor R.J. Berry's autobiography.

Wallace, Victor Hugo, 1927–1977, 77/65. The Eugenics Society of Victoria Minute Book, 2/1/3.

2. Canada

2.1 Library and Archives Canada, Ottawa

2.1.1 Record Group 29

Poliomyelitis, 1939/09–1961/07.

Epidemiology: Diseases – Poliomyelitis – Infantile paralysis (Polio) – Kenny Treatment, 1939–1952.

Epidemiology: Diseases – Poliomyelitis – Reference material regarding poliomyelitis, 1949–1953.

Epidemiology: Diseases – Poliomyelitis – Reference material regarding poliomyelitis, 1937–1951.

Epidemiology: Diseases – Poliomyelitis – Epidemics, 1925–1952.

Correspondence 29 April 1949 – 17 October 1949.

3. United States of America

3.1 Franklin D. Roosevelt Library, New York, NY

Franklin D. Roosevelt: Papers as President, Official File, Sister Elizabeth Kenny Institute, File 5188

Papers as President, President's Personal File, National Foundation for Infantile Paralysis, Basil O'Connor to FDR, 1 December 1944, Container 143.

Papers as President, President's Secretary's File, Letters of support for Sister Elizabeth Kenny, National Foundation for Infantile Paralysis, February 1944–1945, Container 143.

3.2 Minnesota Historical Society (MHS), St Paul, Minnesota. Elizabeth Kenny Papers

3.2.1. MHS 143.E.10.3b Box 1

3.2.1.1 Personal correspondence and related papers, 1942–1951

3.2.1.2 Photographs: Elizabeth Kenny, 1943–1945.

3.2.1.3 Administration
Conference on poliomyelitis (Minneapolis), 3–5 December 1945.
Hearn, Richard J., New York Chapter, 1946–1948.
Dayton, Donald C., 1944–1948.
Complimentary letters and parents' appreciation, undated and 1942–1949.
Inventory: Journal articles, papers and letters in 'Kenny's Brown Bag'.
Kenny Institute, Complimentary letters and parents' appreciation, undated and 1942–1949.

3.2.2 MHS 143.E.10.4f Box 2

3.2.2.1 National Foundation for Infantile Paralysis
Gudakunst, Dr Don W., 1941–1944.
O'Connor, Basil, 1940–1947.
Printed Matter.

3.2.2.2 Correspondence
Ray of Light letters: public response to AMA report on Kenny method, 1944.
Requests for treatment, 1942–1945.
Sullivan, Ed, 1946–1947.
Webber, Mrs Charles C., 1941–1945.

3.2.2.2.1 Technicians
Harvey, Valerie, 1942–1946.
Kenny, Mary Stewart, 1942–1947.

3.2.2.3 US Government
Congressional Investigation, Letters of support, undated and 1945.

3.2.2.4 University of Minnesota
Continuation courses in the Kenny Technique, 1942–1945.

3.2.3 MHS 143.E.10.6f Box 4

3.2.3.1 Medical Personnel and Institutions
Australia 1939–1952.
Belgium.
Belgium Red Cross.

Curtis, Dorothy, 1946–1950.
Houdsen, Nora, 1948–1950.
France 1948.
Pakistan.
United States.
Michigan. Calhoun, Dr Ethel T., 1942–1948.
Georgia. Bennett, Dr Robert L, Georgia Warm Springs Foundation, 1942–1943; Miscellaneous, 1944–1946.
Illinois. Levine, Dr Herbert, 1946–1948; Lewin, Dr Philip, 1943, 1946; Miscellaneous, 1943–1944, 1951.
Minnesota. Ghormley, Dr R.K., 1943; Krusen, Dr Frank, 1942–1947; Miscellaneous, 1942–1945.

3.2.4   MHS 143.E.10.8F Box 6

3.2.4.1   Miscellaneous papers
Newspaper clippings, undated and 1941–1982, 9 folders.
Poliomyelitis (article reprints), undated and 1941–1964.
Kenny Institute 50th anniversary, patient letters, 1991–1992.

3.2.5   MHS 143.E.10.9b Box 7

3.2.5.1   Miscellaneous Papers
Kenny Institute 50th anniversary, patient letters, 1991–1992.

3.2.5.2   Henry, James
Scrapbooks 1940–1952, 1986.
Henry, James, Personal correspondence and related papers, undated and 1943–1976.

3.2.5.3   Biographers' Research papers
Wade Alexander Papers, undated and 1862–1951, 2001 (bulk 1940–1951).
Victor Cohn Papers, Sister Elizabeth Kenny Foundation Records.
Elizabeth Kenny, correspondence, reports and other papers, undated and 1941–1951.
Dr Frank H. Krusen's Elizabeth Kenny file, 1941–1944.

3.2.6   MHS 146.K8.5B.8

3.2.6.1   Elizabeth Kenny Polio Treatment
Reports and papers on (by others). Australia, 1937–1938; United States and Europe, 1941, 1949.
Elizabeth Kenny Institute and Sister Elizabeth Kenny Foundation.
Newspaper and magazine articles regarding Elizabeth Kenny, Australia, undated and 1940–1954.
Australia, undated and 1916–1952.
United States, undated and 1940–1954.
Kenny's death, Australia and the United States 1952–1955.

3.2.7   MHS 146.K.8.6f Box 9

Victor Cohn's Elizabeth Kenny research notes, transcriptions, correspondence and other papers, interviews and other sources, A-W, 1940–1970.

Brand, J., *The History of the National Foundation for Infantile Paralysis, The Response to Developing Problems of Medical Care, 1940–46.*

Selected chronology, undated and 1951–1955.

Elizabeth Kenny letters, 1937–1952.

Interviews and other sources, A–W, 1940s–1970s.

Additional research correspondence, 1953–1974

Photographs of Elizabeth Kenny.

Australia, undated and c.1890–1952.

United States, 1940–1952.

Miscellaneous correspondence and other papers regarding Elizabeth Kenny, 1953–1996.

3.3   National Library of Medicine

3.3.1   Sophia Smith Collection, Smith College. Florence Rena Sabin Papers

3.4   Rockefeller Archive Center (RAC), Tarrytown, NY

3.4.1   Rockefeller Family Archives

3.4.1.1   Office of the Messrs. Rockefeller records RG2

Series K, Medical Interests, Polio. Box 14, Folder 114.

National Foundation for Infantile Paralysis, 1937–1949.

Series K, Medical Interests, Polio. Box 15, Folder 118.

Sister Kenny Foundation, 1944–1960.

3.4.1.2   Commonwealth Fund Records, Administration, Officers Files, 1918–1980, SG1

Series 2, Box 24, Folder 210.

Harkness Report and Sister Elizabeth Kenny Foundation Inc., December 10 1947 – December 17 1948.

National Research Council, Report of Special Committee.

3.4.2   Rockefeller Institute for Medical Research Series 1/1.2

Simon Flexner papers, American Philosophical Society. Correspondence between Simon Flexner and Jean Macnamara, 1929–1933, Microform reel 70.

3.4.3   Rockefeller University Records, Scientific staff, Biographical files

Box 20, Folder 23, Macnamara, (Dr) Jean (Australia).

3.4.4 Rockefeller Foundation records, fellowships, fellowship recorder cards, RG10.2

Medical and Natural Sciences, Drawer 2, Macnamara, (Dr) Jean (Australia).

3.4.5 A guide to Rockefeller Foundation records, projects RG1.1

Series 410, Australia 1924-1961.

Carter, William S. Box 1, Folder 3, Medical Education in Australia 1926.

Hall Institute. Kellaway, Charles H, Box 1, Folder 4, Travel, Pathology 1931–1933.

Hall Institute, Apperly, F.L, Box 1, Folder 4, Travel, Pathology 1931–1933.

Hall Institute Correspondence between Dr Kellaway and Dr Alan Gregg, 1934, Box 2, Folder 15.

Commonwealth Fund Archives. National Research Council. Report of Special Committee, 8 November 1944.

University of Melbourne. Berry, Richard, J.A., Box 1, Folder 7, Visit, Medical Center Development, 1922–1926; 1927–1929.

3.4.5.1 Dean Rusk papers, 1950–1969, Rockefeller Foundation, Series 200

Address by Dean Rusk, President, the Rockefeller Foundation, 1954.

3.4.6 Rockefeller Foundation records, Field Offices, Paris, RG6, SG1, 1933–1976

O'Brien, D., Diaries of Daniel O'Brien (1931–1932).

3.5 Reports

Almoner's report 1939, 'Tasmanian Society for the Care of Crippled Children', Parliamentary Papers (Hobart: Tasmaniana Library, Heritage Collection, State Library of Tasmania).

Commonwealth Department of Health, 'Report of the Australian Conference on Crippled Children' (Canberra: Commonwealth of Australia, 1936).

Commonwealth of Australia, 'Reports of the Director General of Health for the Years 1954–1956' (Canberra: Government Printer, 1956).

———, 'Reports of the Director General of Health for the Years 1961–1962' (Canberra: Government Printer, 1956).

———, 'Public Health and Related Institutions', Reports of the Director General of Health for the years 1947–1958 (Canberra: 1947–1958).

Commonwealth Statistician, 'Year Book of the Commonwealth of Australia' (Canberra: Commonwealth Bureau of Census and Statistics, 1951, 1953, 1954, 1956, 1957, 1958, 1960, 1961, 1962, 1963, 1964, 1965).

Crosby, N.D., 'Reflections on the Epidemiology of the 1947–1948 Epidemic in South Australia', National Health and Medical Research Council (Adelaide: 1952).

Department of Public Health New South Wales, 'Notification of Infectious Diseases', Report of the Director General of Public Health (Sydney: Government Printer, 1915–1918).

———, 'Notification of Infectious Diseases', Report of the Director General of Public Health (Sydney: Government Printer, 1919–1921; 1922–1925; 1926–1929; 1930–1933; 1934–1937; 1938–1941; 1941–1946, 1955).

Department of Public Health Queensland, 'Annual Statement of Notifiable Diseases During Calendar Year', Annual Report of the Commissioner of Public Health (Brisbane: 1914).

———, 'Annual Statement of Notifiable Diseases During Calendar Year', Annual Report of the Commissioner of Public Health (Brisbane: 1916, 1920, 1921, 1922, 1923, 1924, 1925, 1926, 1927, 1928, 1929, 1930, 1932).

———, 'Anterior Poliomyelitis', Annual Report on the health and medical services of the State of Queensland, Vol. 1 (Brisbane: Government Printer, 1935–1938; 1939–1945).

Director General of Health, 'Report, July 1 1961 to June 30 1962' (Canberra: Commonwealth of Australia, 1962).

Kennedy, M.V. and Somerset, H.C.D, 'Bringing up Crippled Children' (Wellington: New Zealand Council for Educational Research, 1951).

Miles, J.R., 'Present Knowledge of the Virus in Relation to Epidemiology', National Health and Medical Research Council (Adelaide: 1952).

Parliament of New South Wales, 'Parliamentary Papers Relating to Public Health' (Sydney: Government Printer, 1868–1903).

Public Health Department of Western Australia, 'Report of the Commissioner of Public Health' (Perth: 1954).

Queensland Bush Children's Health Scheme, 'Annual Reports for the Years 1938–1960' (Brisbane: 1938–1960).

Reverend Drummond, S.G., 'Country Surveys, and the Work of the Far West Children's Health Scheme', Report of the Australian Conference on Crippled Children (Canberra: Commonwealth of Australia, 1936).

Snow, D.J.R. 'Appendix viii: The Poliomyelitis Epidemic: 1954', Report of the Commissioner of Public Health for the year 1954 (Perth: 1956), pp.48–65.

Tasmanian Society for the Care of Crippled Children, Annual Report, Parliamentary Papers (Hobart: Tasmaniana Library, Heritage Collection, State Library of Tasmania, 1939).

The Parliament of the Commonwealth of Australia, 'Report of the Administration of the Northern Territory', Report of the District Officer, Alice Springs (Canberra: Government printer, 1937–1938–1939). Weekly Epidemiological Record, *Bulletin of the World Health Organization*, Vol. 82/39.

3.6   Official Reports

Borchardt, D.H., 'Part V Queensland', Checklist of Royal Commissions: select committees and boards of inquiry (Brisbane: 1970).

Establishment of Royal Commission into the Elizabeth Kenny Method of Treating Paralysis, Queensland Government Gazette, 1935.

Thelander, C.A., Duhig, J.V., Nye, J., Patterson, A.E. and Lahz, R.S., 'Report of the Queensland Royal Commission on Modern Methods for the Treatment of Infantile Paralysis' (Brisbane: 1937).

US Public Health Service, 'Technical Report on the Salk Poliomyelitis Vaccine Produced by the Cutter Laboratories', *US Department of Health, Education and Welfare* (1955).

'Weekly Epidemiological Record. Vaccine Derived Poliovirus in Nigeria'. *Bulletin of the World Health Organization* Vol. 82/39. Geneva: World Health Organization, 2007.

Bibliography

4. Journals

The American Journal of the Care for Cripples, 1914.
The American Journal of Epidemiology, 1959.
The American Journal of Nursing, 1900s to 1956.
The American Journal of Public Health, 1955.
The American Journal of Sociology, 1956.
Australasian Journal of Philosophy, 1923, 1931.
The Australasian Nurses' Journal, 1900s to 1930s.
Australian Economic History Review, 1984.
Australian Historical Studies, 1993, 1997, 2000.
Australian Journal of Experimental Biology and Medical Science, 1939.
The Australian Journal of Physiotherapy, 1955.
The Australian Municipal Journal, 1956.
The British Journal of Nursing, 1915.
British Medical Journal, 1998.
Bulletin of the History of Medicine, 1997, 2000, 2001.
Health and History, 2000, 2002.
The Historical Journal, 1982.
Historical Studies, 1967, 1976, 1986.
Illinois Medical Journal, 1942.
International Journal of Epidemiology, 1983.
Journal of the American Medical Association, 1944.
The Journal of Bone and Joint Surgery, 1943.
Journal of Educational Sociology, 1933.
Journal of Experimental Medicine, 1900s to 1930s.
Journal of the History of Medicine, 1974.
Journal of the History of Medicine and Allied Sciences, 2005.
Journal of Immunology, 1935.
Journal of Orthopaedic and Sports Physical Therapy, 2004.
Labour History, 1988, 2001.
Medical History, 1972.
Medical Journal of Australia, 1900s to 1960s.
New England Journal of Medicine, 2005.
Osiris, 1995.
Physical Therapy Review, 1953.
Proceedings of the American Philosophical Society, 1954.
Proceedings of the Society for Experimental Biology and Medicine, 1936, 1949.
Public Health, 1932.
Science, 1916, 1961.
Scientific American, 1952, 1955.
Social History of Medicine, 2008.
US Department of Health, Education and Welfare, 1955.

5. Newspapers

Adelaide Advertiser
The Advertiser
The Age
The Argus
Associated Press
Clifton Courier
The Courier Mail
The Guyra Argus
Minneapolis Morning Tribune
Moorabbin News
The New York Times
Ottawa Evening Journal
The Settler and South Queensland Pioneer
Smith's Weekly
The Sun
The Sunday Mail
The Sydney Morning Herald
The Sydney Telegraph
The Telegraph
Toowoomba Chronicle
Townsville Daily Bulletin
The Truth
The Weekend Australian
The West Australian

6. Polio Perspectives

'Your Stories', edited by Mary-Ann Liethof, Collingwood: PolioNetwork, a service of Paraquad Victoria.

AAP., 'Polio outbreak in Nigeria sparked by vaccine, experts say', Summer 2007, p.4.

Associated Press. 'Belgium Threatens to Jail Parents Who Refuse to Vaccinate Children', Vol. 20, no. 2, Winter 2008.

Bazley, P. 'Pauline's Polio Story', Autumn 2008, Ibid.

Bruno, R.L. 'Thanks to One Unvaccinated Student, Australia Has Its First Case of Polio in 21 Years'. October 2007, p.8.

Corrigan, P. 'Polio Story', Summer 2006, Ibid.

Gillan, H.R. 'My Polio Experience', Autumn 2008, Ibid.

Heath, V.M. 'Polio Story', Winter 2006, Ibid.

Kosseck, M. 'Polio Story', 2006, Ibid.

Medlyn-White, L. 'Your Stories', Summer 2005, Ibid.

Metter, B. 'Polio Story', 2006, Ibid.

Murray, E. 'Polio Story', Autumn 2002, Ibid.

Pickering, J. 'Jill's Polio Story', 2002, Ibid.

Pruscino, L. 'Legend of East Gippsland, Autumn 2007, Ibid.

Smith, J. 'Your Stories – Joan's Journey', Summer 2007, Ibid.
Smythe, E. 'Polio Story', 2006, Ibid.
Swann, J.M. 'Polio Story', Autumn 2002, Ibid.
Van Delft, J. 'Polio Story', Autumn 2006, Ibid.
Watson, B. 'Polio Story', Autumn 2008, Ibid.
Whitthread, K. 'Polio Story', 2002, Ibid.

7. Post-Polio Network (NSW) Inc.

Member Stories, Kensington: Post-Polio Network (NSW) Inc.
Atkinson, H. 'My Story', no. 26,
Barnett, S. 'A Story', no. 7, Ibid.
Bernstein, C. 'Mazzy Meets the Dragon', no. 3, Ibid.
Buchanan, G. 'I Used to Jump Puddles', no. 7, Ibid.
Buchanan, G. "I Used to Jump Puddles.' (now known as Polio NSW), Summer 2012.
Ellis, L. 'Post-Polio Post', No. 37, Ibid.
Falconer, M. 'Spectrum of Polio Infection Effects in Australian Population'. *Post-Polio Network (NSW) Inc. Network News*, February 2004, p.5.
Featherstone, P. 'Life's Good?' no. 4, Ibid.
Gaumond, J. 'Immunisation', no. 6, Ibid.
Hasemer, M. 'A Working Holiday in London', no. 9, Ibid.
O'Reilly, G. 'Post-Polio Post', no. 48, Ibid.
Solomon, P. 'Living in a Country Town', no. 8, Ibid.
Thomas, G, ed., 'A Story to Break the Silence', No. 45. Ibid.

8. Conference Proceedings

Papers and Discussions Presented at the First International Poliomyelitis Conference, Philadelphia: J.B. Lippincott Company, 1949.
Papers and Discussions Presented at the Third International Poliomyelitis Conference, Philadelphia: J.B. Lippincott Company, 1955.

9. Papers

Anderson, J.A. 'Diagnosis and Treatment of Poliomyelitis in the Early Stage'. Paper presented at the First International Poliomyelitis Conference, New York, 1948, pp.109–19.
Barriére-Borchard, A. 'Selection of Methods in Physical Medicine for Poliomyelitis'. Paper presented at the Third International Poliomyelitis Conference, Rome, 1954, pp.314–19.
Colville, P. 'Reports of Official Delegates: Australia'. Paper presented at the Third International Poliomyelitis Conference, Rome, 1954, pp.27–30.
Greene, W.T. 'The Management of Poliomyelitis: The Convalescent Stage'. Paper presented at the First International Poliomyelitis Conference, New York, 1948, pp.165–86.
Keefer, C.S. 'Social Aspects of Poliomyelitis: United States'. Paper presented at the Third International Poliomyelitis Conference, Rome, 1954, pp.13–18.
Lépine, P. 'Epidemiology and Pathogenesis of Poliomyelitis: Present State of the Problem'. Paper presented at the Third International Poliomyelitis Conference, Rome, 1954, pp.129–37.

McQuarrie, I. 'The Evolution of Signs and Symptoms of Poliomyelitis'. Paper presented at the First International Poliomyelitis Conference, New York, 1948, pp.57–62.

Paul, J.R. 'Future Prospects'. Paper presented at the Third International Poliomyelitis Conference, Rome, 1954, pp.420–23.

Payne, A.M. 'Poliomyelitis as a World Problem'. Paper presented at the Third International Poliomyelitis Conference, Rome, 1954, pp.393–400.

Smith, F.B. 'The Victorian Poliomyelitis Epidemic 1937–1938'. Paper presented at the Health Transition Workshop, Canberra, 15–19 May 1989.

Southwood, A. 'Reports of Official Delegates: Australia'. Paper presented at the Third International Poliomyelitis Conference, Rome, 1954.

Weller, T., Robbins, F. and Enders, J. 'Cultivation of Poliomyelitis Virus in Cultures of Human Foreskin and Embryonic Tissues'. Paper presented at the Proceedings of the Society for Experimental Biology and Medicine, October 1949, p.153.

Wilson, J.R. 'Lessons from Sister Kenny's enterprise: intellectual openness, political assertiveness and a tolerance of difference', presented at the Fifth Elizabeth Kenny Oration, Townsville, August 1995.

Zanoli, P.R. 'Orthopaedics and Physical Medicine: A Summary'. Paper presented at the Third International Poliomyelitis Conference, Rome 1954, pp.411–15.

Secondary Sources

Books

Ackerknecht, E.H. *A Short History of Medicine*. Rev. ed. Baltimore: Johns Hopkins University Press, 1982.

Alexander, W. *Sister Elizabeth Kenny: Maverick Heroine of the Polio Treatment Controversy*. Rockhampton: Central Queensland University Press, 2003.

Anderson, W. *The Cultivation of Whiteness: Science, Health and Racial Destiny in Australia*. Melbourne: Melbourne University Press, 2005.

Anderson, W.K. *Fever Hospital: A History of Fairfield Infectious Diseases Hospital*. Melbourne: Melbourne University Press, 2002.

Aronowitz, R. 'From Myalgic Encephalitis to Yuppie Flu: A History of Chronic Fatigue Syndromes'. In *Framing Disease: Studies in Cultural History*, edited by C.E. Rosenberg and J. Golden. New Brunswick, NJ: Rutgers University Press, 1992, pp.155–81.

Barclay, J. and Chartered Society of Physiotherapy (Great Britain). *In Good Hands: The History of the Chartered Society of Physiotherapy 1894–1994*. Oxford: Butterworth Heinemann, 1994.

Barry, H. *Orthopaedics in Australia: The History of the Australian Orthopaedic Association*. Sydney: Australian Orthopaedic Association, 1983.

Bassett, J. *Guns and Brooches: Australian Army Nursing from the Boer War to the Gulf War*. Melbourne: Oxford University Press, 1997.

Beisser, A.R. *Flying without Wings: Personal Reflections on Being Disabled*. 1st ed. New York: Doubleday, 1989.

Benison, S. *Tom Rivers: Reflections on a Life in Medicine and Science. An Oral History Memoir*. Cambridge, Mass.: MIT Press, 1967.

Bennington, J.L., Brecher, G., Lee, W.S., Mackay, B. and Smith, N.J., eds. *Saunders*

Bibliography

Dictionary and Encyclopedia of Laboratory Medicine and Technology. Philadelphia: W.B. Saunders, 1984.

Bentley, P. and Dunstan, D. *The Path to Professionalism: Physiotherapy in Australia to the 1980s*. Melbourne: Australian Physiotherapy Association, 2006.

Berry, R. and Gordon, R. *The Mental Defective: A Problem in Social Inefficiency*. London: Kegan Paul, Trench and Tribner, 1931.

Bigland, E. *The True Story About Sister Kenny*. London: Shakespeare Head, 1956.

Black, K. *In the Shadow of Polio: A Personal and Social History*. Cambridge, Mass.: Perseus Publishing, 1996.

Bollet, A.J. *Plagues & Poxes: The Impact of Human History on Epidemic Disease*. New York: Demos Medical Publishing, 2004.

Bolton, G.C. *A Fine Country to Starve In*. Nedlands: University of Western Australia, 1972.

Boughton, C.R. *A Coast Chronicle: The History of the Prince Henry Hospital*. 2nd ed. Sydney: Knudsen Printing, 1981.

Bourke, J. *Dismembering the Male: Men's Bodies, Britain and the Great War*. London: Reaktion Books, 1996.

Brogan, A.H. *Committed to Saving Lives: A History of the Commonwealth Serum Laboratories*. South Yarra, Vic.: Hyland House, 1990.

Brown, E.R. *Rockefeller Medicine Men*. Berkeley: University of California Press, 1979.

Bruno, R.L. *The Polio Paradox: Understanding and Treating 'Post-Polio Syndrome' and Chronic Fatigue*. New York: Time Warner, 2002.

Burnet, F. Macfarlane. *Changing Patterns: An Atypical Autobiography*. Melbourne: William Heinemann, 1968.

Burnet, F. Macfarlane and White, D.O. *Natural History of Infectious Disease*. 4th ed. Cambridge: Cambridge University Press, 1972.

Burnet, F. Macfarlane. *Walter and Eliza Hall Institute, 1915–1965*. Melbourne: Melbourne University Press, 1971.

Butler, A.G. *The Official History of the Australian Army Medical Services in the War of 1914–1918*. Melbourne: Australian War Memorial, 1930.

Bynum, W., Lock, S. and Porter, R. *Medical Journals and Medical Knowledge: Historical Essays*. (The Wellcome Institute Series in the History of Medicine.) London: Routledge, 1992.

Carmichael, G.J. *Hospital Children: Sketches of Life and Character in the Children's Hospital Melbourne*. 2nd ed. Main Ridge, Vic.: Loch Haven Books, 1891. Reprint, 1991.

Clarke, J. *All on One Good Dancing Leg*. Sydney: Hale & Iremonger, 1994.

Cohn, V. *Sister Kenny: The Woman Who Challenged the Doctors*. St Paul: University of Minnesota Press, 1975.

Colbeck, M. *Sister Kenny of the Outback*. London: Edinburgh House, 1965.

Coles, K.F. *The History of the New South Wales Society for Crippled Children*. Sydney: New South Wales Society for Crippled Children, 1976.

Cooter, R. *Studies in the History of Alternative Medicine*. New York: St. Martin's Press, 1988.

———. *Surgery and Society in Peace and War: Orthopaedics and the Organization of Modern Medicine, 1880–1948*. London: Macmillan Press, 1993.

Cox, F. *A Review of Recent Literature on Typhus Fever and Acute Anterior Poliomyelitis*. Melbourne: Albert J. Mullett, Government Printer, 1917.

Creager, A. *The Life of a Virus*. Chicago: University of Chicago Press, 2002.

Crofford, E. *Healing Warrior: A Story About Sister Elizabeth Kenny.* San Francisco: Carolrhoda Books, 1989.
Cumpston, J.H.L. *Health and Disease in Australia: A History.* Introduced and edited by M.J. Lewis. Canberra: AGPS, 1989.
Daniel, T. 'Polio and the Making of a Doctor'. In *Polio*, edited by T.M. Daniel and F.C. Robbins. Rochester: University of Rochester, 1997, pp.79–96.
Daniel, T.M. and Robbins, F.C. eds., *Polio.* Rochester: University of Rochester, 1997.
Davis, F. *Passage through Crisis: Polio Victims and Their Families.* Indianapolis: Bobbs-Merrill Company, 1963.
Davis, L.J. *Bending over Backwards: Disability, Dismodernism, and Other Difficult Positions.* New York: New York University Press, 2002.
———. *Enforcing Normalcy: Disability, Deafness and the Body.* London: Verso, 1995.
Davison, G., Dunstan, D. and McConville, C. *The Outcasts of Melbourne.* Sydney: George Allen & Unwin, 1985.
Dickerson, M. and Mason, C. *Hospitals and Politics: The Australian Hospitals Association 1946–1986.* Canberra: Australian Hospitals Association, 1986.
Docker, E.W. *Sister Kenny.* Sydney: WC Penfold, 1969.
Duffin, J. *History of Medicine: A Scandously Short Introduction.* Toronto: University of Toronto Press, 1999.
Dyason, D. 'The Medical Profession in Colonial Victoria, 1834–1901'. In *Disease, Medicine, and Empire: Perspectives on Western Medicine and the Experience of European Expansion*, edited by R.M. Macleod and M.J. Lewis. London: Routledge, 1988, pp.194–216.
Facey, A.B. *A Fortunate Life.* Fremantle: Fremantle Arts Centre Press, 1981.
Fenner, F. *History of Microbiology in Australia.* Canberra: Brolga Press, 1990.
Finger, A. *Elegy for a Disease: A Personal and Cultural History of Polio.* New York: St. Martin's Press, 2006.
Fishbein, M., Salmonsen, E. and Kektoen, L., eds. *A Bibliography of Infantile Paralysis, 1789–1949.* (National Foundation for Infantile Paralysis.) Philadelphia: JB Lippincott, 1951.
Fisher, F.G. *Raphael Cilento: A Biography.* St Lucia: University of Queensland Press, 1994.
Fisher, P. *The Polio Story.* London: William Heinemann, 1967.
Foley, J.D. *In Quarantine: A History of Sydney's Quarantine Station 1828–1984.* Kenthurst, NSW: Kangaroo Press, 1995.
Ford, E. *Bibliography of Australian Medicine 1790–1900.* Sydney: Sydney University Press, 1976.
Foucault, M. *The Birth of the Clinic: An Archaeology of Medical Perception.* London: Routledge, 1973.
Foucault, M. and Gordon, C. *Power/Knowledge: Selected Interviews and Other Writings, 1972–1977.* New York: Harvester Wheatsheaf, 1980.
Fox, C. *Working Australia.* Sydney: Allen and Unwin, 1991.
Freeman, J. *Lights and Shadows of Melbourne Life.* London: Sampson, Low, Marston, Searle and Rivington, 1888.
Frischer, R.E. 'Waiting for Society to Catch Up'. In *Polio*, edited by T.M. Daniel and F.C. Robbins. Rochester: University of Rochester, 1997, pp.67–78.
Gallagher, H. *Black Bird Fly Away: Disabled in an Able-Bodied World.* Arlington: Vandamere Press, 1998.

Bibliography

———. *FDR's Splendid Deception*. New York: Dodd, Mead & Company, 1985.

Gandevia, B. 'Medicine in the Local Newspaper: The Early Australian Gazettes'. In *New Countries and Old Medicine: Proceedings of an International Conference on the History of Medicine and Health*, edited by L. Bryder and D. Dow. Auckland: Pyramid Press, 1994, pp.178–183.

———. ed., *Bibliography of Australian Medicine and Health Services to 1950*. 4 vols, Canberra: AGPS, 1988.

———. *Tears Often Shed: Child Health and Welfare in Australia from 1788*. Rushcutters Bay, NSW: Pergamon Press, 1978.

Gandevia, B., Simpson, S., Holster, A. and Royal Australasian College of Physicians. *An Annotated Bibliography of the History of Medicine and Health in Australia*. Sydney: Royal Australasian College of Physicians, 1984.

Gillespie, J. *The Price of Health, Australian Governments and Medical Politics 1910–1960*. Cambridge: Cambridge University Press, 1991.

Gould, T. *A Summer Plague: Polio and Its Survivors*. New Haven: Yale University Press, 1995.

Granshaw, L.P. and Porter, R. *The Hospital in History*. (Wellcome Institute Series in the History of Medicine.) London; New York: Routledge, 1989.

Gregory, A. *The Ever Open Door: A History of the Royal Melbourne Hospital 1848–1998*. South Melbourne: Hyland House, 1998.

Hyslop, A. *Sovereign Remedies: A History of Ballarat Base Hospital, 1850s to 1980s*. Sydney: Allen & Unwin, 1989.

Inglis, K. *Hospital and Community: A History of the Royal Melbourne Hospital*. Carlton: Melbourne University Press, 1958.

Jones, C. and Porter, R. *Reassessing Foucault: Power, Medicine, and the Body*. (Routledge Studies in the Social History of Medicine.) London: Routledge, 1994.

Kenny, E. *Infantile Paralysis and Cerebral Diplegia, Methods Used for the Restoration of Function*. Sydney: Angus and Robertson, 1937.

———. *My Battle and Victory: A History of the Discovery of Poliomyelitis as a Systemic Disease*. London: Robert Hale, 1955.

———. *Poliomyelitis: Findings in Investigations of Evidence Concerning Poliomyelitis, with Special Reference to the Kenny Concept of the Disease and Its Treatment from 1937 to 1947*. Brisbane: [s.n.], 1948.

———. *The Treatment of Infantile Paralysis in the Acute Stage*. Minneapolis: Bruce Publishing, 1941.

Kenny, E. and Ostenso, M. *And They Shall Walk*. 8th ed. New York: Dodd, Mead and Company, 1943. Reprint, 1946.

Kenny, E. and Pohl, J.E. *The Kenny Concept of Infantile Paralysis and Its Treatment*. Minneapolis: Bruce Publishing, 1943.

Kessler, H.H. *The Crippled and the Disabled: Rehabilitation of the Physically Handicapped in the United States*. New York: Columbia University Press, 1935.

Kewley, T.H. *Social Security in Australia: The Development of Social Security and Health Benefits from 1900 to the Present*. Sydney: Sydney University Press, 1965.

Killalea, A. *The Great Scourge: The Tasmanian Infantile Paralysis Epidemic*. Sandy Bay, Tas.: Tasmanian Historical Research Foundation, 1995.

King, A.D. *Buildings and Society: Essays on the Social Development of the Built Environment*. London: Boston: Routledge & Kegan Paul, 1980.

Kita, A. and Durfee, P. *Dr. Noguchi's Journey: A Life of Medical Search and Discovery*. Tokyo: Kodansha International, 2005.

Klein, A.E. *Trial by Fury: The Polio Vaccine Controversy*. New York: Charles Scribner's Sons, 1972.

Kübler-Ross, E. *On Death and Dying*. London; New York: Routledge, 1989.

Lawes-Gilvear, N. *Living with Polio: The Laughter and the Tears*. Launceston: Self-published, 1992.

Levine, H. *I Knew Sister Kenny: A Story of a Great Lady and Little People*. Boston: The Christopher Publishing House, 1954.

Lewis, M.J., *The People's Health: Public Health in Australia, 1950 to the Present*. London: Praeger, 2003.

Loudon, I., ed. *An Illustrated History of Western Medicine*. Oxford: Oxford University Press, 1997.

Lupton, D. *Medicine as Culture: Illness, Disease and the Body in Western Societies*. London: Sage, 1994.

Mackenzie, W.C. *The Treatment of Infantile Paralysis: A Study on Muscular Action and Muscle Regeneration*. Melbourne: [s.n.], 1910.

Marshall, A. *I Can Jump Puddles*. Sydney: Halstead Press, 1955.

Marshall, N. *The Yooralla Story: A History of the Yooralla Hospital School for Crippled Children, 1918–1977*. Melbourne: Yooralla Society of Victoria, 1978.

Martyr, P. *Paradise of Quacks: An Alternative History of Medicine in Australia*. Paddington, NSW: Macleay Press, 2002.

Mayne, A.J.C. *Fever, Squalor and Vice: Sanitation and Social Policy in Victorian Sydney*. St Lucia: University of Queensland Press, 1982.

McCalman, J. *Sex and Suffering: Women's Health and a Women's Hospital: The Royal Women's Hospital, Melbourne*. Carlton: Melbourne University Press, 1998.

McKellar Hall, R.D. *Reflections of an Orthopaedic Surgeon*. Perth: Hesperian Press, 1983.

McNally, R.J. *Remembering Trauma*. Cambridge, Mass.: Belknap Press of Harvard University Press, 2003.

Mee, C.L. *A Nearly Normal Life*. Boston: Little, Brown and Company, 1999.

Mitchell, A.M. and Alfred Hospital Melbourne. *The Hospital South of the Yarra: A History of Alfred Hospital Melbourne from Foundation to the Nineteen-Forties*. Melbourne: Alfred Hospital, 1977.

Molony, J.N. *The Penguin History of Australia*. Ringwood, Vic.: Penguin, 1988.

New York Department of Health. *A Monograph on the Epidemic of Poliomyelitis (Infantile Paralysis) in New York City in 1916*. New York: Department of Health, 1917.

Norris, A.M., ed. *The Society: Being Some Account of the Victorian Society for Crippled Children and Adults*. South Melbourne: Victorian Society for Crippled Children and Adults, 1974.

Numbers, R., 'Physicians, Community and the Qualified Ascent of the American Medical Profession'. In *Major Problems in the History of American Medicine and Public Health*, edited by J.H. Warner and J.A. Tighe. Boston: Houghton Mifflin, 2001, pp.298–303.

Oldstone, M.B.A. *Viruses, Plagues, and History*. New York: Oxford University Press, 1998.

Oshinsky, D.M. *Polio: An American Story*. New York: Oxford University Press, 2005.

Overheu, V. *It Helps to Be Stubborn*. Perth: St George's Books, 1984.

Bibliography

Palmer, G. and Short, S. *Health Care and Public Policy*. Melbourne: McMillan, 1994.

Parker, H.T. *Crippled Children in Tasmania*. (Australian Educational Series, no. 14.) Melbourne: Melbourne University Press, 1932.

Patel, K. and Rushefsky, M.E. *The Politics of Public Health in the United States*. Amonk, NY: M.E. Sharpe, 2005.

Patrick, R. *A History of Health & Medicine in Queensland 1824–1960*. St Lucia: University of Queensland Press, 1987.

Paul, J.R. *A History of Poliomyelitis*. New Haven: Yale University Press, 1971.

Pearn, J. *Pioneer Medicine in Australia*. Brisbane: Amphion Press, 1988.

Peltier, L.F. *Orthopaedics: A History and Iconography*. San Francisco: Norman Publishing, 1993.

Pensabene, T.S. *The Rise of the Medical Practitioner in Victoria*. (Health Research Project, Research Monograph Series.) Canberra: Australian National University, 1980.

Portelli, A. 'What Makes Oral History Different'. In *The Oral History Reader*, edited by R. Perks and A. Thomson. London: Routledge, 1998, pp.32-42.

Porter, R. *The Greatest Benefit to Mankind: A Medical History of Humanity from Antiquity to the Present*. London: Harper Collins, 1997.

Porter, R. and Bynum, W. *Companion Encyclopedia of the History of Medicine*. 2 vols. London: Routledge, 1993.

Priestly, M. *Disability: A Life Course Approach*. Cambridge: Polity Press, 2003.

Queensland Society for Crippled Children. *Souvenir of Government House Fete in Aid of Qld Society for Crippled Children*. Brisbane: Queensland Society for Crippled Children.

Richards, W. *His Majesty's Territorial Army*. London: Virtue and Company, 1911.

Riska, E. and Wegar, K., eds. *Gender, Work and Medicine: Women and the Medical Division of Labour*. (Sage Studies in International Sociology.) London: Sage Publications, 1993.

Rogers, N. *Dirt and Disease: Polio before FDR*. New Brunswick, NJ: Rutgers University Press, 1992. Reprint, 1996.

———. *Polio Wars: Sister Kenny and the Golden Age of American Medicine*. New York: Oxford University Press, 2014.

———. 'Sister Kenny Goes to Washington: Polio, Populism and Medical Politics in Postwar America'. In *The Politics of Healing*, edited by R.D. Johnston (New York: Routledge, 2004), pp.91–116.

Rosenberg, C.E. *Explaining Epidemics and Other Studies in the History of Medicine*. Cambridge: Cambridge University Press, 1992.

Rosenberg, C.E. 'Florence Nightingale on Contagion: The Hospital as Moral Universe'. In *Healing and History: Essays for George Rosen*, edited by C.E. Rosenberg. New York: Science History Publications, 1979, pp.90–108.

Rosenberg, C.E. and Golden, J., eds. *Framing Disease: Studies in Cultural History*. (Health and Medicine in American Society.) New Brunswick, NJ: Rutgers University Press, 1992.

Russell, K. *The Melbourne Medical School*. Melbourne: Melbourne University Press, 1977.

Sandow, E. *The Construction and Reconstruction of the Human Body*. London: Bale and Sons, 1907.

Seavey, N.G., Smith, J.S. and Wagner, P. *A Paralyzing Fear: The Triumph over Polio in America*. New York: TV Books, 1998.

Sexton, C. *The Seeds of Time*. 2nd ed. Melbourne: Oxford University Press, 1999.

Sherson, S. *Being There: Nursing at 'the Melbourne' Victoria's First Hospital*. Melbourne: The Graduate Nurses' Association of the Royal Melbourne Hospital, 2005.

Silver, J. and Wilson, D. *Polio Voices: An Oral History from the American Polio Epidemics and Worldwide Eradication Efforts*. (Praeger Series on Contemporary Health and Living.) Westport, Connecticut: Praeger, 2007.

Smith, F.B. *Florence Nightingale: Reputation and Power*. London: Croom Helm, 1982.

———. *The People's Health: 1830–1910*. Canberra: Australian National University Press, 1979. Reprint, 1990.

Smith, J.S. *Patenting the Sun: Polio and the Salk Vaccine*. New York: William Morrow, 1990.

Snow, D.J.R. *The Progress of Public Health in Western Australia, 1829–1977*. Perth: University of Western Australia, 1981.

Snyder, S.L. and Mitchell, D.T. *Cultural Locations of Disability*. Chicago: University of Chicago Press, 2006.

Spencer, M. *John Howard Lidgett Cumpston, 1880–1954: A Biography*. Tenterfield: Self-published, 1987.

Spurr, N. *Spurr of the Moment: The Story of Noel Spurr OAM*. Burwood East, Vic.: Memoirs Foundation, 2007.

Starr, D. *Blood*. New York: Harper Collins, 2002.

Starr, P. *The Social Transformation of American Medicine*. New York: Basic Books, 1982.

Stephens, H.D. *Summary of an Epidemic of 135 Cases of Acute Poliomyelitis Occurring in Victoria in 1908*. Melbourne: 1908.

Strauss, A. 'The Structure and Ideology of American Nursing', *The Nursing Profession: Five Sociological Essays*, edited by F. Davis, New York: John Wiley, 1966, pp.60–104.

Templeton, J. *Prince Henry's: The Evolution of a Melbourne Hospital 1869–1969*. Melbourne: Robertson and Mullens, 1969.

Tesh, S.N. *Hidden Arguments: Political Ideology and Disease Prevention Policy*. New Brunswick, NJ: Rutgers University Press, 1988.

The Institute. *The Sydney Norland Institute: A Training College for the Training of Educated Women in Nursery Nursing*, Woollahra, NSW: [s.n.], 1911.

Thomas, H. *Sister Elizabeth Kenny, Lives to Remember*. London: Adam and Charles Black and Sons, 1958.

Topley, W.W.C., Parker, M. and Wilson, G. *Principles of Bacteriology, Virology and Immunity*. 8th ed. London: Edward Arnold, 1990.

Tosh, J. and Lang, S. *The Pursuit of History*. 4th ed. Harlow, UK: Pearson Longman, 2006.

Towns, J, 'A Bird's Eye View of Poliomyelitis in Victoria', in Brodribb, B., and Harris, R., eds, *Polio Papers*, Australian Polio Network, Hawthorn: Citadel Press, 1991, pp.35–50.

Turner, B.S. *Medical Power and Social Knowledge*. London: Sage Publications, 1987.

Vagabond and Cannon, M. *The Vagabond Papers*. Abridged ed. Melbourne: Melbourne University Press, 1969.

Vogel, M.J. and Rosenberg, C.E., eds. *The Therapeutic Revolution: Essays in the Social History of American Medicine*. Philadelphia: University of Pennsylvania Press, 1979.

Warner, J.H. and Tighe, J.A. *Major Problems in the History of American Medicine and Public Health: Documents and Essays*. Boston: Houghton Mifflin, 2001.

Welsh, F., ed. *Federation, Great Southern Land: A New History of Australia*. London: Penguin Books, 2004.

Westbrook, M. *An Australian Survey of the Late Effects of Polio*, in Brodribb, B., and Harris, R., eds, *Polio Papers*, Australian Polio Network, Hawthorn: Citadel Press, 1991, pp.35–50.

White, K. *Joseph Lyons*. Melbourne: Penguin Books, 1987.

Wicksteed, J.H. *The Growth of a Profession: Being the History of the Chartered Society of Physiotherapy, 1894–1945*. London: E. Arnold, 1948.

Williams, H.E., ed. *Caring for Disabled Children, From Charity to Teaching Hospital: Ella Latham's Presidency 1933–1954, the Royal Children's Hospital, Melbourne*. Glenroy, Vic.: Book Generation, 1989.

Willis, E. *Medical Dominance: The Division of Labour in Australian Health Care*. Sydney: Allen & Unwin, 1989.

Wilson, D.J. *Living with Polio: The Epidemic and Its Survivors*. Chicago: University of Chicago Press, 2005.

Wilson, J.R. *Through Kenny's Eyes: An Exploration of Sister Elizabeth Kenny's Views About Nursing*. Townsville: The Townsville Regional Group, Royal College of Nursing, James Cook University of North Queensland, 1995.

Woodruff, P. *Two Million South Australians*. Adelaide: Peacock Publications, 1984.

Wright, W.G. *Muscle Training in the Treatment of Infantile Paralysis*. Boston: Ernest Gregory, 1916.

Yule, P. *The Royal Children's Hospital: A History of Faith, Science and Love*. Rushcutters Bay, NSW: Halstead Press, 1999.

Zola, I.K. *Missing Pieces: A Chronicle of Living with a Disability*. Philadelphia: Temple University Press, 1982.

Zwar, D. *The Dame: The Life and Times of Dame Jean Macnamara, Medical Pioneer*. Melbourne: Macmillan, 1984.

Electronic Sources

Personal websites

Vickers-Willis, J. 'Footprint: From the Iron Lung'. http://vickers-willis.com/html/homefromtheironlung.htm.

Spurr, N., http://hometown.aol.com.au/noelspurr/myhomepage/club.html

www.post-polionetwork.org.au/news/ppn48.html

www.post-polionetwork.org.au/stories/coonabrabran.html

www.post-polionetwork.org.au/stories/dragon.html

www.post-polionetwork.org.au/news/ppn45.html

Others

ABC Catalyst, www.abc.net.au/catalyst/stories/2576978.htm

Australian Dictionary of Biography, www.adb.online.anu.edu.au

Australian Institute of Health and Welfare, www.aihw.gov.au/publications/phe/motca/motca.pdf.

Australian Government and Medicare Australia. 'Immunisation Register'. http://www1.hic.gov.au/general/acircirgacir.

Australian Light Horse Association, www.lighthorse.org.au/personal-histories/personal-histories-boer-war-ww1-1/personal-histories-william-henry-harold-kenny

Australian War Memorial, https://www.awm.gov.au/encyclopedia/homefront/us_forces/

Centre for Disease Control, www.cdc.gov/EID/content/15/1/63.htm.

Documenting Democracy, www.foundingdocs.gov.au/area-aid-8.html
Encyclopaedia of Australian Science, www.eoas.info/bib/ASBS01644.htm
Guardian Newspaper, www.guardian.co.uk/footandmouth/story/0,,2215280,00.html.
International Ventilator Users Network, www.ventusers.org/edu/valnews/val10-1a.html.
Nobel Prize, http://nobelprize.org/nobel_prizes/medicine/laureates/1954/index.html.
National Library of Medicine, www.nlm.nih.gov/medlineplus/print/ency/article/001402.htm

Television Broadcast

Nicholls, B., Carlton, M., and Jarvis, G. *Time Frame*. Episode 11, 'Polio Days'. Australia: Australian Broadcasting Commission, Social History Unit, 1997. Broadcast 6 March 1997.

Journal Articles

Anderson, G.L., 'Dr Lorenz and the Crippled Children of the Southwest: A Demonstration of the Value of Publicity and a Splendid Demonstration of Professional Cooperation', *The American Journal of Nursing* Vol. 22, no. 9 (1922): pp.708–12.

Anon., 'Anti-Polio Campaign', *The Australian Municipal Journal* (1956): p.344.

Anon., 'Health Act Amendment Act of 1911, Queensland', *The Australasian Nurses' Journal* Vol. 10, no. 2 (1912).

Anon., 'No Vaccine for the Scaremongers', *Bulletin of the World Health Organization* Vol. 86 (2008): pp.425–26.

Anon., 'State Registration', *The Australasian Nurses' Journal* Vol. 10, no. 4 (1911), pp.110–111.

Anon., 'Nursing Legislation in Queensland', *The Australasian Nurses' Journal* Vol. 10, no. 2 (1912), pp.38–39.

Anon., 'Starting A Hospital', *The Australasian Nurses' Journal*, Vol., 12 (March 15, 1913), pp.80–82.

Anon., 'Acute Poliomyelitis', *The Australasian Nurses' Journal* (October 15, 1914), pp.350–352.

Anon., 'Poliomyelitis in Hobart, *The Australasian Nurses' Journal* Vol. 28 (1931), pp.156–157.

Anon., 'Poliomyelitis in Tasmania, *The Australasian Nurses' Journal* Vol. 29 (1932), pp.58–60.

Anon., 'Poliomyelitis Vaccine', *Australian Journal of Pharmacy*, 30 May (1956): pp.510–11.

Anon., 'The Iron Lung in Australia', *The Hammer: Newsletter of the Health and Medicine Museums* (2003), p.20.

Armstrong, L.E., 'Massage in English War Hospitals', *The Australasian Nurses' Journal* Vol. 12, 14 February (1917), pp.46–47.

Australasian Massage Association, 'Special General Meeting of the Queensland Branch to Consider the Matter of Miss Kenny', *The Australasian Nurses' Journal* Vol.32, No.9,(1934), p.203.

Bachelard, P.M., 'Can We Diagnose Feeble-Mindedness in Children?' *Australasian Journal of Philosophy* Vol. 9, no. 2 (1931): pp.120–30.

Baker, R. and McCullough, L., 'Appropriation of Moral Philosophy: The Case of the Sympathetic and the Unsympathetic Physician', *Kennedy Institute of Ethics Journal* Vol. 17 (2007): pp.3–18.

Bibliography

Benison, S., 'International Medical Cooperation: Dr Albert Sabin, Live Poliovirus Vaccine and the Soviets', *Bulletin of the History of Medicine* Vol. 56, no 4 (1982): pp.460–83.

———, 'Poliomyelitis and the Rockefeller Institute: Social Effects and Institutional Response', *Journal of the History of Medicine* Vol. 29 (1974): pp.74–93.

Bingham, R., 'The Kenny Treatment for Infantile Paralysis: A Comparison of Results with Those of Older Methods of Treatment', *The Journal of Bone and Joint Surgery* Vol. 25, no. 3 (1943): pp.647–50.

Brodie, M., 'A Comparison between Convalescent Serum and Non-Convalescent Serum in Poliomyelitis', *Journal of Experimental Medicine* Vol. 56, no.4 (1932): pp.507–19.

———, 'The Role of Convalescent Serum in Preparalytic Poliomyelitis', *Journal of Immunology* Vol. 28 (1935): pp.353–61.

Bull, H.W., 'Poliomyelitis in the City of Melbourne 1937–1938', *Medical Journal of Australia* Vol. 1, no. 23 (1940): pp.809–12.

Burgess, M., *NSW Public Health Bulletin* (2003): pp.5–8.

Burnet, F. Macfarlane, 'Current Thought on the Prophylaxis of Poliomyelitis', *Medical Journal of Australia* Vol.1, No.8 (1954): pp.192–94.

———, 'The Epidemiology of Poliomyelitis with Special Reference to the Victorian Epidemic of 1937–1938', *Medical Journal of Australia* Vol. 1, no. 10 (1940): pp.325–35.

———, 'Immunological Recognition of Self', *Science* Vol. 133, no. 3449 (1961): pp.307–11.

———, 'Influenza Virus Infections of the Chick Embryo Lung', *British Journal of Experimental Pathology* Vol. 21 (1940): p.147–155.

———, 'The New Laboratory Approach to Poliomyelitis', *Medical Journal of Australia* Vol. 2, no. 14 (1952): pp.481–82.

———, 'A Review of Poliomyelitis', *Medical Journal of Australia*, vol.2, no.14 (1952) pp.481–84.

Burnet, F. Macfarlane and Dora Lush, 'Studies on Experimental Herpes Infection in Mice, Using the Chorioallantoic Technique', *The Journal of Pathology and Bacteriology* Vol. 49, no. 1 (1939): pp.241–59.

Burnet, F. Macfarlane and Macnamara, J., 'The Activity of Stored Antipolymyelitic Serum in Experimental Poliomyelitis', *Medical Journal of Australia* Vol. 2, no. 5 (1929).

Burnet, F. Macfarlane and Macnamara. J., 'Immunological differences between strains of poliomyelitic virus.' *British Journal of Experimental Pathology* Vol.12, No.2 (1931): p.57.

Burnet, F. Macfarlane, Jackson, A.V. and Robertson, E.G., 'The Use of *Macacus Cynomolgus* as an Experimental Animal', *Australian Journal of Experimental Biology and Medical Science* No. 17 (1939): pp.375–91.

Byrne, E. and Roberts, A., 'Polio Epidemic of 1950–51 in the Newcastle Area', *Medical Journal of Australia* Vol.2, no. 1 (1952): pp.10–12.

Calderwood, C., 'Nursing Care in Poliomyelitis: Orthopedic Care of Patients in the Acute Stage of Poliomyelitis', *The American Journal of Nursing* Vol. 40, no. 6 (1940): pp.624–31.

Cameron, D. and Jones, I.G., 'John Snow, the Broad Street Pump and Modern Epidemiology', *International Journal of Epidemiology* Vol. 12, no. 4 (1983): pp.393–96.

Cameron, R.G.B., 'Observations on Poliomyelitis of Epidemiological Interest', *Medical Journal of Australia* Vol. 1, no. 19 (1951), p.705.

Casely, E., 'Physiotherapy in South Australia', *The Australian Journal of Physiotherapy* Vol. 1, no. 4 (1955): pp.164–69.

Cawte, M., 'Craniometry and Eugenics in Australia: R.J.A. Berry and the Quest for Social Efficiency', *Historical Studies* Vol. 22, no. 86 (1986): pp.35–53.

Curtis, A., 'The Crippled Childrens' School', *The American Journal of Nursing* Vol. 1, no. 6 (1901): pp.427–28.

Dale, J., 'The Epidemiology of Poliomyelitis', *Medical Journal of Australia* Vol. 2, no. 9 (1928): pp.258–62.

———, 'Letter to the Editor', *Medical Journal of Australia* Vol. 2 (1935): p.641.

Davis, F., 'Definitions of Time and Recovery in Paralytic Polio Convalescence', *The American Journal of Sociology* Vol. 61, no. 6 (1956): pp.582–87.

Dawson, L., 'The Salk Polio Vaccine Trial of 1954: Risks, Randomization and Public Involvement in Research', *Clinical Trials* Vol. 1 (2004): pp.122–30.

Denton, M., 'Further Comments on the Elizabeth Kenny Controversy', *Australian Historical Studies* Vol. 114 (2000): pp.152–58.

Dickey, B., 'The Labor Government and Medical Services in New South Wales 1910–1914', *Historical Studies* Vol. 12 (19672).

Duffy, J., 'Franklin Roosevelt: Ambiguous Symbol for Disabled Americans', *Midwest Quarterly* Vol. 29 (1987): pp.113 35.

Duhig, J., 'Pathology of Poliomyelitis', *Medical Journal of Australia* Vol. 2, no. 10 (1922).

Editorial, 'Poliomyelitis', *Medical Journal of Australia* Vol. 1, no. 8 (1930): pp.257–58.

———, 'Poliomyelitis', *Medical Journal of Australia* Vol. 1, no. 7 (1918).

———, 'Poliomyelitis in Melbourne', *Medical Journal of Australia* Vol. 1, no. 23 (1940): pp.809–12.

———, 'Gamma Globulin in the Prophylaxis of Paralytic Poliomyelitis', *Medical Journal of Australia* Vol. (1954): pp.299–300.

Elson, M., 'Editorial. Sister Elizabeth Kenny', *Physical Therapy Review*, Vol. 33 (1953): p.81.

Fairchild, A., 'The Polio Narratives: Dialogues with FDR', *Bulletin of the History of Medicine* Vol. 75 (2001): pp.488–534.

Feery, B., 'Impact of Immunisation on Disease Patterns in Australia', *Medical Journal of Australia* Vol., no. 22 August (1981): pp.172–76.

Fine, P., Eames, K. and Heymann, D.L., 'Herd Immunity: A Rough Guide', *Clinical Infectious Diseases*, Vol. 52, no. 7 (2011): pp.911–16.

Flexner, S., 'A Note on the Serum Treatment of Poliomyelitis (Infantile Paralysis)', *Science* Vol. 44, no. 1130 (1916): pp.259–61.

———, 'Respiratory vs Gastro-Intestinal Infection in Poliomyelitis', *Journal of Experimental Medicine* Vol., 64, no. 2 (1936): p.209–226

Flexner, S. and Amoss, H.L., 'The Relation of the Meninges and Choroid Plexus to Poliomyelitic Infection', *Journal of Experimental Medicine* Vol. 25, no. 4 (1917): pp.525–37.

Flexner, S. and Lewis, P.A., 'Experimental Epidemic Poliomyelitis in Monkeys', *Journal of Experimental Medicine* Vol. 12, no.2 (1910): pp.227–55.

Flexner, S. and Noguchi, H., 'Experiments on the Cultivation of the Microorganism Causing Epidemic Poliomyelitis', *Journal of Experimental Medicine* Vol. 18, no. 4 (1913): pp.461–85.

Ford, E., 'Some Early Australian Medical Publications', *Medical History* Vol. 16 (1972), pp.205–255.

Francis, T., Korns, R., Voight, R., Boisen, M. and Hemphill, R., 'An Evaluation of the 1954 Poliomyelitis Vaccine Trials: A Summary Report', *American Journal of Public Health* Vol. 45, no. 5 (Part 2) (1955): pp.1–63.

Bibliography

Galbraith, D., 'Rehabilitation in Poliomyelitis', *Medical Journal of Australia* Vol. 2, no. 14 (1952): pp.483.

Geary, L., 'Australian Medical Students in 19th Century Scotland', *Proceedings of the Royal College of Physicians Edinburgh* Vol. 26 (1996): pp.472–86.

Ghormley, R., Compere, E., Dickson, J., Funston, R., Key, J., McCarroll, H. and Schumm, H., 'Evaluation of the Kenny Treatment of Infantile Paralysis', *Journal of the American Medical Association* Vol. 123, no. 7 (1944): pp.406–09.

Gillespie, J.A., 'Medical Markets and Australian Medical Politics', *Labour History* Vol. 54 (1988): pp.30–46.

Gleeson, B., 'Domestic Space and Disability in Nineteenth-Century Melbourne, Australia', *Journal of Historical Geography* Vol. 27 (2001): pp.223–40.

Goodman, G., Hirschman, J., Hepps, D. and Rudy, L., 'Children's Memory for Stressful Events', *Merrill-Palmer Quarterly* Vol. 37 (1991), pp.109–157.

Graham, F.W., 'Letter: Byrne and Roberts Article on Polio in Newcastle Area', *Medical Journal of Australia* Vol.4 (1952): p.176.

Hamilton, A., 'Letter: Byrne and Roberts Article on Polio in Newcastle Area', *Medical Journal of Australia* Vol.4 (1952): p.175.

Hammon, W., 'Gamma Globulin in Poliomyelitis', *Scientific American* Vol. (1952).

Hardy, A., 'Poliomyelitis and the Neurologists: the View from England, 1896–1966', *Bulletin of the History of Medicine* Vol. 71, no. 2 (1997): pp.249–72.

———, 'Straight Back to Barbarism: Antityphoid Inoculation and the Great War', *Bulletin of the History of Medicine* Vol. 74, no. 2 (2000): pp.265–90.

Heintzelman, R.A., 'The Crippled Child and the Curriculum Guide: Content of the Revised Curriculum Guide for Schools of Nursing as It Relates to Nursing Services in the Expanded Program for Crippled Children', *The American Journal of Nursing* Vol. 39, no. 7 (1939): pp.774–80.

Henderson, D.A., White, J., Morris, L. and A. Langmuir, 'Paralytic Disease Associated with Oral Polio Vaccines', *Journal of the American Medical Association*, Vol. 190, no. 1, pp.41–48.

Honesty, E.T., 'The Handicapped Child', *The Journal of Negro Education* Vol. 1, no. 2 (1932): pp.304–24.

Hooker, C., 'Diphtheria, Immunisation and the Bundaberg Tragedy: A Study of Public Health in Australia', *Health and History*, Vol. 2, no. 1 (2000): pp.52–78.

Horstmann, D.M., et al, 'The Trial Use of Sabin's Attenuated Type 1 Poliovirus Vaccine in a Village in Southern Arizona', *American Journal of Epidemiology* Vol. 70 (1959): pp.169–84.

Hull, B.P. and McIntyre, P.B. 'Mapping Immunisation Coverage and Conscientious Objectors to Immunisation in NSW' *NSW Public Health Bulletin*, Vol 14 (2003): pp.8–12.

Ingram, M.L., 'Trends in Education of Crippled Children', *Journal of Educational Sociology* Vol. 6, no. 6 (1933): pp.339–47.

Ingram, W., 'The Treatment of Paralysis at the Elizabeth Kenny Clinic, Royal North Shore Hospital of Sydney, [Report of Commission of Inquiry], in *Medical Journal of Australia* Vol. 2, no. 20 (1937): pp.888–94.

Jones, G., 'Eugenics and Social Policy between the Wars', *The Historical Journal* Vol. 25, no. 3 (1982): pp.717–28.

Kapp, C. 'Surge in Polio Spreads Alarm in Northern Nigeria. Rumours About Vaccine Safety in Muslim-run States Threaten WHO's Eradication Programme', *Lancet* Vol. 362, no. 9396 (2003), pp.1631–32.

Kenny, E., 'Infantile Paralysis', *Medical Journal of Australia* Vol. 2, no. 2 (1946): pp.70–71.

Kent Hughes, W., 'Letter to Editor', *Medical Journal of Australia*, 18 March (1939).

Koven, S., 'Remembering and Dismemberment: Crippled Children, Wounded Soldiers and the Great War in Great Britain', *The American Historical Review* Vol. 99, no. 4 (1994): pp.1167–1202.

Lancaster, H.O., 'Epidemics of Poliomyelitis in New South Wales', *Medical Journal of Australia* Vol. 1, no. 8 (1954): pp.245–46.

Lewin, P., 'Kenny Treatment of Infantile Paralysis During the Acute Stage', *Illinois Medical Journal* Vol. (April, 1942) Vol. 81, pp.281–96.

Linker, B., 'The Business of Ethics: Gender, Medicine, and the Professional Codification of the American Physiotherapy Association, 1918–1935', *Journal of the History of Medicine and Allied Sciences* Vol. 60, no. 3 (2005): pp.320–54.

Longmore, P.K. and Goldberger, D., 'The League of the Physically Handicapped and the Great Depression: A Case Study in the New Disability History', *Journal of American History* Vol. 87, no. 3 (2000): pp.888–922.

Lovell, H.T., 'The Tasmanian Mental Deficiency Act', *Australasian Journal of Philosophy* Vol. 1, no. 4 (1923): pp.285–89.

MacDonald, L., 'The Treatment of Poliomyelitits', *Medical Journal of Australia* Vol. 1, no. 19 (1938): pp.797–800.

Mackenzie, W., 'Section on Diseases in Children. Australasian Medical Congress, Brisbane', *Medical Journal of Australia* Vol. 2, no. 12 (1920): p.285.

Macintosh, A.M., 'The Treatment of Acute Poliomyelitis', *Medical Journal of Australia* Vol. 2, no.2 1954). p.417.

Macnamara, J., 'After-Care of Poliomyelitis', *Medical Journal of Australia* Vol. I, no. 5 (1925): pp.616–17.

———, 'Treatment of Poliomyelitis During the Acute and Convalescent Phase', *Medical Journal of Australia* Vol. II, no. 9 (1928).

———, 'The Treatment of Acute Poliomyelitis by Means of Human Immune Serum.' *Medical Journal of Australia*, Vol. 2 (1929) pp.838–840.

———, 'The Care of the Paralysis of Poliomyelitis', *Medical Journal of Australia* Vol. 2, no. 17 (1946): pp.577–80.

———, 'The Early Treatment of Poliomyelitis', *Medical Journal of Australia* Vol. 2 (1935): pp.374–77.

———, 'Letter to Editor', *Medical Journal of Australia* Vol. 2 (1932).

———, 'Preventative Orthopaedics and the Physiotherapist', *Medical Journal of Australia*, Vol. 1 (1951): pp.293–98.

———, 'The prevention of Crippling following Poliomyelitis', *Medical Journal of Australia*, Vol.2, Issue 1, pp.4–8.

Macnamara, J., & Morgan, F. G. (1932). Poliomyelo-encephalitis in Victoria (1925–1931): Treatment by Human Immune Serum', *The Lancet*, 219(5661), pp.469-472.

Madsen, W., 'Early 20th Century Untrained Nursing Staff in the Rockhampton District: A Necessary Evil?' *Journal of Advanced Nursing* Vol. 51, no. 3 (2005): pp.307–13.

Martin, I., 'When Needs Must: The Acceptance of Volunteer Aids in British and Australian Military Hospitals in World War I', *Health and History* Vol. 4, no. 1 (2002) pp.88–98.

Martyr, P., 'A Response to Margaret Denton', *Australian Historical Studies* Vol. 114 (2000): pp.159–62.

———, 'A Small Price to Pay for Peace: The Elizabeth Kenny Controversy Re-Examined', *Australian Historical Studies* Vol. 108 (1997): pp.47–65.

Bibliography

McCloskey, B., 'Report of an Investigation into an Outbreak of Poliomyelitis in a Small Town Remote from Melbourne', *Medical Journal of Australia* Vol.1, No.17 (1951): pp.612–613.

McMurtrie, A.K., 'Nursing Care of Crippled Children in the United States', *The American Journal of Nursing* Vol. 16, no. 2 (1915): pp.115–18.

McMurtrie, D.C., 'Notes on the Early History and Care for Cripples', *American Journal of Care for Cripples* Vol. I (1914).

Mead, S., 'A Century of the Abuse of Rest', *Journal of the American Medical Association* Vol. 182 (1962): pp.344–45.

Meldrum, M., 'A Calculated Risk: The Salk Polio Vaccine Field Trials of 1954', *British Medical Journal* Vol. 317, no. 7167 (1998): pp.1233–36.

Melnick, J.A., 'A New Era in Polio Research', *Scientific American* Vol. 193 (1955).

Metcalfe, R., 'A Critical Evaluation of the Kenny Treatment', *The Medical Press and Journal* (1954): pp.477–80.

Miles, J., 'Observations on Serum from Aborigines in the Northern Territory of Australia', *Medical Journal of Australia* Vol. 2, no. 21 (1953): pp.773–76.

Morgan, F., 'The Preparation of Serum from Human Donors Recovered from Poliomyelitis', *Medical Journal of Australia* Vol. 2, no. 3 (1928): pp.264–67.

National Health and Medical Research Council, 'Poliomyelitis in Australia: Report of the Poliomyelitis Subcommittee of the NHMRC', *Medical Journal of Australia* Vol. 1, no. 25 (1964): pp.935–40.

Neumann, D.A., 'Polio: Its Impact on the People of the United States and the Emerging Profession of Physical Therapy', *Journal of Orthopaedic and Sports Physical Therapy* Vol. 34, no. 8 (2004): pp.479–92.

Nichol, W., 'The Medical Profession in New South Wales', *Australian Economic History Review* Vol. 24, no. 2 (1984).

Park, W., 'Serum Treatment in Poliomyelitis', *Public Health* Vol. 45 (1932): pp.284–86.

Parson, M., 'The Nursing Care of Orthopedic Children', *The American Journal of Nursing* Vol. 32, no. 2 (1932): pp.135–37.

Paul, J. and Trask, J., 'Detection of Poliomyelitis Virus in So-Called Abortive Types of the Disease', *Journal of Experimental Medicine* Vol. 56 (1933): pp.319–43.

Potts, F.J., 'The Shriners' Hospitals: A General Outline of the History of the Founding of the Shriners' Hospitals for Crippled Children', *The American Journal of Nursing* Vol. 26, no. 10 (1926): pp.745–52.

Pritchard, D.G., 'The Development of Schools for Handicapped Children in England During the Nineteenth Century', *History of Education Quarterly* Vol. 3, no. 4 (1963).

Report by Board of Directors of Royal North Shore Hospital, Sydney, 'The Treatment of Paralysis at the Elizabeth Kenny Clinic, Royal North Shore Hospital of Sydney', *Medical Journal of Australia* Vol. 2, no. 20 (1937): pp.888–94.

Rivers, T.M., 'The Story of Research on Poliomyelitis', *Proceedings of the American Philosophical Society* Vol. 98, no. 4 (1954): pp.250–54.

Robertson, E., 'An Examination of the Olfactory Bulbs in Fatal Cases of Poliomyelitis During the Victorian Epidemic of 1937–38', *Medical Journal of Australia* Vol. 1, no. 9 (1940), pp.156–162

Roe, M., 'The Establishment of the Australian Department of Health: Its Background and Significance', *Historical Studies* 17 (1976): pp.188–189.

Rogers, N., 'The Debate Considered', *Australian Historical Studies* No. 114 (2000): pp.163–66.

———, 'Silence Has Its Own Stories: Elizabeth Kenny, Polio and the Culture of Medicine', *Social History of Medicine* Vol. 21, no. 1 (2008): pp.145–61.

Sabin, A. and Olitsky, P., 'Cultivation of the Poliomyelitis Virus in Vitro in Human Embryonic Nervous Tissue', *Proceedings of the Society of Experimental and Biological Medicine* Vol. 34 (1936): pp.357–59.

Scholes, F., 'A Review of Poliomyelitis', *Medical Journal of Australia* Vol.2, No. 14 (1952), p.484.

Scofield, E.C., 'Schools for Segregation of Crippled Children: A May Day Celebration', *The American Journal of Nursing* Vol. 30, no. 4 (1930): pp.469–70.

Searle, G.R., 'Eugenics and Politics in Britain in the 1930's', *Annals of Science* Vol. 36, no. 2 (1979): pp.159–69.

Serotte, B., 'Contagious', *Fourth Genre: Explorations in Non-fiction* Vol. 5, no. 1 (2003), pp.118–35.

Snow, D.J.R., 'Crowds and Poliomyelitis: With Special Reference to a Recent Epidemic in Western Australia', *Medical Journal of Australia* Vol.1, no. 1 (1955): pp.2–5.

———, 'Poliomyelitis and Atmospheric Conditions in Certain Australian Cities', *Medical Journal of Australia* Vol. 2, no. 1 (1952): pp.17–19.

———, 'The Spot-Map in Epidemiology: A Note on the Use of Spot-Maps During Two Epidemics of Poliomyelitis in Western Australia', *Medical Journal of Australia* Vol. 43, no. 17 (1956), pp.702–704

Southby, R., 'Acute Poliomyelitis in Victoria', *Medical Journal of Australia* Vol. 1 (1925), pp.9–10.

———, 'Treatment of Acute Anterior Poliomyelitis in the Early Stages', *Medical Journal of Australia* (1935): pp.367–73.

Southcott, R.V., 'Studies on a Long-Range Association between Bulbar Poliomyelitis and Previous Tonsillectomy', *Medical Journal of Australia* Vol., no. 8 (1953): pp.281–98.

Southcott, R.V., Crosby, N.D. and Stenhouse, N.S., 'Studies on the Epidemiology of the 1947–1948 Epidemic of Poliomyelitis in South Australia', *Medical Journal of Australia* Vol. 2, no. 14 (1949): pp.482–96.

Spencely, G., 'The Minister for Starvation: Wilfrid Kent Hughes and the Unemployment Relief (Administration) Act of 1933', *Labour History* Vol. 81 (2001): pp.135–54.

Stanley, N.F., 'Poliomyelitis: The Experimental Approach to Its Prevention', *Medical Journal of Australia* Vol.2, no. 11 (1954): pp.417–21.

Stephen, D., 'Poliomyelits', *Medical Journal of Australia* Vol. 1, no. 14 (1918).

Stevenson, J.L., 'After-Care of Infantile Paralysis', *The American Journal of Nursing* Vol. 25, no. 9 (1925): pp.729–33.

———, 'The Kenny Method: Nursing Responsibilities in Relation to the Kenny Method of Treatment for Infantile Paralysis', *The American Journal of Nursing* Vol. 42, no. 8 (1942): pp.904–10.

Stokes, J., 'Observations on Serum from Aborigines in the Northern Territory of Australia: Iii Antibodies against Brunhilde (Type 1) and Leon (Type 3) Poliomyelitis Viruses', *Medical Journal of Australia* Vol. 2, no. 12 (1955): pp.433–38.

Thelander, C.A., Duhig, J.V., Nye, J., Patterson, A.E. and Lahz, R.S., 'Report of the Queensland Royal Commission on Modern Methods for the Treatment of Infantile Paralysis', *Medical Journal of Australia* Vol. 1, no. 5 (1938), pp.187–224.

Tomes, N.J, 'Epidemic Entertainments: Disease and Popular Culture in Early-Twentieth-Century America', *American Literary History* Vol. 14, no. 4 (2002): pp.617–24.

Tomes, N.J., 'American Attitudes Toward the Germ Theory of Disease: Phyllis Allen Richmond Revisited', *Journal of the History of Medicine and Allied Sciences* Vol. 52, no. 1 (1997), pp.17–50.
Vickers, W., 'Report on the Education and Treatment of Cripples in the United States of America', *Medical Journal of Australia* Vol. 2, no. I (1925): pp.9–10.
Warner, J.H., 'The History of Science and the Sciences of Medicine', *Osiris* Vol. 10 (1995): pp.164–93.
Webster, R., 'Scientific', *Medical Journal of Australia*, Vol. 1, no. 14 (1918), pp.292–294.
Webster, R., 'Anterior Poliomyelitis', *Medical Journal of Australia* Vol. 1, no. 18 (1918).
Weller, T., Robbins, F. and Enders, J., 'Cultivation of Poliomyelitis Virus in Cultures of Human Foreskin and Embryonic Tissues', *Proceedings of the Society for Experimental Biology and Medicine* Vol. 72 (1949): p.153–155.
Wilkinson, M., 'Poliomyelitis Epidemic 1937: A Recollection', *Australian Paediatric Journal* Vol. 24, no. 2 (1988): pp.112–13.
Wilkinson, R.S, 'Letter: Epidemiology of 47–48 Polio Outbreak in South Australia', *Medical Journal of Australia* Vol.2, no. 17 (1949).
Williams, S., 'Obituary – Annie Jean Macnamara', *Medical Journal of Australia*, Vol. 6 (1970), pp.472-475.
Willis, E., 'Sister Elizabeth Kenny and the Evolution of the Occupational Division of Labour in Health Care', *Australian and New Zealand Journal of Sociology* Vol. 15, no. 3 (1979): pp.30–38.
Wilson, D.J., 'Braces, Wheelchairs, and Iron Lungs: The Paralyzed Body and the Machinery of Rehabilitation in the Polio Epidemics', *Journal of Medical Humanities* Vol. 26, no. 2/3 (2005), pp.173–190.

Unpublished Theses and Other Sources

Anon., Sister Elizabeth Kenny: Testimonials for Sister Kenny, self-published by the Sister Elizabeth Kenny Memorial Museum, Nobby, Queensland (n.d.).
Buxton, A.J.G. 'Poliomyelitis in South Australia 1937–1956'. BA (Hons) History, Adelaide University, 1977.
Highley, K. 'For Want of a Cake of Soap and a Towel: A Study of Epidemic Poliomyelitis in Mid Twentieth Century Australia'. BA (Hons), Australian National University, 2004.
Highley, K. 'Mending Bodies: Polio Treatment in Australia'. PhD, Australian National University, 2009.
Martyr, P. 'The Professional Development of Rehabilitation in Australia 1870–1981'. PhD, University of Western Australia, 1994.
Ross, J.C. 'A History of Poliomyelitis in New Zealand'. Master of Arts in History, University of Canterbury, 1993.
Smith, J.H. 'Fear, Frustration and the Will to Overcome: A Social History of Poliomyelitis in Western Australia'. PhD, Edith Cowan University, 1997.
Thame, C. 'Health and the State: The Development of Collective Responsibility for Health Care in Australia in the First Half of the Twentieth Century'. PhD, Australian National University, 1974.

INDEX

AAH *see* Australian Auxiliary Hospitals
Aboriginal people, polio incidence   44–5
adult sufferers   11–13, 31–2
after-care   125–43
  New South Wales   131–2
  Victoria   129–31, 139
Aikens, T.   69, 86
almoners *see* medical social workers
alternative medicine, Australia   4, 47, 68, 140, 175
  United States   68
  see also folk remedies; homeopathy
AMA *see* American Medical Association
American Medical Association   68, 97–8, 99–101
Anthony, H.L.   32
antibodies *see* natural immunity
anti-Semitism   100, 163
anti-vaccinationists   162–3, 173
Apperly, Frank   47–8
ATNA *see* Australasian Trained Nurses' Association
atrophy of muscles *see* muscle atrophy
Australasian Trained Nurses' Association   74, 75
Australian Auxiliary Hospitals (UK)   77–8
Australian Jockey Club   133
Australian Orthopaedic Association   50
bacteriology, history   144–5

Bazeley, Percival   158, 162
bedsores   28–9, 35
Bendigo Base Hospital   35
Berry, R.J.A.   56
Blue Sisters *see* Kenny-trained therapists
BMA *see* British Medical Association
Both, Edward   27
Brisbane General Hospital   80–1, 82–3, 92–3, 102
British Association of Physical Medicine   103
British Medical Association   4, 47, 50, 60, 68, 69, 81, 82, 89, 92, 129, 163–4
British Orthopaedic Association   90

Brodie, Maurice   58, 156
bulbar polio sufferers   28
Burnet, Frank Macfarlane   52, 56, 57, 59, 105, 107, 150, 151–4, 155–6, 157, 160–1, 164
Burstall, Aubrey   27

Canonbury, Sydney (NSW)   133
Champonnière, Just Lucas- *see* Lucas-Champonnière, Just
charitable hospitals, exclusion of patients   21
charitable institutions, dependence on   47, 52, 117, 125, 126–7
Children's Hospital, Boston   26
Children's Hospital, Hampton *see* Hampton Children's Hospital
Children's Hospital, Melbourne *see* Royal Children's Hospital
Children's Hospital, Perth   89, 104
Chuter, Charles   80–2, 84, 87, 91, 92, 93, 96, 102, 103, 105, 106
Cilento, Raphael W.   82–6, 88, 102
Clifton, Queensland   74–5, 79
Commonwealth Serum Laboratory   59, 158, 162
concealment, of crippled children   127–8
Connaught Laboratories (Canada)   165
Consultative Council on Poliomyelitis (Vic)   139
convalescence *see* rehabilitation
Cooper, Leila   83–4, 85
country children *see* rural children
Country Women's Association, support for Kenny   105, 106
Crawford, Harold   82–3, 88
Cregan, Daphne, treated by Kenny   79
cripple, as label   42
crippled children, Australia   79–80
  1928 survey   127
  care of   49, 87, 125–34
  education   125, 126, 132–4
Crippled Children's Association (SA)   139
CSL *see* Commonwealth Serum Laboratory
cuirass respirator   27, 116

– 257 –

Cumpston, J.H.L. 24, 83, 87
Cutter Laboratories (US) 160, 161, 165
CWA *see* Country Women's Association

Davis, Fred 17
death rate, from polio 24, 42
deaths, of respirator patients 29
deformity, attitudes to 62–3, 142–3
  see also concealment; disability, attitudes to; exhibition
depression 111
diphtheria, decline 24
  immunisation programs 164–5
disability, attitudes to 115, 116, 117, 119, 125, 126–7, 133–4
  see also concealment; deformity; exhibition
disability allowances, Australia 32, 128
disabled, care of 125–6
disabled children *see* crippled children
diseases, aetiology 144–5
doctors, case loads 24, 26
Drinker, Philip 27
Drinker respirator *see* respirators
Drummond, S.G. 131–2
Duncan Hospital (NZ) 123

early intervention, in Kenny treatment 68, 72, 108, 123, 170
Elizabeth Kenny Institute, Minneapolis 97–101, 105, 120, 123
embryonic tissue *see* foetal tissue
employment, of sufferers 139, 143
employment-oriented rehabilitation 125, 127, 132, 133–4
Enders, John 155, 157, 160
epidemics 5, 57
  Australia 2, 5, 26, 39–44, 89
    1937–8 23–4, 42, 63, 152–3, 154, 163, 171
    1961–2 165–6
    government response 43–4
  New Guinea 57
  Sweden 145, 146
  United States, 1916 40–1
epidemiology, of polio 39–45, 172–3
eugenics 6–7, 56, 154
exhibition, of crippled children 128
experimental medicine, and polio *see* poliovirus, research
Experimental Muscle Re-Education Clinic 83–6

faecal matter, and poliovirus 146, 150, 154, 172
Fairfield Hospital, Melbourne 23–4, 35, 36, 37, 48, 63, 112, 113, 114, 116, 121, 124, 136, 139–40

family life, disruption of 19–20, 31, 33, 135, 143
  see also parents; relationships
Far West Children's Health Scheme (NSW) 131–2
feeding tubes 37
financial impact, of polio 31–2
First World War, nurses and 75–6
  and orthopaedics 49–50
Fishbein, Morris 94, 99–100
Flexner, Simon 52, 56–7, 148–50, 152
foetal tissue, in poliovirus research 154, 156, 157
folk remedies 14, 15, 150
  see also alternative medicine
Forgan Smith, William 82, 94
Frankston Hospital 129, 131, 133
frog breathing 38, 116
Fryberg, Abraham 92

Galbraith, Douglas 87, 170
gastrointestinal illness 11, 147
general practitioners, and immunisation programs 163–4
germ theory 145
  vs. miasma theory 5–6
Ghormley, R.K. 99, 101
Golden Casket lottery, Queensland 80
GPs *see* general practitioners
Grueber, Alison 24–5
Guinane, James 86

Hall, R. McKellar 88–9, 104
Hampton Children's Hospital, Melbourne 93, 118, 122, 129
handicrafts, in rehabilitation 132, 133, 134, 139
Hanlon, E.M. 81–2, 83, 87, 102, 105
Heine, J. von 145
Heine-Medin disease *see* polio
heliotherapy 51
Helms, Karen 58
herd immunity 173–4
Hobart Hospital 133
Hodge, Isobel 56
home care, of sufferers 120, 121–2, 137–9, 140
homeopathy 4, 14, 140
hospitalisation 3, 8, 18, 20, 111
hospitals 21–38
  food 35, 36–7
  Melbourne 47–8
    infectious diseases policy 48
  Queensland 80–1
  schooling in 132–4
  see also names of hospitals, *e.g.* Brisbane General Hospital; Royal Children's Hospital, Melbourne

Index

hot packs, in pain relief 66, 72, 81, 92, 98, 108, 118, 119–20, 171
Hughes, Billy *see* Hughes, W.M.
Hughes, W.M. 43, 86–7, 90
Hughes, W.S.K. *see* Kent Hughes, W.S.
human tissue, and virus culture 154, 156
hydrotherapy 95, 96, 117
hypersensitivity, of skin 19

immigrants, and polio transmission 5, 41
immobilisation, as treatment 19, 35, 49, 50, 63, 96, 104, 108, 123, 124, 139, 169, 170–1
  see also plaster casts; splints
immunisation programs *see* Salk immunisation programs
immunisation rates, Australia 163, 174
immunity *see* herd immunity; natural immunity
indigenous Australians *see* Aboriginal people
infant mortality, Australia 4, 11
infantile paralysis *see* polio
Institute of Physico-Chemical Biology, Paris 57–8
insurance, against polio 32–3
iron lungs *see* respirators
isolation, in hospitals 22–3, 25, 31, 48, 50
  transition from 111–2

James, Henry 103
Joint State and Municipal Campaign Against Poliomyelitis (Vic) 52–3
Journal of the American Medical Association 9

Kendall, F. 96
Kendall, H. 96
Kenny, Elizabeth 1, 2, 3–4, 8, 38, 51, 65–109, 169, 170, 175–7
  acknowledgement of pain 18, 19
  communication skills 96–7
  death 106
  education 70, 71
  family 69–73
  and the First World War 75–8
  Infantile Paralysis and Cerebral Diplegia 89
  My Battle and Victory 106
  nursing training 73–4
  popularity in the US 106
  as potato buyer 73
  and Queensland government 80–8, 91–2, 105–6
  treatment methods *see* Kenny treatment
  The Treatment of Infantile Paralysis in the Acute Stage 96–7
Kenny, Mary 69–70
Kenny, Mary Stewart 94, 103
Kenny, Michael 69–70
Kenny clinics, Queensland 74–5, 82–9, 92, 101–2
  see also names of clinics, e.g. Sister Kenny Clinic and Training School
The Kenny Concept of the Disease of Infantile Paralysis (film) 103
Kenny Foundation 98, 106, 107
Kenny Institute *see* Elizabeth Kenny Institute
Kenny-trained therapists 24–5, 120–1, 123, 140
Kenny treatment 81
  American acceptance of 67, 68, 94–109, 169
  Australian rejection of 67–8, 88–92, 93, 96, 103–4, 107, 121–2, 124
  evaluation of 83–9, 95–6, 99, 171
  as evidence-based medicine 175–6
  New Zealand acceptance of 67, 123–4
  popular defence of 89–90, 99–101, 120
  in the United Kingdom 90, 103, 122–3
Kent Hughes, W.S. 52
Knapp, Miland 94–5
Koch, Robert 51–2
Kolmer, John 156
Kuhn, Stanley 79

Landsteiner, Karl 146
Launceston Hospital 24, 26, 35–6
Leake, James P. 156
Levaditi, C. 150
Lewin, Philip 99, 102–3
Love, J.S., support of Kenny clinic 82
Lovett, Robert 104–5, 170
Lucas-Championnière, Just 49
Luddy, Mary 92–3
lumbar puncture 12, 21–2, 53–4, 147
Lush, Dora 154, 155
Lyons, Enid 58
Lyons, Joe 58, 87

Macfarlane Burnet, F. *see* Burnet, Frank Macfarlane
MacKenzie, Colin 50, 51
Mackinnon, Eleanor 86–7
Macnamara, Jean 1, 2, 38, 45–6, 48, 50, 51, 52–64, 88, 89, 91, 104–5, 130–1, 139, 151–2, 169–70
marriage *see* relationships
massage therapy 49, 51, 79
  First World War 77–8
  see also physiotherapy
McDonnell, Aeneas 71–2, 74, 76, 77
Medical Act of 1908 47
Medical Journal of Australia 58, 89
medical practitioners 9
  see also general practitioners; doctors
medical profession 3–4, 14, 66, 124
  history in Australia 46–7
  see also British Medical Association

– 259 –

medical social workers 56
Medin, K.O. 145–6
Melbourne, public health 47
Melbourne Hospital *see* Royal Melbourne Hospital
Melbourne Ladies Benevolent Society 127
meningitis, symptoms 16
mental illness, and physical disability 6, 42
  see also depression; psychological trauma
Menzies, Frederick 90, 91
miasma theory 35
  vs. germ theory 5–6
micro-organisms 5, 144–5, 148
Middleton, June 95, 136
misinformation 15, 18
monkeys, in poliovirus research 53, 146, 148, 150, 151
mortality *see* death rate; deaths; infant mortality
muscles, atrophy 147
  re-education 50, 51, 66, 79, 175
  strength testing 96, 124
myxomatosis, Macnamara's support for 64

nasal cavity, as entry point 60, 148–9, 150–1, 153–4, 157
nasal spray, as prophylactic 60
National Foundation for Infantile Paralysis (US) 94, 95, 97, 98–101, 106, 155, 159, 160–1, 167
National Health and Medical Research Council 162, 163, 167
National Information Bureau (US) 98–9
National Research Council (US) 98
natural immunity 16, 39, 44
Netter, Arnold 52
New South Wales Society for Crippled Children 129, 132
New Zealand Crippled Children's Society 126
New Zealand Department of Health 123–4
newspapers, role of *see* press coverage
NFIP *see* National Foundation for Infantile Paralysis
NHMRC *see* National Health and Medical Research Council
Nightingale, Florence 65
Noguchi, Hideyo 149
Norland Institute *see* Sydney Norland Institute
notifiable diseases, Australia 40
nurses, case loads 23, 25
  and the medical profession 65–6
  registration, Queensland 74–5
  training, Australia 75
nursing care 50, 112
  of respirator patients 28–9
  standards of 34
Nye, Jarvis 93

O'Brien, Daniel 60–1
occupational therapy 130, 132, 133
O'Connor, Basil 94, 98, 159, 160
Olitsky, Peter 153
oral vaccines *see* Sabin vaccine
orthopaedic medicine 49–50, 61
orthoses, affordability 128
Osborne, Pauline 108
ostracism, of sufferers 18, 135–6
  of sufferers' families 17–18, 33–4
  see also stigma
outpatient care 92, 130, 139

Page, Earle 86, 107
pain, acknowledgement of 18, 19
  experience of 18–19, 114–5, 118–9, 141
  relief, by heat application 66, 72, 81, 92, 98, 108
paralysis 1, 5, 6, 147
parents, of sufferers 17 18, 19 20, 22, 23, 31, 33, 36, 113, 114, 121–2
Park, W.H. 58, 156
passive exercise 49, 72, 81, 92–3, 108
Pasteur, Louis 148
Pasteur Institute 150
Paul, John 108
personal narratives 7–9
personal relationships *see* relationships
Perth Children's Hospital *see* Children's Hospital, Perth
physical disability, and mental illness 6, 42
physiotherapy 51, 118–9, 124, 176–7
  history of 117
  see also massage therapy
plaster casts 50, 66, 104, 108, 124, 131, 141–2
Plastridge, Alice L. 95
pneumonia, and polio sufferers 35–36
polio, aetiology 5–6, 15, 43, 16
  in Australia 39–45, 179–80
  declining notifications 165, 172
  diagnosis 12–14, 16–17, 53–4, 147
  effect on different age groups 5
  as endemic disease 16, 39, 44–5, 172–3
  epidemics *see* epidemics
  as infectious disease 2–3
  incidence 2, 178–80
  misdiagnosis 12–14
  as notifiable disease 39–40
  onset 1, 10–14, 16–17
  prognosis 147
  progression 2–3, 11–12, 147
  public attitudes to 4–5, 17–18, 33, 41, 42, 113
  rehabilitation 3, 38, 110–43
  symptoms 1, 6, 11–12
  treatment *see* treatment

Index

Polio Aunts 139
poliomyelitis *see* polio
poliovirus, in the 21st century 172–4
   as enterovirus 146
   ignorance of transmission 43
   research 144–68
   transmission 2, 5, 6, 15, 18, 40–1, 60, 146–7, 148–55, 171–2
   variant strains 152–3, 155, 158
Popper, Erwin 146
Port Lincoln, epidemic 39
post-polio syndrome 171
poverty 4, 128
Powell, Mostyn 59
power failure, and respirators 31
PPS *see* post-polio syndrome
press coverage, Australia 15–16, 43, 55
Prince Henry Hospital, Sydney 34, 112, 166
Prince Henry's Hospital, Melbourne 4
privacy, patients' lack of 112
psychological trauma, of sufferers 111, 115, 116
public health, administration, Queensland 81
   advances 145
   Australia 4
   Melbourne 47
   see also sanitation, improvement
public trust, in medicine 14
Pye, Aubrey 93

quarantine
   Melbourne 48
   New York 40–1
Queen Mary's Hospital, Carshalton (UK) 90, 103, 108–9, 122–3
Queen's Memorial Fund Hospital *see* Fairfield Hospital
Queensland Nurses' Registration Board 75

rabbit control, and J. Macnamara 64
rehabilitation 3, 38, 110–43
reintegration, into society 142–3
relationships, of sufferers 19, 135–8, 143
respirators 26–31, 115–6, 136, 147
respiratory muscles, atrophy of 147
respiratory transmission, theory of 148–9, 150, 153–5
Rivers, Tom 149–50
Robbins, Frederick 155
Robertson, E. Graeme 153–4
Robertson, Walter 123
Rockefeller, John D. 98–9
Rockefeller Foundation 47–8, 57, 60–1, 153
Rockefeller Institute, New York 52, 57, 61, 148–50
rocking beds 38, 116
Roosevelt, Franklin D. 41, 94, 116–7, 134, 150, 159

Rotary Club, Sydney survey 127–8
Rountree, J. 92
Royal Alexandra Hospital for Children, Sydney 132
Royal Children's Hospital, Melbourne 48, 51, 56, 114, 130–1
Royal Commission, into Kenny treatment 88, 89, 90, 91–2, 93
Royal Melbourne Hospital 48
Royal North Shore Hospital, Sydney 87, 89–90, 91
Royal Society of Medicine 103
rural cases, of polio 45
rural children, access to care 113, 131–2, 140

Sabin, Albert 153, 157, 161, 166–1
Sabin vaccine 1, 158, 161, 166–8, 173
saline baths 50, 124
Salk, Jonas 157–9, 163
Salk immunisation programs 1, 159–60, 161–7
   opposition to 162–3
Salk vaccine 157–61, 165
   effectiveness 160, 161, 166
   production in Australia 161–2
Sandow, Eugene 72
sanitary systems, deficiency of 16
sanitation, improvement 16, 40
scarlet fever, decline in 24
Scholes, F.V. 23–4
schools, closure of 40, 43
   and polio sufferers 34, 142–3
   see also hospitals, schooling in
self-image, of sufferers 116, 136–7
self-pity 112
serum collection, Victoria 53, 55–6, 59
serum therapy 45, 51–5, 58–9
   opponents of 58–9
   research 53, 152
Simpson, George 154
Sister Elizabeth Kenny Foundation *see* Kenny Foundation
Sister Kenny Clinic and Training School, Brisbane 92
slums 5–6
   New York 41
Society for the Care of Crippled Children (Tas) 131, 133
Southby, Robert 59
spinal cord, and poliovirus 145, 146
spinal tap *see* lumbar puncture
splints 2, 21, 35, 37, 38, 49, 62, 104, 124, 137
St George Hospital, Sydney 118
Starr, Kenneth 102
Steele, Annie 83–4, 85
Stephen, Douglas 54
stigma, of polio 4–5
   see also ostracism; polio, public attitude to

– 261 –

stretching, as therapy 81, 118, 121, 123
subversive behaviour, of patients 37
sunstroke, as cause of polio 15
superstition 15
support groups 8
surgery, to correct deformity 66, 140–2
Swan, Charles 153–4
Swan, Evelyn 84
Sydney Norland Institute 73, 75
Sylvia stretcher, development of 79, 80

Tasmanian Education Department 133, 134
Tasmanian Society for the Care of Crippled Children *see* Society for the Care of Crippled Children
Thomas splint *see* splints
treatment 3–4, 49–51, 110–24
　in Australia 45
　debates 2, 4, 8, 9, 38
　see also treatment methods, e.g.
　　immobilisation; Kenny treatment
tuberculosis, compared with polio 32

University of Melbourne 47–8
University of Minnesota, and Kenny treatment 97
University of Pittsburgh 157, 158

vaccination *see* Salk immunisation programs
　rates *see* immunisation rates
vaccines, development of 156–61
VAD *see* Voluntary Aid Detachment
van Riper, Hart E. 108
verandahs, and patient care 25, 35
Victorian Education Department 134
Victorian Society for Crippled Children and Adults 134
viruses 145, 149–50
visiting hours, restriction of 33, 110, 113
Voluntary Aid Detachment (UK) 76

Walter and Eliza Hall Institute, Melbourne 56, 57, 151–4, 155–6, 157
Warm Springs, Georgia 95–6, 98–9, 117
　Macnamara's visit to 62, 95
Webster, Reginald 53, 54, 150–1
Weller, Thomas 155
Wickman, Ivar 146
World War I *see* First World War
Wright, Wilhelmine 72

xenophobia, and polio 5

Yooralla Hospital School, Melbourne 126, 134, 136